ADVANCED APPLICATIONS
OF CURRICULUM-BASED MEASUREMENT

The Guilford School Practitioner Series

EDITORS

STEPHEN N. ELLIOTT, PhD   JOSEPH C. WITT, PhD
University of Wisconsin–Madison   Louisiana State University, Baton Rouge

Recent Volumes

Advanced Applications of Curriculum-Based Measurement

♦♦♦

Edited by

Mark R. Shinn

♦

THE GUILFORD PRESS
New York London

© 1998 The Guilford Press
A Division of Guilford Publications
72 Spring Street, New York, NY 10012

http://www.guilford.com

Printed in the United States of America

This book is printed on acid-free paper.

Last digit is print number: 9 8 7 6 5 4 3 2

Library of Congress Cataloging-in-Publication Data

Advanced applications of curriculum-based measurement / edited by Mark
   R. Shinn.
      p.   cm. — (The Guilford school practitioner series)
   Includes bibliographical references and index.
   ISBN 1-57230-257-7
   1. Curriculum-based assessment—United States.   I. Shinn, Mark R.
2. Educational counseling—United States—Case studies.   3. Student
II. Series.
LB3060.32.C74A38   1998
371.26'4—dc21   97-33494
                                                                  CIP

Contributors

◆

Scott K. Baker, PhD, College of Education, University of Oregon; Eugene Research Institute, Eugene, OR

Suzanne Bamonto, Doctoral Candidate, School Psychology Program, Department of Applied Behavioral and Communications Sciences, University of Oregon, Eugene, OR

Vicki L. Collins, PhD, Department of Special Education, Northern Illinois University, DeKalb, IL

Christine A. Espin, PhD, College of Education and Human Development, University of Minnesota, Minneapolis, MN

Lynn S. Fuchs, PhD, Department of Special Education, Peabody College, Vanderbilt University, Nashville, TN

Susan Gallagher, PhD, LaGrange Area Department of Education, LaGrange, IL

Roland H. Good III, PhD, School Psychology Program, College of Education, University of Oregon, Eugene, OR

Jeff Grimes, MS, Consultant, Department of Education, State of Iowa, Des Moines, IA

Lisa Habedank Stewart, PhD, School Psychologist, Fergus Falls Area Special Education Cooperative, Fergus Falls, MN

Gretchen Jefferson, Doctoral Candidate, School Psychology Program, College of Education, University of Oregon, Eugene, OR

Ruth A. Kaminski, PhD, School Psychology Program, College of Education, University of Oregon, Eugene, OR

Vivian Lezcano-Lytle, MA, Consultant, St. Paul Public Schools, St. Paul, MN

Judith Plasencia-Peinado, MS, Doctoral Candidate, School Psychology Program, College of Education, University of Oregon, Eugene, OR

Kelly A. Powell-Smith, PhD, School Psychology Program, Department of Psychological and Social Foundations, College of Education, University of South Florida, Tampa, FL

Mark R. Shinn, PhD, School Psychology Program, Department of Applied Behavioral and Communications Sciences, University of Oregon, Eugene, OR

W. David Tilly III, PhD, Consultant, Department of Education, State of Iowa, Des Moines, IA

Gerald Tindal, PhD, College of Education, University of Oregon, Eugene, OR

Acknowledgments

♦

This book contains chapters that represent additions to knowledge and practice regarding the use of Curriculum-Based Measurement in a Problem-Solving Model. The book is dedicated to the memory of our colleague and friend, Caren Wesson, PhD. Among our cohorts at the University of Minnesota during the late 1970s and early 1980s, it was Caren who steadfastly represented the needs of students with learning problems and their teachers. Her commitment was combined with a contagious sense of optimism and an infectious laugh that is sorely missed. Chapter authors of this book have donated their share of royalties to the Caren Wesson Memorial Fund at the University of Wisconsin at Milwaukee. The Memorial Fund is designed to support the education of future teachers.

This book also could not have been produced without the support of my son, Peter, who constantly reminds me about the joys of being a father, and without the mentorship of Stanley Deno, who remains my teacher. Thanks are also offered to Kristin Peterson, doctoral candidate in school psychology, who painstakingly proofread these chapters prior to publication.

Contents

♦

CHAPTER 1

◆◆◆

Advanced Applications of Curriculum-Based Measurement: "Big Ideas" and Avoiding Confusion

◆

MARK R. SHINN
SUZANNE BAMONTO

Curriculum-Based Measurement (CBM) is a set of standard simple, short-duration fluency measures of reading, spelling, written expression, and mathematics computation. CBM was developed to serve as Dynamic Indicators of Basic Skills (DIBS; Shinn, 1995) or general outcome indicators (Fuchs & Deno, 1991) measuring "vital signs" of student achievement in important areas of basic skills or literacy. In other words, they were designed to function as "academic thermometers" to monitor students' growth in important skills domains relevant to school outcomes. CBM consists of the following core testing strategies:

1. In reading, students read aloud from basal readers for 1 minute. The number of words read correctly constitutes the basic decision-making metric. Maze, a multiple choice cloze reading technique, also has been validated as a CBM testing strategy (Fuchs & Fuchs, 1992b). The number of correct word choices per 5 minutes is the primary metric.
2. In spelling, students write words that are dictated at specified intervals (either 5, 7, or 10 seconds) for 2 minutes. The number of correct letter sequences and words spelled correctly is counted.
3. In written expression, students write a story for 3 minutes after being given a story starter (e.g., "Pretend you are playing on the playground and a spaceship lands. A little green person comes

1

out, calls your name, and . . .""). The number of words written, spelled correctly, and/or correct word sequences is counted.
4. In mathematics, students write answers to computational problems via 2- to 5-minute probes. The number of digits written correctly is counted.

CBM is used by individual special education and general education teachers and school psychologists in public schools throughout the United States. It is used system wide in a Problem-Solving model in a number of schools and school districts in this country. In one state, Iowa, CBM forms a cornerstone of special education systems reform using a Problem-Solving approach. See Reschly and Grimes (1991) and Tilly and Grimes (Chapter 2, this volume) for information on this statewide use of CBM.

This chapter, like this book, is *not* intended for the novice reader to acquire basic information about CBM and its use in a Problem-Solving model. Instead, that reader is referred to Shinn (1989), Shinn (in preparation), or a variety of professional articles on CBM (e.g., Deno, 1986; Fuchs & Deno, 1991; Shinn, 1995). This chapter is intended for the reader who is generally familiar with the measurement tools and the basic framework for the Problem-Solving model as conceptualized by Deno (1989). Its purpose is to provide a brief history of CBM and review the "big ideas" in its use. The chapter also is intended to review these "big ideas" in the context of some of the criticism directed at CBM as a measurement instrument and as part of a change in the role of school psychologists.

BRIEF HISTORY OF CBM

CBM has evolved through a number of phases and names for its testing strategies, beginning with Stanley Deno's attempts in the early 1970s to provide his special education student teachers with efficient yet accurate ways of assessing the effects of their instruction. Building on the accumulating body of knowledge from behavioral assessment of social behaviors in the budding field of applied behavior analysis, Deno sought to give his teacher trainees academic measures that could be (1) collected daily, if necessary; (2) graphed; and (3) evaluated for evidence of student learning within short periods of time. See Deno (1992) for more information on this early history. Deno's development and field-testing efforts in public school special education programs with Phyllis Mirkin led to the first formal conceptualization of CBM as *Data-Based Program Modification* (DBPM; Deno & Mirkin, 1977).

The *validation and enrichment phase* of CBM began in earnest in 1978, when Deno was awarded a contract from the then U.S. Bureau of the Educationally Handicapped (BEH) as coprincipal investigator of the University of Minnesota Institute for Research on Learning Disabilities (IRLD). One of the principal aims of the IRLD was to develop and validate simple methods of writing Individualized Education Plan (IEP) goals that could be used formatively to assess student progress. Graduate students, including Lynn Fuchs, Jerry Tindal, Doug Marston, Steve Robinson, Caren Wesson, and Mark Shinn were instructed to search the professional literature for potential academic or social behavioral tasks that showed promise as simple measures of student improvement. The potential measures were vigorously examined with school-aged children, with and without disabilities, regarding their technical properties (e.g., reliability, concurrent validity) as well as their logistics features (e.g., ease of administration). Although the core measures included some of the tools of DBPM (e.g., oral reading fluency), the IRLD research identified other technical tools such as fluency-based spelling and written expression assessment. See Deno, Mirkin, and Chiang (1982) as an example of these early validation efforts. The validated tools were referred to as "simple" measures.

After extensive investigations of technical adequacy, the use of the simple measures in educational decision making became the focus of study. In the Pine County Special Education Cooperative under the direction of Gary Germann, teachers were trained, students' progress was assessed over time, and decision-making outcomes were evaluated (e.g., Germann & Tindal, 1985). The use of the descriptor "simple measures" to represent the emerging measurement technology proved unsatisfactory, in large part because the term only described one broad and perhaps less relevant feature (i.e., the fact that the measures were not complicated) of the measurement system. Data-Based Assessment was the next descriptor that was used. It tapped into a more salient feature about the measurement system in that educational progress decisions were to be data based, but eventually this term was discarded in preference to Curriculum-Based Assessment (CBA) around 1983 (e.g., Marston & Magnusson, 1985). This descriptor appeared to represent one of the measurement technology's more important features and was responded to favorably by educators.

Interest in the general topic of CBA exploded in the mid-1980s with a decrease in confidence in prevailing assessment practices in special education and school psychology (i.e., test-and-place using commercial, nationally norm-referenced tests) and an increased interest in seeking alternative testing approaches. CBA as a viable alternative was promoted by the publication of a special issue of *Exceptional Children* on the topic edited by Tucker (1985), and an edited book by Idol, Nevin, and Paolucci-Whitcomb (1986). These summary articles and book chapters also were accompanied by a rapidly expanding professional literature with research-based investigations of features of CBA.

However, it was clear when reading the mid-1980s professional literature that there were a number of *different* approaches to assessing student performance with curriculum materials. CBA was *not* a unified method of testing and, in fact, the approaches grouped together under this general term differed considerably. In an effort to set its testing practices apart from other CBA models, a consistent use of the descriptor "Curriculum-Based Measurement" (CBM) was undertaken around 1986 in Deno's seminal article in *School Psychology Review* on formative evaluation (Deno, 1986). The differences in CBA models were laid out explicitly in a special issue of *School Psychology Review* (Shinn, Rosenfield, & Knutson, 1989). Two of the most salient differences among the CBA models were the (1) purposes of assessment, and (2) research support for testing practices and decision making.

CBM from the late 1980s and through today has seen continued support from the U.S. Department of Education for preservice graduate training and research and development. CBM has also served as a dependent measure in a number of federally funded research projects. See Chapter 4 by Fuchs and Chapter 9 by Powell-Smith and Habedank-Stewart in this book and Shinn, Powell-Smith, and Good (1996) for examples of this federally funded research.

The general acceptance of CBM as a viable assessment tool is evidenced in a number of other ways, including its prominence in task force documents on assessment and special education reform. Among the most visible federal documents in recent years was *The National Agenda for Achieving Better Results for Children and Youth with Disabilities* (U.S. Department of Education, 1994). The document, compiled by assessing interdisciplinary focus groups of educators, parents, and advocates, emphasized the role of CBM by name and the type of measurement characterized by CBM (e.g., continuous progress measures, measuring student results, assessments to maintain and support appropriate teaching) as potential solutions to the accepted problems of conventional "test-and-place" assessment activities. Similar content was included in the National Association of School Psychologists document (1994) entitled *Assessment and Eligibility in Special Education: An Examination of Policy and Practice with Proposals for Change.*

As mentioned earlier in this chapter, adoption of CBM and using it in a Problem-Solving model continues at a high-level pace. An interesting shift in focus has occurred since the mid-1990s, however. Although one of the inherent messages in using CBM in a Problem-Solving model is the linkage to what is taught in general education classrooms and the need to make special education decisions in the context of general education expectations, most adoption historically has been stimulated by special education assessment reform interests. In particular, alternative assessment implementation using CBM has been spearheaded by school psychologists. It appears that adoption now is being stimulated much more frequently by general educators, most typically principals who are seeking ways of documenting the progress of their students in the basic skills areas. We see this avenue as the most promising for facilitating the improvement of basic skills and literacy for all children, including students who receive special education.

"BIG IDEAS" ABOUT CBM

Advances in cognitive psychology have demonstrated the importance of "big ideas" as a mechanism for enhancing understanding of key concepts in a body of knowledge (Carnine, 1994). The maturation of CBM as both an assessment technology and, in a sense, as part of an ideology, has come about as the "big ideas" have crystallized. Three "big ideas" about CBM stand out:

1. CBM measures are validated for use as "dynamic indicators of basic skills," or *DIBS,* for purposes of formative evaluation (Deno, 1986; Fuchs & Deno, 1991; Fuchs & Deno, 1992a, 1992b).
2. The principal purpose of CBM is in formative evaluation.
3. CBM can be used more comprehensively in a Problem-Solving model to make a variety of decisions (Deno, 1989; Shinn, 1995).

Fully understanding these "big ideas" is helpful and arguably necessary for continued inroads to be made for using CBM in better, more functional assessment activities.

CBM as DIBS

A major big idea of CBM is its use as *dynamic indicators* of *basic skills* to facilitate timely, formative evaluation for the purpose of improving achievement outcomes. In fact, we encourage persons to use this "big idea" in the form of the acronym DIBS to facilitate understanding.

Dynamic

The "D" in DIBS represents the key concept of the *dynamic* nature of a measure. Dynamic means sensitive to differences. Sensitivity encompasses two dimensions, sensitivity to differences (1) *among* individuals (i.e., persons with a skill should be discriminated from persons without a skill), and (2) *within* persons over time (i.e., persons improving in a skills area should show higher test scores over time). Commercially available norm-referenced achievement tests are constructed to be sensitive to differences *among* individuals. For example, a good commercial reading test should be able to distinguish good readers from poor readers. CBM, like commercially available tests, also is sensitive to differences among individuals (Shinn & Marston, 1985; Shinn, Tindal, Spira, & Marston, 1987). However, unlike commercial norm-referenced achievement tests, CBM is dynamic (i.e., sensitive) to differences *within* a person over time. They are designed to be sensitive to the short-term effects (i.e., 4–6 weeks) of instruction. When a student's skills change, the measures will detect this growth. For example, in general education classrooms, pupils typically improve about one to three words read correctly per week on a CBM oral reading measure (Fuchs, Fuchs, Hamlett, Walz, & Germann, 1993). This sensitivity allows for a student's learning to be detected and documented.

Indicators

The "I" represents the second key concept in the "big idea" of DIBS, that of the *indicator.* In education, the concept of indicators for purposes of assessment and decision making is not as common as it is in other areas such as medicine or business. In medicine, for example, almost every visit to a physician results in routine data collection on weight, blood pressure, and temperature. In hospital settings, temperature is seen as such an important indicator that this information is collected via a thermometer around the clock, regardless of the nature of the hospital stay.

The specification of any measure as an indicator is based on empirical data. As mentioned earlier in this chapter, beginning in 1978, an extensive program of research was undertaken to identify key behaviors that would meet the technical requirements to serve as indicators of academic performance. CBM has been validated to be correlates of key behaviors indicative of overall performance in the academic areas of reading, mathematics computation, written expression, and spelling. The technical evidence for this conclusion is beyond the scope of this chapter, however, and the reader is encouraged to see Marston (1989) or Good and Jefferson (Chapter 3, this volume) for specific validity evidence.

Knowing students' scores on the indicator can give one an accurate picture of their performance on a *broader* number of tasks in the same domain. For example, counting the number of words read correctly from text under standardized 1-minute testing conditions is an excellent indicator of general reading achievement, including comprehension for most students. Similarly, counting the number of correct letter sequences written under standardized 2-minute testing conditions is an excellent indicator of general spelling skills.

Because CBM is designed to serve as indicators and this concept is unfamiliar to educators, including educational measurement specialists, it is important to recognize potential confusions it may cause. As an indicator, it is important to recognize up front that CBM measures do not, nor were they intended to, sample *all* behaviors in an academic domain. In reading, for example, they will *not* provide direct information about whether a student can separate fact from fiction or identify the compellingness of an author's argument. It is important also to recognize explicitly that because a measure is used as an important indicator, it does not mean that the indicator should be the only information collected. Using an indicator does not preclude using other specific skills measures of interest. Should a teacher be interested in a student's fact versus fiction skills, a measure that assesses this specific skill would be appropriate.

Basic Skills

The "BS" represents the third key concept in the "big idea" of DIBS, that of the *basic skills*. The measures are designed *only* to assess student performance in the basic skills areas of reading, spelling, mathematics computation, and written expression. The measures were not designed to assess student performance in content areas such as science or social studies, or even to assess a student's reading skills in the written materials in these subjects. Although this constraint to particular domains may appear limited, the role of basic skills to learning and success in content-area courses is well documented. In addition, the idea of mastery of basic skills is synonymous with literacy, one of the prerequisites for successful employment beyond the schooling years.

   This basic skills focus allows CBM a key role in assessing student performance in acquisition of reading, spelling, written expression, and mathematics computation skill for general education students through the end of third grade. Although a significant proportion of general education students past third grade may have already mastered basic skills, CBM remains useful for assessing student progress for low performing or at risk general education students through sixth grade. Nearly all special education students through high school have serious basic skills or literacy deficits. See Chapter 8, this volume, by Espin and Tindal for more information. The utility of using CBM to assess student progress with students in special education in these key areas is well established.

CBM and Formative Evaluation

Historically, CBM has been used by special education and general education teachers "for the primary purpose of evaluating the effects of their instructional programs" (Shinn, 1995, p. 547). Too often, the effectiveness of an individual student's instructional program is evaluated at the *end* of an instructional period, when it is too late to change the program (i.e., *summative* evaluation). In contrast, CBM is used in formative evaluation (Deno, 1986), in which student performance is assessed continuously *during* instruction, and regular decisions are made about whether student progress is satisfactory or unsatisfactory. Should the former conclusion be reached, the instructional program typically is maintained. Should the latter conclusion be reached, the instructional program is changed in some meaningful way with the goal of improving student outcomes (Deno, 1985, 1986; Fuchs & Deno, 1991).

Earlier in this chapter, a metaphor of CBM as an academic thermometer was employed. Thermometers are excellent tools in formative evaluation of health interventions. Consider a situation in which parents are giving their child Tylenol to reduce a high fever. Taking the child's temperature on an ongoing basis after giving the medication and observing a decrease in temperature would suggest that Tylenol was an effective intervention. Observing no change in temperature or an increase in temperature would suggest a need for a change in intervention strategy.

An example of a general education teacher's use of CBM in formative evaluation is presented in Figure 1.1. Jennifer, a first grader, was referred by her classroom teacher because of serious academic concerns. A new reading program was implemented in the general education classroom in consultation with the building school psychologist. This program was evaluated twice per week using CBM, in which Jennifer read random-

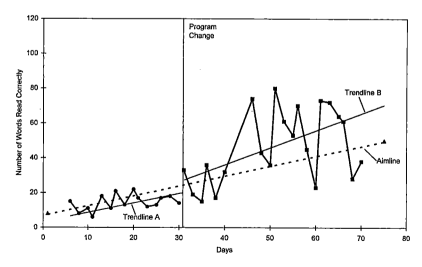

FIGURE 1.1. A graph of Jennifer's rate of progress regarding oral reading fluency.

ly selected passages from Macmillan Level 1. After about 6 weeks of instruction and formative evaluation, it was concluded that the student was
not making the rate of progress necessary for the instructional program to
be considered effective. This decision was reached by comparing the expected rate of progress (the aimline) with the student's actual rate of
progress (the trendline). Therefore, an instructional change was made, and
progress again was evaluated formatively. The change was beneficial for
the student as the rate of progress improved dramatically. In fact, the actual rate of progress exceeded the expected rate of progress.

The failure to recognize the "big idea" that CBM's principal use is as
a formative evaluation tool leads some to fail to understand some of its
measurement features. To support formative evaluation, tests must be (1)
standardized, (2) logistically feasible, and (3) sensitive to improvement.
These features are not independent.

Formative evaluation tools must be standardized (i.e., administered,
scored, and interpreted in consistent ways) so that changes in test scores
are attributable to student improvement rather than changes in testing
conditions. Formative evaluation also requires that information about student performance be collected on a repeated basis. Therefore, the testing
tools must be logistically feasible (i.e., doable). Efficiency is the key so that
significant amounts of precious instructional time are not lost to testing.
Efficiency is also apparent in the time frame necessary for decision making
about instructional program effects; that is, teachers need to make decisions about the effectiveness of a particular instructional program as *quickly as possible* so that ineffective programs can be "detected" and modified.
When ineffective programs are maintained, again, precious instructional
time is lost. This aspect of efficiency is most critical when students are significantly behind, as teachers have not a moment to waste. The goal in logistically feasible formative evaluation is to collect the *most* and *best* data in
the *shortest period of time.*

Finally, the tools in formative evaluation must be sensitive to change.
Sensitivity to change requires a relation between the content of the test
and what is taught (i.e., the curriculum). The degree of this relation is influenced by two extremes. On one extreme, a test could be very sensitive
by testing exactly what is taught. Unfortunately, this "sensitivity" may be
contaminated by a practice effect. The question becomes, "Is the student
doing better on this particular passage, or is the student a better *reader*
now?" On the other extreme is a test with little or no relationship to what
is taught. Even if a student learned what was taught, scores on a test with
no relation to what is taught may not reflect this growth. This is one difficulty in using commercial achievement tests to measure student growth.
In other words, the teaching-test content overlap must not be so high as to
allow for a practice effect or be so low as not to include items taught.

Given CBM's principal use as tests to be used in formative evaluation, some of its more "unusual" features make sense. CBM uses standardized testing practices with short-duration fluency tests (e.g., 1 to 3 minutes) for each of the basic skills areas. The standardized feature is easily understood. The unusual emphasis on short-duration fluency measures makes sense in the context of time efficiency and repeatability of formative evaluation. Short tests allow teachers to collect repeatable information without serious distractions from teaching.

However, this time efficiency would lack utility if the score from the test did not allow for accurate decisions about an individual student's progress over time (e.g., Is the student a better reader now than 2 weeks earlier?). Accurate decisions could not be made without suitably sensitive measures. CBM is unusual in that in formative evaluation, students typically are not tested on *exactly* what they are being taught. Instead, they may be tested using a long-term measurement approach (Fuchs & Deno, 1991) with material in which they would be expected to be performing in a year. For example, a student receiving reading instruction in Level 3 in the *Scribner* series might be tested continuously in Level 4 or 5 of the *Scribner* series. This high, but not perfect, relation between what is taught and what is tested allows for better decisions to be made about student growth and effective instruction. See Fuchs and Shinn (1989) or Fuchs and Deno (1991) for more information on this topic.

CBM and Its Use in a Problem-Solving Model

The big idea discussed in the previous section was the use of CBM as a formative evaluation tool equivalent to a thermometer in ascertaining the effectiveness of a medical intervention; CBM is used typically to determine the effectiveness of an *instructional* intervention in the basic skills areas. However, thermometers are used to make more than just decisions about whether a medical intervention is effective (i.e., a reduced temperature to 100.3°F after Tylenol). Using a thermometer, physicians can make four other decisions: (1) whether there is a health problem that warrants further investigation (e.g., a temperature of 102.5°F), (2) whether the problem is serious and may require special treatment (e.g., a temperature of 104°F is more severe than 101°F), (3) what the goals are for the specialized treatment (reduce temperature to 98.6°F), and (4) whether the specialized treatment is no longer necessary (the goal temperature of around 98.6°F has been reached). It is important to note that a thermometer typically does not tell you directly what is wrong or what has caused a high temperature. This deficiency does not diminish its utility as an important health indicator. These four additional uses of a thermometer in health evaluation and its use in deciding medical treatment effectiveness are presented in the first column in Table 1.1.

Although the primary purpose of CBM has been to evaluate the effects of basic skills instructional programs, it routinely has been used as a locally normed achievement test to make other decisions with students. Initially, CBM was used in the decision-making model proposed by Salvia and Ysseldyke (1978). The core decisions of the Salvia–Ysseldyke model consisted of screening, eligibility, intervention planning, and progress monitoring. This model could be conceptualized as *procedural* in nature, where a sequence of differentiated decisions were driven rationally by the sequence in which they were to be made. See Marston and Magnusson (1985) for more detail on the use of CBM in the Salvia–Ysseldyke deci-

TABLE 1.1. Comparison of Health and Reading Problem Decisions and Problem-Solving Model

Health problem	Reading problem	Problem-Solving model
There is a *health* problem that warrants further investigation (e.g., a temperature of 102.5°F).	There is a *reading* problem that may warrant further investigation (e.g., the student reads significantly more slowly than same-grade peers).	Problem Identification
The *health* problem is serious and may require special treatment (e.g., a temperature of 104°F is more severe than 101°F).	The *reading* problem is serious and may require a special treatment (e.g., the student's reading skills and instructional needs fall outside of the range of typical treatments).	Problem Certification/ Validation
Setting goals for the specialized treatment (reduce temperature to 98.6°F.)	Setting the goals of the specialized reading program (read the same number of words correctly as peers in 1 year).	Exploring Solutions Goals Intervention Content Intervention Process
Deciding whether a given intervention is effective during the treatment process (a reduced temperature to 100.3°F after aspirin).	Determining if the specialized reading intervention is effective during the course of treatment (the student is improving oral reading fluency at the rate projected by the goal).	Evaluating Solutions
If a specialized treatment is no longer necessary (the goal temperature of around 98.6°F has been reached).	If the specialized reading program is no longer necessary (the student's reading skills fall within the range of typical peers).	Problem Solution

sion-making model. The Salvia–Ysseldyke procedural model offered an advantage of an assessment process dictated by the decision one is trying make rather than what we call the "big bang" test-and-place model, in which lots of information is collected in an undifferentiated manner at the time of special education eligibility determination. Unfortunately, the procedural model also was inherently atheoretical, with few underlying assumptions, especially with respect to *who* should be assessed and why.

Significant improvements in educational decision making occurred when the shift to a Problem-Solving model took place. The Problem-Solving model, as laid out by Deno (1989) is sequential like the Salvia–Ysseldyke procedural model. Each of the five decisions, Problem Identification, Problem Certification, Exploring Solutions, Evaluating Solutions, and Problem Solution, also is followed by another rationally. These decisions are listed in the third column of Table 1.1. This table also shows the parallel in problem-solving decisions between the analogy of a child with temperature and a student with a reading problem.

The Problem-Solving model offers the procedural advantages of the Salvia–Ysseldyke model of sequenced and differentiated assessment and decision making. However, it also offers the advantage of being *theory-driven* by a series of underlying assumptions. Foremost among these assumptions is the definition of a problem as *situational* rather than person driven. A problem is defined as a discrepancy between what is expected and what is occurring in a *specific* (i.e., situational) context. For example, a reading problem would be defined as a discrepancy between how a particular student reads compared to a particular local standard (i.e., from a school or community) rather than a national, decontextualized standard. Inherent in this conception is the need to assess *situations* in addition to students.

Deno's (1989) Problem-Solving model also clearly specifies the relation of special programs, including special education, as problem-solving systems designed to meet the unmet needs of some students in the general education system. Conversely, if students' needs are met within the general education system, there is no need for special programs. A *sociological* versus psychological focus as the basis for entitlement is explicit. What constitutes the need for specific programs is driven by societal values (e.g., the need for literacy skills) rather than personal characteristics (e.g., mental retardation). Finally, the Problem-Solving model holds as an implicit cornerstone the need to examine the effects of interventions, because they can never be known in advance. Most importantly, intervention effects are evaluated frequently and at the individual-student level.

It is the use of CBM in a Problem-Solving model, with all of its underlying assumptions, that must be made clear for full understanding of what the measurement tools can and cannot do. It also is important to know that a Problem-Solving model is robust. It is broader than just academic problems and certainly may employ broader tools than just CBM. For example, the Problem-Solving model is applicable for students' problem social behaviors when they are viewed within a situation-centered perspective and measurement activities are valid and consistent with the model's assumptions.

CONFUSION ABOUT CBM

The second major purpose of this chapter is to examine what critics have said about CBM. We believe that some of the limited criticism that has been published comes from a failure to understand the "big ideas." Other criticisms come from differences in philosophy.

By and large, Curriculum-Based Assessment (CBA) in general, and CBM in particular, has not been the subject of frequent criticism in the professional literature. In fact, few articles have been published about CBA at all. What literature has been published in recent years on CBA has been tied to Shapiro's CBA work (1996; Shapiro & Derr, 1990). This CBA approach is "CBM-like"; that is, problems are considered to be an interaction of the child's skills and the environment, CBM-like measurement procedures (e.g., reading aloud for 1 minute) are recommended for assessing student skills, and intervention efforts are focused on the remediation of observable academic skills (Shapiro & Derr, 1990). However, testing usually occurs with the immediate instructional materials in contrast to CBM's long-term measurement approach. Another key difference is Shapiro's emphasis on the specific skill measured (e.g., reading aloud) rather than the construct measured (general reading achievement). There is no evidence that data are used as DIBS, nor is there any attention to a Problem-Solving model.

Professional writing on CBM and research using CBM as dependent measures continues at a healthy pace. It is estimated that over 150 articles have been published since 1988. However, this professional writing remains tied to a few of the original CBM authors (e.g., Deno, L. Fuchs, D. Fuchs, Tindal, Marston) or their students (e.g., Allinder, Habedank, Stecker). It is difficult to explain the lack of independent research and whether it reflects a general acceptance of the research being done by the CBM researchers, disinterest in CBM, or a lack of background in time-series, idiopathic research methodology. What little *critical* literature has been published is largely opinion pieces (e.g., Hargis, 1993) and/or in nonrefereed sources such as state newsletters (e.g., Lombard, 1988a).

Criticisms of CBM within this literature have been directed to philosophical and technical issues, ranging from topics of technical adequacy to disagreements over how to define a disability. An analysis of the published critiques (e.g., Hargis, 1993; Lombard, 1988a, 1988b; Mehrens & Clarizio, 1993; Taylor, Willits, & Richards, 1988) has revealed three explicit themes: (1) confusion over technical issues, (2) model discriminations (i.e., failure to discriminate between models of CBA and unfamiliarity with the Problem-Solving model), and (3) disagreement over conceptual issues (i.e., how to define a disability and what to expect from students). Implicit in these critiques also may be a resistance to changing existing assessment practices, whether these practices require modification or not.

An overview of the common criticisms of CBM in the existing literature is provided in Tables 1.2, 1.3, and 1.4. In the first column of each table, criticisms of CBM are provided in the authors' own words. The second column contains our interpretation of each first-column quote. The third column contains our hypothesis for why the authors might have reached their conclusion.

Confusion over Technical Issues

The first group of criticisms of CBM outlined in Table 1.2 appears to stem from confusion over technical issues. By technical issues, we mean concerns regarding the specific nature and purposes of testing and utility of procedures versus broad concerns over the paradigms in which the technology is used. Each issue will be discussed in the order of appearance in Table 1.2.

Intended CBM Focus

Several authors (Lombard, 1988a, 1988b) and most recently Mehrens and Clarizio (1993) fail to understand the "big idea" of CBM as DIBS. Instead, they appear to have made the assumption that CBM is intended to be used for assessing each and *every* academic content domain. The presumption is that CBM is intended to replace *all* existing achievement tests. For example, as shown in Table 1.2, Mehrens and Clarizio (1993) stated, "We submit that the teachers' curriculum is far broader than the domains sampled by CBM and the measures do not have curricular validity for the elementary school curriculum. . . . Their measures sample the elementary school curriculum, but the sample is obviously not representative" (p. 246). In other words, any test is not useful or valid unless it samples the *total* curriculum. Perhaps the first author's expertise with group achievement tests led him to this erroneous conclusion. Because group achievement tests are most often used to make *general* program evaluation decisions and comparisons across schools, districts, and states, regardless of the curriculum used, such tests may be judged on their coverage of the general domain of elementary-school achievement. It is more desirable to use *group*

TABLE 1.2. Confusion over Technical Issues Regarding CBM

Their words . . .	What they mean . . .	Why they may have reached that conclusion . . .
"We submit that the teachers' curriculum is far broader than the domains sampled by CBM and the measures do not have curricular validity for the elementary school curriculum. . . . Their measures sample the elementary school curriculum, but the sample is obviously not representative" (Mehrens & Clarizio, 1993, p. 246).	As a rule, assessment systems are not useful unless they sample the total curriculum. CBM does not sample the total curriculum, therefore it cannot be useful.	The expertise of the first author with group achievement tests may have led to this belief. Comprehensive curricular sampling is desirable given the uses of group achievement tests, but may not be necessary for making decisions about individual students with specific achievement problems.
"Proponents seem to have overstated the potential of CBM and inappropriately promoted it as a megatesting technology, a one-size-fits-all measurement system that will answer all the important questions about specialized education" (Lombard, 1988a, p. 20).	According to proponents, CBM is useful for assessing every type of academic concern, and can, in the absence of any other information, answer all important assessment questions with regard to specialized education.	This author attempts to overgeneralize the use of CBM to include purposes for which it was not designed.
"Perhaps the most crucial point . . . is the obvious poverty of content in such narrow sampling of behavior as 'words read out loud.' . . . The proper assessment of reading involves the interrelated proficiency of a complex of skills, such as 'word decoding, semantic access, sentence processing and discourse analysis' " (Lombard, 1988a, p. 20).	The number of words read out loud cannot be a valid measure of reading because it is too simple.	Insufficient regard for or knowledge of the research base on CBM technical adequacy.
". . . the rationale for the CBM model is based, in part, on supposed technical inadequacies of (PNATs)." (Mehrens & Clarizio, 1993, p. 244). "Given the argument of CBM proponents that tests are more useful if tied to the local set of objectives, it is difficult to know why they almost invariably use (PNATs) as a criterion in their validity studies" (p. 247).	CBM proponents use faulty logic by criticizing published, norm-referenced achievement tests (PNATs) as inadequate while using these tests as criteria by which they attempt to validate their technology.	The authors appear to have overlooked the *specific* criticisms of PNATs by CBM proponents, attending only to the fact that PNATs are criticized.

(continued)

15

TABLE 1.2. *Continued*

Their words . . .	What they mean . . .	Why they may have reached that conclusion . . .
"An important consideration is that CBA can be no better than the curriculum selected for instruction" (Taylor et al., 1988, p. 17). "Even if a local curriculum is good, restricting assessment to only that local curriculum is misleading to those who make inferences to the broader domain if the local curriculum departs significantly from the national curriculum" (Mehrens & Clarizio, 1993, p. 243).	If a curriculum is not valid, it follows logically that assessment drawn from that curriculum also would not be valid. It would not be useful to assess student performance in a curriculum that is not "valid," even if it is the one students are expected to master.	Confusion over curricular validity and its relation to validity of measurement procedures.

achievement tests that cover as much of the curriculum as possible, so that comparisons on general constructs such as reading and science can be made across settings. However, this curriculum coverage is *not* a necessary feature of *all* assessment devices, particularly those like CBM, which are designed primarily for use as DIBS with individual students having specific achievement difficulties within specific curriculum skills areas.

Perhaps Mehrens and Clarizio would be surprised to discover that we agree that basic skills do not comprise the total elementary-school curriculum. However, the fact that basic skills are not the entire curriculum does not diminish their importance as an integral *part* of the elementary curriculum. We hold that it is imperative for students to master basic skills if they are to become successful and contributing members of society (see Deno, 1989, for a discussion of cultural imperatives and cultural electives). Because of this importance, basic skills acquisition should be assessed routinely using CBM as a dynamic indicator of these basic skills.

Technical concerns regarding the intended focus of CBM also were expressed by Lombard (1988a), who criticized proponents for having "overstated the potential of CBM and inappropriately promoted it as a megatesting technology, a one-size-fits-all measurement system that will answer *all* the important questions about specialized education" (p. 20, italics added). CBM authors have made explicit statements about its assessment focus on basic skills for use in a Problem-Solving model (e.g., Knutson & Shinn, 1991; Shinn, 1989). Sufficient evidence of its utility for these purposes abounds (e.g., Shinn, 1989; Fuchs, 1993). It is a good indi-

TABLE 1.3. Model Confusions

Their words . . .	What they mean . . .	Why they may have reached that conclusion . . .
"It is important that researchers and practitioners not waste time discovering the same appropriate purposes and making the same faulty assumptions about CBA that have been made about CRT" (Taylor et al., 1988, p. 15).	All models of CBA are essentially criterion-referenced testing and should be treated as such in the literature and the schools.	Failure to discriminate among models of CBA and failure to realize that CBM is *not* criterion-referenced testing.
"Many times educators and the public do not wish to make inferences just about the specific content that has been taught. In those situations, one should not have a perfect match between instruction and assessment. We do not believe this whole issue has been addressed adequately by the CBM advocates" (Mehrens & Clarizio, 1993, p. 244).	A perfect match between assessment and instruction occurs when using a CBM approach.	Confusion of CBM and CBA. Failure to recognize that CBM utilizes a long-term measurement approach, which does not include a perfect match between assessment and instruction, as opposed to a short-term measurement approach utilized by other CBA approaches.
"The use of CBM has exacerbated the inadequacy of the mainstream educational system by providing a short-cut, pseudostatistical eligibility system for special education programs. This practice moves school districts away from the more proper goal of improving the mainstream so it is more hospitable . . . to a diverse population of students . . ." (Lombard, 1988a, p. 20).	CBM is used primarily for determining eligibility for special education services. This practice will lead schools to place all low-achieving students into special education programs, taking away the impetus to improve general education so it accommodates a range of learners.	Failure to discriminate between use of CBM as a tool (i.e., for determining eligibility) and in a model (i.e., problem-solving assessment, where special education services are only one of a range of intervention options).
"The treatment utility of CBM is severely limited by its failure to be prescriptive with respect to (a) *what* to change, and (b) *how* best to instruct the child" (Mehrens & Clarizio, 1993, p. 252).	To be useful in linking assessment and intervention, techniques must specify, *a priori*, what and how to teach as well as when to modify instruction.	This thinking follows a diagnostic–prescriptive model of service delivery rather than a Problem-Solving model.

TABLE 1.4. Disagreements over Conceptual Issues Related to CBM

Their words . . .	What they mean . . .	Why they may have reached that conclusion . . .
Situation-centered definition of disability: (1) " . . . means that a student with a disability in one school district may not have a disability in another because the relevant variable is the *local* context or environment"; (2) " . . . ignores a child's characteristics that may be useful in explaining *why* a child can or cannot perform, and focuses only on the situation" (Mehrens & Clarizio, 1993, p. 242, italics in original).	Disabilities are within-child characteristics that are influenced minimally by the environment. To be useful, assessment techniques must identify students with these internal disabilities rather than identify students who are in need of help but may not have such disabilities.	These authors are arguing from a disability model of service delivery. Their argument is based on three assumptions: (1) that there is a clearly identifiable population of children with learning disabilities, (2) current assessment techniques can help identify these children with a high degree of reliability, and (3) between-district variability does not exist regarding "type of student" served in special education.
"Data gathered throughout the decades support the fact that students learn at different rates and it is unreasonable to establish the same time-dependent future goals for everyone" (Mehrens & Clarizio, 1993, p. 251).	Students in special education have less of a capacity to learn than the average student, therefore cannot hope to catch up to their peers in terms of achievement. Setting goals too high in this way would be setting the student up for failure.	Assumes that rate of progress is independent of instruction, that observed performance discrepancies are more a function of the child than the environment.
"Academic expectations should be child centered, not norm centered. Trying to make children conform to lock-step norm standards causes the flood of basically normal children into special education and produces most of our drop-outs" (Hargis, 1993, p. 282).	It is not appropriate to compare students to each other. The expectation that students should perform at roughly equivalent levels leads to school failure and drop-outs. The instruction and curriculum rather than the child is what needs to be assessed and modified.	Conceptual disagreement over assumptions about student learning, when and how to intervene, and what expectations should be set for students.

cator of overall proficiency in the basic skills areas, and is sensitive to changes in this proficiency over time. CBM can be used in a Problem-Solving model to assist with the five decisions for students at risk for problems in the *basic skills* areas. Therefore, within the context of basic skills assessment, CBM can be useful in addressing *many* of the important questions about specialized education. It may *not* be useful for addressing questions about students who have exclusive needs outside the domain of basic skills (e.g., content knowledge, study skills, higher order thinking skills). It is not realistic or even desirable to expect a single system of assessment to cover all types of academic problems encountered in the schools, nor is it appropriate to use systems for purposes other than those for which they were designed.

Limited Behavior Sample

At first glance, it may seem illogical that very-short-duration fluency measures of a particular behavior would provide a meaningful measure of a construct. For example, at *first glance,* one would wonder about the meaningfulness of counting the number of words read correctly in 1 minute as a measure of reading. Lombard (1988a) expressed concern about a limited behavior sample when he said, "Perhaps the most crucial point . . . is the obvious poverty of content in such narrow sampling of behavior as 'words read out loud.' How much can legitimately be inferred about a student from such limited measures?" (p. 20). Similarly, Hargis (1993) stated that CBM procedures "produce only numbers" (p. 282).

We would agree with the "first glance" perspective. However, such a perspective is unscientific in that it fails to attend to the research base establishing the CBM measures as technically adequate for the constructs assessed. This "first glance" perspective appears to rely on face validity, not other recognized strategies to evaluating whether a test measures what it is supported to measure. Ample evidence is available using well-established techniques and state-of-the-art strategies to evaluate the technical properties of CBM.

Concerns about limited behavior samples also are put forth in the context of what appears to be a task analysis perspective. For example, Lombard stated a perspective that "the proper assessment of reading involves the interrelated proficiency of a complex of skills such as word decoding, semantic access, sentence processing and discourse analysis" (1988a, p. 20). These are examples of component skills involved in the reading process, from which overall reading ability would be inferred.

This method of reading assessment is based on two assumptions: (1) that a test must assess all possible component skills for good decision making, and (2) that the only way the "whole" can be measured is by summing the parts. Although appealing, this task-analytic approach has not been validated (Salvia & Ysseldyke, 1995) and at the least would ensure cumbersome, time-consuming testing. Again, it is useful to understand the "big idea" of CBM as DIBS in addressing this concern. The selection of potential dynamic indicators was driven by an interest in measuring behavior as *holistically* as possible; that is, attempts were made to select terminal behaviors that included as many of the important subcomponents, so that by directly assessing the global skill of interest, inferences could be drawn about a number of specific behaviors.

Using Published Achievement Tests to Validate CBM

The third technical point of confusion is centered on the criticisms of published, norm-referenced achievement tests (PNATs) by CBM authors. Proponents of CBM have been criticized for denouncing PNATs as inadequate while using them as criteria in validity studies. For example, Mehrens and Clarizio (1993) stated that "given the argument of the CBM proponents that tests are more useful if tied to the local set of objectives, it is difficult to know why they almost invariably use NSTs [nationally standardized tests] as a criterion in their validity studies" (p. 247).

These authors appear to have made the assumption that CBM is presented as an alternative to PNATs solely because the latter tests are technically inadequate. This assumption is inaccurate. As educational measurement specialists, proponents of CBM recognize that many PNATs generally are well constructed and may be suitable for some purposes, assuming that the sample of students of interest matches the characteristics of the normative sample. For example, group achievement tests can provide reliable, accurate information on how students perform on generic and important skills domains (e.g., reading, science) relative to a national sample. This information can allow for school-to-school, district-to-district, and state-to-state comparisons of scores on these tests. PNATs also may be appropriate for large-scale screening efforts to identify those students who might be at risk for academic problems.

Because many PNATs are technically adequate general measures of skills such as reading and mathematics, they make very appropriate comparisons for use in criterion-related validity studies. For example, scores on CBM reading probes *should* be correlated highly with scores obtained with well-constructed reading tests, if 1 minute oral reading tests measure general reading achievement.

The primary criticism of PNATs in the CBM literature centers on their limited utility in a *Problem-Solving* model. As stated earlier, a Problem-Solving model defines problems situationally and attempts to remedy these problems. The situational definition of a problem requires a local normative context, as will be discussed further later in this chapter. Student performance is compared to a local norm, and these local comparisons are used to determine the severity of the problem, set goals, plan interventions, and evaluate the effectiveness of these interventions. To be useful in problem solving, measurement procedures must be *logistically feasible,* so that local normative data can be collected and individual student performance can be evaluated over time, and *sensitive* to small changes in student performance, so that program modifications can be made in a timely fashion. CBM meets these criteria, but most PNATs do not. Typical PNATs are not logistically feasible; it would be impractical to administer these tests on a frequent basis. Typical PNATS also are not sensitive to small changes in student performance. For more detail on these issues, see Marston (1989), or Howell, Fox, and Morehead (1993).

Importance of a "Good" Curriculum

The final technical issue pertains to confusion over the relation between curriculum quality and CBM measures. In at least two sources, concerns are raised with regard to the "validity" or "appropriateness" of the local curriculum, and how that might affect the validity of the inferences or appropriateness of the decisions made using CBM. The presumption is that if a curriculum is inappropriate, then measurement derived from the curriculum will be faulty. For example, Taylor, Willits, and Richards (1988) asserted that "the most crucial concern regarding the use of CBA is the validity of the curriculum being used" (p. 17). Similarly, Mehrens and Clarizio (1993) stated that "there are many problems with limiting achievement inferences to the local curricular domain. Obviously a curriculum could be 'good or poor, boring or engaging, racist or sexist, outdated or updated'" (p. 243).

It is unclear what Taylor et al. (1988) mean by "curriculum validity," but one can infer that it has to do with its social validity or effectiveness. These issues of effective *treatment* are very different from test validity. Our principal answer to this important concern does not deal with CBM. Instead, we argue that should there be evidence that a general education curriculum lacks "curriculum validity" (it is ineffective, racist, outdated, etc.), educators should *change* it. The importance of using a validated instructional curriculum cannot be overemphasized, and this importance has little or nothing to do with CBM. But if general education expects students to *learn* a particular general education curriculum, we should examine student performance in learning it. Perhaps the outcomes would provide the necessary evidence to change or retain the curriculum!

We would argue that, again, critics go back to the big idea of DIBS. CBMs are designed to assess basic skills (e.g., reading) first and foremost, whether the curriculum is Scribner, Scott-Foresman, or Reading Mastery. The premise of "Curriculum-Based" versus "Curriculum Measurement" is that the closer the relation between what is taught and what is measured, the better the decision, especially with respect to student progress. This relation need not be perfect for good educational decision making, especially in formative evaluation. See Fuchs and Deno (1992a) for more detail on this topic. Other features of CBM such as the use of standard, important tasks of about-equal difficulty in a formative evaluation model outweigh the magnitude of the relation of the test to the curriculum.

Model Confusions

The second group of broad confusions presented in Table 1.3 appears to arise out of a general lack of distinction between *models* of assessment. See Taylor et al. (1988) and Mehrens and Clarizio (1993). One type of model confusion is a failure to discriminate among different CBA models. The second type of model confusion is a lack of familiarity with the Problem-Solving model in which CBM is used.

Discrimination among CBA Models

The lack of recognized discrimination among different models of CBA is exemplified in a quote from a recently published textbook on educational psychology. In the context of a half-page summary of CBA, Travers, Elliot, and Kratochwill (1993) state, "Although each form of CBA has some unique characteristic, they are more alike than different" (p. 488).

Each model claims utility in improving student achievement outcomes in some way. Each model uses curriculum as the source of testing materials. Some models of CBA *are* similar in that they utilize short-duration tests drawn from the curriculum. Some also purport to assess student progress over time (Shapiro & Derr, 1990). These commonalities should not be overgeneralized, however, to suggest that CBA models are more alike than different. For example, one could claim that commercial, norm-referenced achievement tests improve achievement outcomes, use curriculum for test materials, and can be used to measure student progress.

The lack of distinction on very important dimensions promotes confusion rather than advances informed choices about measurement systems. Other than being defined by what they are *not* (i.e., published, norm-referenced achievement tests), CBA models have little in common with respect to purpose, test construction, technical adequacy, efficacy, utility, or research support.

Examples in the work of Taylor, Willits, and Richards (1988) are illustrative. In their article, they treat five models of CBA as one approach

(Shinn & Good, 1993). Their criticisms are based on the weaknesses of criterion-referenced tests (CRT), but only two of five CBA models can be classified as CRTs. Interestingly, CBM is not among them.

A major dimension on which these differences between models appear is the amount of overlap between the curriculum and the testing material. In their critique of CBM, Mehrens and Clarizio (1993) made several references to the match between teaching and testing material, and the problems associated with "teaching the test" that may occur when using CBM procedures. It is important to note that "teaching to the test" is a potential problem with *any* achievement test. It is not unique to CBA procedures. However, the likelihood of teaching to the test is diminished with CBM focus on a long-term measurement approach in which students are tested in materials designed to represent the general outcomes they are expected to achieve over the entire year. Probes are selected from the *annual* curriculum in which the student is expected to reach a given level of proficiency, not what the student was taught that day, that week, or even that month. Any teaching to the test in CBM is obvious, as the testing material is not equal in content and difficulty to the current instructional material.

Unfamiliarity with the Problem-Solving Model

It has been suggested in this chapter that CBM be used as either a dynamic indicator in formative evaluation or in a Problem-Solving model. However, some educators appear to be confused about how CBM can be used and instead attempt to incorporate CBM as an "add-on" into their existing assessment practices and test-and-place service delivery. Examples of this confusion are shown in Table 1.3. This lack of familiarity appears to lead some critics to view CBM technology as a proposed replacement for all traditional assessment in a test-and-place assessment model. Because CBM is validated for use within the framework of a Problem-Solving model, it is especially important to address this confusion.

The most obvious example of unfamiliarity with the Problem-Solving model is Mehrens and Clarizio (1993). These authors make statements throughout their critique that illustrate this unfamiliarity at many stages of the Problem-Solving model. For example, with regard to screening (Problem Identification), they state that "there is simply too little evidence available at the current time to conclude that this approach would lead to better decisions than more conventional screening criteria" (p. 251). When discussing the issue of norms, they state that "CBM is not superior to (PNATs) with respect to the norming issue. They are equal with respect to local norms . . ." (p. 250). These and similar statements are used to argue that CBM is *no better* than PNATs in many respects, without considering that the advantage of CBM lies in its utility as a continuous measurement system for making several types of decisions about students (i.e., its use in a Problem-Solving model). As discussed earlier, PNATs are not adequate for these purposes. Therefore, with all other technical characteristics being equal, CBM is arguably more useful than PNATs for making decisions about students.

Another example of the unfamiliarity of Mehrens and Clarizio with the Problem-Solving model lies at the Exploring and Evaluating Solutions stages. When evaluating the treatment utility of CBM, these authors state that "the treatment utility of CBM is severely limited, however, by its failure to be prescriptive with respect to (a) *what* to change and, (b) *how* best to instruct the child" (p. 252, italics in original). This statement is not entirely accurate, because error analyses based on performance on CBM probes do provide valuable information for identifying a student's specific skills and a starting point for instruction. See Fuchs (1993) and Fuchs, Chapter 4, this volume, as examples. However, the main point is that Mehrens and Clarizio appear to expect CBM to be useful within a diagnostic–prescriptive model of service delivery. This model has been rejected by proponents of CBM due to its lack of empirical validation (Deno, 1985). In fact, the failure of the aptitude-by-treatment-interaction approach is one of the factors that provided an impetus for the development of CBM in the first place.

Disagreements over Conceptual Issues

It would be erroneous to assert that all the criticisms about CBM stem from misunderstandings. A few issues taken up by critics appear to result from philosophical disagreements about the way things are or *should* be. Table 1.4 contains quotes relevant to these issues. Two major areas of contention center on (1) the definition of a problem (or "disability") and (2) what expectations to place on children who experience achievement difficulties.

Definition of a Problem

The Problem-Solving model is explicitly tied to a needs-based service delivery system rather than a "medically" or organically based disability model. Problems are defined as an *interperson* discrepancy between expectations for other students in the same environment and the behavior of a specific student. This way of viewing and subsequently measuring problems is in stark contrast to the prevailing *intrapersonal* perspectives that underlie most conventional assessment practices. For example, special education testing typically examines *within*-person discrepancies between ability and achievement. Extensive assessment is designed to identify solely within-child variables such as "processing" as explanations for problems and targets for intervention. According to this model, a child's achievement difficulties are thought to be due to some internal disability, such as mental retardation or learning disabilities.

This conceptual shift not surprisingly is challenging to educators who have conceptualized problems as solely within-the-child. Many of the criticisms echo this challenge. Mehrens and Clarizio (1993) argue that practice based on a situational definition of a problem will lead to variability between schools in the identification of students who are eligible for special education. "Acceptance of this situation-centered definition . . . means that a student with a disability in one school may not have a disability in another because the relevant variable is the *local* context or environment" (p. 242, italics in original). These authors are correct but fail to recognize that such variability *already* exists from school to school, community to community, and state to state (Singer, Palfrey, Butler, & Walker, 1989; U.S. Department of Education, 1995). In fact, we would argue that schools implicitly employ a needs-based service delivery system. There is considerable evidence that schools identify and serve the lowest performing students in a particular school or community in special education (Shinn & Marston, 1985; Shinn, Tindal, & Spira, 1987; Shinn, Tindal, Spira, & Marston, 1987; Shinn, Tindal, & Stein, 1988). Furthermore, there is no *contradictory* evidence that schools do not use deviance from local performance standards as the basis for special education service delivery. The unfortunate situation is that the within-person assessment and decision-making system does not match the service delivery system.

Expectations for Students

A second conceptual disagreement concerns the expectations that should be placed on students who experience achievement difficulties. Table 1.4 contains two quotes with respect to this topic. Both express concerns about the level of expectations placed on students who experience academic problems, with the implication that these expectations are unduly high or unrealistic.

The concerns expressed by Hargis (1993) center on the "normative" aspect of setting expectations. In his critique of CBM, he wrote, "Academic expectations should be child centered, not norm centered. Trying to make children conform to lock-step norm standards *causes* the flow of basically normal children into special education and produces most of our drop-outs" (p. 282, italics added). Hargis comes from an antimeasurement perspective, and he believes that if his instructional procedures are followed, students will achieve to the best of their own ability. From his perspective, it is damaging to place expectations on individual children based on the performance of other students. His perspective on the importance of mastery of basic skills "by a certain age" is unclear. Also missing in his commentary is any empirical support for his claims on (1) the deleterious effects of norm-centered academic expectations, or (2) the achievement outcomes for students when his recommended measurement and instructional procedures are followed.

The concerns about academic expectations expressed by Mehrens and Clarizio (1993) come from a different perspective than those expressed by Hargis. These authors state, "The (goal) was set independent of other student characteristics such as measured aptitude in spite of the wealth of data across decades indicating that such data predict future performance quite well" (p. 249). Mehrens and Clarizio assume here that students with achievement problems may have less of a capacity to learn than typically achieving students. The role of effective instruction is undermined in this statement. Also implied is that aptitude data will identify those students who indeed have a limited capacity to learn, and that for students with lower measured aptitude, goals should be more conservative than for those with higher aptitude scores.

Several problems are inherent in this argument. First, the correlation between aptitude and achievement at a given time is by no means a perfect one, so a wide range of achievement scores are possible within any given aptitude level. In a chapter on best practices on intellectual assessment, Reschly and Grimes (1991) stated that using an IQ test to set limits on an individual student's potential to acquire new information is inappropriate. Furthermore, aptitude test results are *reasonably* good predictors of achievement (1) in the absence of interventions, and (2) for students scoring within the average range on aptitude and achievement measures (Salvia & Ysseldyke, 1995).

The argument by Mehrens and Clarizio that goals set using CBM procedures may be unrealistic also can be refuted on empirical grounds. Fuchs (1993) summarized research supporting the idea that goal ambitiousness is linked to student achievement. Students with moderately or highly ambitious goals demonstrated greater achievement gains than students whose goals were not ambitious. Whether students attained their goals had no bearing on achievement. Therefore, the practice of setting unambitious goals in response to aptitude data might actually limit the potential of students to acquire basic skills in a timely manner rather than enhance the achievement of these students.

SUMMARY

In this chapter, we have attempted to review three big ideas about CBM that we believe are essential to advance implementation of this measurement technology and increase the likelihood that educators may implement a Problem-Solving model. CBM is designed to (1) serve as DIBS, or Dynamic Indicators of Basic Skills; (2) be used in a formative evaluation approach; and (3) be an integral tool in a Problem-Solving model. We have attempted to show how failure to understand these "big ideas" can explain some of the limited criticism that has been directed at the technology.

Understanding these "big ideas" is insufficient for explaining *all* of the criticism of CBM. We believe that some of the criticisms are part of the inevitable resistance to change in assessment practices and corresponding changes in conceptions of what defines a problem. Of the criticisms, some come from the field of school psychology. Most school psychologists have been trained to administer, score, and interpret only published, norm-referenced tests. Most have been taught to look almost exclusively within the child for disabilities and that this information is the key "unlock the gate" into special education for those students demonstrating some evidence of a "disability." The problems with this approach have been discussed in detail in the school psychology and special education literature, and will not be reiterated here. The need for a change in assessment practices is evident, and the technology now is available to address some of the problems with the traditional assessment paradigm. However, creating and validating the technology is only a small part of the change process. As Erickson (1986) put it:

> Old paradigms are rarely replaced by falsification. Rather the older and the newer paradigms tend to coexist, as in the survival of Newtonian physics, which can be used for some purposes, despite the competition of the Einstenian physics, which for other purposes has superseded it. Especially in the social sciences, paradigms don't die; they develop varicose veins and get fitted with cardiac pacemakers. (p. 120)

This quote is especially relevant to the assessment paradigms within school psychology and special education. Fagan and Wise (1994) criticized CBM proponents for "too zealously selling their ideology" (p. 283). Bracken (1993) expressed concern over the "religious fervor" with which leaders the field of school psychology have been promoting "alternative assessment." Inherent in each of these expressions of concern is an unwillingness of practitioners and trainers to abandon the traditional practice of administering nationally norm-referenced tests for the purposes of labeling and categorizing students. Some professionals may be unwilling to (1) adopt a new paradigm regarding the delivery of services to students at risk, (2) learn the skills required to implement this new approach, and (3) discard the old paradigm under which they have been trained and practicing for varying numbers of years, and the practices within that paradigm. Doing these three things requires a change in thinking and a change in behavior, which may mean more work for many practitioners and trainers, most of whom already are overworked. However, for many practitioners, these changes will mean an improvement in the quality of services they deliver to students in their districts and greater satisfaction with the impact they are making on students' lives.

ACKNOWLEDGMENTS

The development of this chapter was supported, in part, by Grant No. H029D60057 from the U.S. Department of Education, Special Education Programs to provide leadership training in Curriculum-Based Measurement and its use in a Problem-Solving model. The views expressed within this chapter are not necessarily those of the U.S. Department of Education. The student performance graph in Figure 1.1 was contributed by Chris Parker, obtained while he was a school psychologist in New Bedford, Massachusetts. Mr. Parker is now obtaining his doctoral degree from the University of Oregon.

REFERENCES

Bracken, B. A. (1993). School psychology and the debate over assessment: Issues of fire and brimstone. *Michigan Psych Report, 22*(1), 1, 15–16.

Carnine, D. W. (1994). Introduction to the mini-series: Diverse learners and prevailing, emerging, and research-based educational approaches and their tools. Special section: Educational tools for diverse learners. *School Psychology Review, 23*, 341–350.

Deno, S. L. (1985). Curriculum-based measurement: The emerging alternative. *Exceptional Children, 52*, 219–232.

Deno, S. L. (1986). Formative evaluation of individual student programs: A new role for school psychologists. *School Psychology Review, 15*, 358–374.

Deno, S. L. (1989). Curriculum-based measurement and alternative special education services: A fundamental and direct relationship. In M. R. Shinn (Ed.), *Curriculum-based measurement: Assessing special children* (pp. 1–17). New York: Guilford Press.

Deno, S. L. (1992). The nature and development of curriculum-based measurement. *Preventing School Failure, 36*(2), 5–10.

Deno, S. L., & Mirkin, P. (1977). *Data-based program modification: A manual.* Reston, VA: Council for Exceptional Children.

Deno, S. L., Mirkin, P., & Chiang, B. (1982). Identifying valid measures of reading. *Exceptional Children, 49*(1), 36–45.

Erickson, F. (1986). Qualitative methods in research on teaching. In M. C. Wittrock (Ed.), *Handbook of research on teaching* (3rd ed., pp. 161–199). New York: Macmillan.

Fagan, T. K., & Wise, P. S. (1994). *School psychology: Past, present, and future.* New York: Longman.

Fuchs, L. S. (1993). Enhancing instructional programming and student achievement with curriculum-based measurement. In J. Kramer (Ed.), *Curriculum-based measurement* (pp. 65–104). Lincoln, NE: Buros Institute of Mental Measurements.

Fuchs, L. S., & Deno, S. L. (1991). Paradigmatic distinctions between instructionally relevant measurement models. *Exceptional Children, 57*(6), 488–500.

Fuchs, L. S., & Deno, S. L. (1992a). Effects of curriculum within curriculum-based measurement. *Exceptional Children, 58*(3), 232–243.

Fuchs, L. S., & Fuchs, D. (1992b). Identifying a measure for monitoring student reading progress. *School Psychology Review, 21*(1), 45–58.

Fuchs, L. S., Fuchs, D., Hamlett, C. L., Walz, L., & Germann, G. (1993). Formulative evaluation of academic progress: How much growth can we expect? *School Psychology Review, 22*(1), 27–48.

Fuchs, L. S., & Shinn, M. R. (1989). Writing CBM IEP objectives. In M. R. Shinn (Ed.), *Curriculum-based measurement: Assessing special children* (pp. 132–154). New York: Guilford Press.

Germann, G., & Tindal, G. (1985). Applications of direct and repeated measurement using curriculum based assessment. *Exceptional Children, 51*(2), 110–121.

Hargis, C. H. (1993). Review of Curriculum-Based Measurement: Assessing special children. *Journal of Psychoeducational Assessment, 11,* 280–284.

Howell, K., Fox, S. L., & Morehead, M. K. (1993). *Curriculum-based evaluation: Teaching and decision making.* Pacific Grove, CA: Brooks/Cole.

Idol, L., Nevin, A., & Paolucci-Whitcomb, P. (1986). *Models of curriculum-based assessment.* Rockville, MD: Aspen.

Knutson, N., & Shinn, M. R. (1991). Curriculum-based measurement: Conceptual underpinnings and integration into problem-solving assessment. *Journal of School Psychology, 29,* 371–393.

Lombard, T. (1988a). Caution urged in embracing CBM assessment. *NASP Communique, 16,* 20.

Lombard, T. (1988b). *Curriculum-based measurement: Megatesting or mctesting.* St. Paul: Minnesota State Department of Education.

Marston, D. (1989). Curriculum-based measurement: What is it and why do it? In M. R. Shinn (Ed.), *Curriculum-based measurement: Assessing special children* (pp. 18–78). New York: Guilford Press.

Marston, D., & Magnusson, D. (1985). Implementing curriculum-based measurement in special and regular education settings. *Exceptional Children, 52,* 266–276.

Mehrens, W. A., & Clarizio, H. F. (1993). Curriculum-Based Measurement: Conceptual and psychometric considerations. *Psychology in the Schools, 30,* 241–254.

National Association of School Psychologists. (1994). *Assessment and eligibility in special education: An examination of policy and practice with proposals for change.* Alexandria, VA: National Association of State Directors of Special Education.

Reschly, D. J., & Grimes, J. P. (1991). State department and university cooperation: Evaluation of continuing education and consultation and curriculum-based assessment. *School Psychology Review, 20,* 522–529.

Salvia, J., & Ysseldyke, J. E. (1978). *Assessment in special and remedial education*. Boston: Houghton Mifflin.

Salvia, J., & Ysseldyke, J. E. (1995). *Assessment* (6th ed.). Boston: Houghton Mifflin.

Shapiro, E. S. (1996). *Academic skills problems: Direct assessment and intervention* (2nd ed.). New York: Guilford Press.

Shapiro, E. S., & Derr, T. F. (1990). Curriculum-based assessment. In T. B. Gutkin & C. R. Reynolds (Eds.), *The handbook of school psychology* (2nd ed., pp. 365–387). New York: Wiley.

Shinn, M. R. (Ed.). (1989). *Curriculum-based measurement: Assessing special children*. New York: Guilford Press.

Shinn, M. R. (1995). Curriculum-based measurement and its use in a problem-solving model. In A. Thomas & J. Grimes (Eds.), *Best practices in school psychology* (pp. 547–568). Silver Spring, MD: National Association of School Psychologists.

Shinn, M. R., & Good, R. H. (1993). CBA: An assessment of its current status and a prognosis for its future. In J. Kramer (Ed.), *Curriculum-based measurement* (pp. 139–178). Lincoln, NE: Buros Institute for Mental Measurements.

Shinn, M. R., & Marston, D. (1985). Differentiating mildly handicapped, low-achieving and regular education students: A curriculum-based approach. *Remedial and Special Education, 6*, 31–45.

Shinn, M. R., Powell-Smith, K. A., & Good, R. H. (1996). Evaluating the effects of responsible reintegration into general education for students with mild disabilities on a case-by-case basis. *School Psychology Review, 25*(4), 519–539.

Shinn, M. R., Rosenfield, S., & Knutson, N. (1989). Curriculum-based assessment: A comparison and integration of models. *School Psychology Review, 18*, 299–316.

Shinn, M. R., Tindal, G., & Spira, D. (1987). Special education referrals as an index of teacher tolerance: Are teachers imperfect tests. *Exceptional Children, 54*, 32–40.

Shinn, M. R., Tindal, G., Spira, D., & Marston, D. (1987). Practice of learning disabilities as social policy. *Learning Disability Quarterly, 10*(1), 17–28.

Shinn, M. R., Tindal, G., & Stein, S. (1988). Curriculum-based assessment and the identification of mildly handicapped students: A research review. *Professional School Psychology, 3*, 69–85.

Shinn, M. R., Ysseldyke, J., Deno, S. L., & Tindal, G. (1986). A comparison of differences between students labeled learning disabled and low achieving on measures of classroom performance. *Journal of Learning Disabilities, 19*, 545–552.

Singer, J. D., Palfrey, J. S., Butler, J. A., & Walker, D. K. (1989). Variation in special education classification across school districts: How does where you live affect what you are labeled? *American Educational Research Journal, 26*, 261–281.

Taylor, R. L., Willits, P. P., & Richards, S. B. (1988). Curriculum-based assessment: Considerations and concerns. *Diagnostique, 14*, 14–21.

Travers, J. F., Elliot, S. N., & Kratochwill, T. R. (1993). *Educational psychology: Effective teaching, effective learning*. Madison, WI: Brown & Benchmark.

Tucker, J. (1985). Curriculum-based assessment: An introduction. *Exceptional Children, 52,* 199–204.

U.S. Department of Education. (1994). *The national agenda for achieving better results for children and youth with disabilities.* Washington, DC: Author.

U.S. Department of Education. (1995). *Implementation of the Individuals with Disabilities Education Act: Seventeenth annual report to Congress.* Washington, DC: Author.

CHAPTER 2

Curriculum-Based Measurement: One Vehicle for Systemic Educational Reform

♦

W. DAVID TILLY III
JEFF GRIMES

Special education in Iowa is engaged in a process of transformation that began in the late 1980s and continues to evolve. Although Curriculum-Based Measurement (CBM) is not the reform, it is an important part of the process in many educational agencies. In this chapter, we will describe the successful change process that has sustained innovation throughout the past 7 years. This chapter is not meant to be a "how to" cookbook. Many right ways to implement system change exist. However, a series of principles and processes that have emerged, in our experience, support successful implementation of specific innovations, such as CBM. These reform principles, processes, and their underlying foundations provide the structure for the first section of the chapter. In this section, we describe the systematic process Iowa used to initiate and sustain a system reform process. The second section of the chapter describes how CBM, as an innovation, has been used to assist in implementing the change process.

THE IOWA CHANGE PROCESS

Too often educators seeking to implement improvements talk about infusing new concepts into the educational *system*, but fail to consider the impact on a system designed to function in absence of the innovation. The long-term result often is diminished support for the new concepts and procedures. In short, the system returns to business as usual. It has been our experience that change can be supported effectively across time only when various components in a system are considered jointly.

Iowa's special education reform, initiated in the late 1980s, was comprehensive. The innovations focused on improved performance for preschoolers, elementary, and secondary students; the behaviors of concern were academic, social, ambulation, vocational, speech and language, and more. The entire range of student needs was addressed, including students with mild, moderate, and severe disabilities. The proposed changes affected general, compensatory, and special education. In addition to educational interventions, improved parent communication and partnership was consider essential to the overall success of the reform. Within this scope of system improvement, we will consider one aspect of the change process, CBM's contribution.

Ongoing Improvement as a Goal

Before a system is changed, persons within that system must have a sense that life is not as they want it to be, and that the work necessary to make things better is warranted. This sense of personal disharmony is the origin of passion for the change process. Educators, parents, and community members want an effective educational system. In postindustrial America, the term "effective educational system" means schools that prepare students to meet the demands of a quickly changing society. In this context, an educated individual must be prepared to respond to changing societal demands of the workplace and community. Educators, parents, and community leaders must consider their definition of an improved educational system when examining the question of whether school improvement is needed. The absence of viewing education in current contexts predictably leads to an inevitable question, "Is the system broke? And if it ain't, don't fix it." That woeful adage invites a reactive, crisis-management mentality rather than a proactive attitude where continuous improvement and early detection of concerns is embraced as a means of maintaining a quality educational system. Moving a system away from the former perspective toward the latter is one of the first tasks of educational reform.

Iowa's initial special education reform efforts occurred at a time when there was limited interest in overall change. That condition has changed. There is a growing interest in Iowa, as well as in America as a whole, for systemic school improvement (Fullan, 1996; Hargreaves, 1994; Shanker, 1995). When these opportunities arise, it is crucial that special education become an integral part of the overall effort. For this to occur, it is incumbent upon leaders to work toward integrated school improvement plans in which special education is a full partner in the change process.

"Systems" include all of its members, and special education will benefit from becoming a partner in an overall reform initiative. Although every state or educational agency will create its own process for educational change, the Iowa experience may be instructive in considering reform initiatives.

Establishment of Broad-Based Support for Reform

When polishing an apple, a point in time occurs when no matter how much additional effort is put forth, there is little possibility of improved luster. A point of diminishing return has been reached. This is not a criticism of the apple, the polisher, or the polishing process. It is a simple fact that there are limits built into the basic design of an apple that allow it to become "only so shiny." Such is the case with most any structure or system. In a comparable way, the people of Iowa determined that the special education service delivery system that emerged through the 1970s and '80s to support prevailing federal and state mandates (Education of All Handicapped Act and subsequently Individuals with Disabilities Act) had developed just about as much "shine" as the system could muster.

Enormous numbers of professionals worked to accomplish the procedural purposes and processes defined by that system. Despite all their positive efforts, the luster did not improve. Iowans expressed concern about the number of students with disabilities who were not making successful post–high school adjustment following graduation (Sitlington, Frank, & Carson, 1993), parent participation was too often limited to legally required contacts, and the degree of student accomplishment on Individualized Education Plan (IEP) goals was virtually unknown. Student progress was monitored most often by annual pre and post-tests thus preventing data-based adjustments to improve educational interventions during the school year. Problem prevention was a concept cautiously approached by special educators.

At the same time, compared to other states, education in Iowa was distinguished by high Scholastic Aptitude Test (SAT) and American College of Testing (ACT) scores, high rates of students proceeding to advanced education, and other benchmarks of a remarkable educational system. Likewise, special education in Iowa was progressive, innovation-oriented, and had much to be proud of. Accolades notwithstanding, the majority of the people in Iowa were not willing to say, "We are doing the best we can and that is good enough to our students with special needs." Quality relative to other states was not considered to be the paramount issue. Instead, the question was whether our system was as good as it could get on an absolute scale. A growing awareness emerged that fundamental change would be required to further enhance outcomes for students with unique educational needs. The polishing process for Iowa's brightly shining apple needed reconsideration. Thus, "reform" from the beginning was framed as an opportunity to improve an already excellent system.

The special education reform process began in Iowa through a process of soliciting input from a broad base of stakeholders prior to taking action. An understanding emerged that change is best conceived when those who are directly affected by the change are engaged in a collaborative process to reconsider educational services. Uniting the energy and imagination of people at all levels of service, including the parents, teachers, support-service providers, administrators, and community representatives lays a strong foundation for supporting change.

It is important to note that policymakers were included as *participants* in these meetings with stakeholders. This framework encouraged discussions to consider students' needs at the local school level rather than in some more abstract, policy conceptualization. The future was conceived as a beginning with a bottom-up orientation, with improved outcomes for students as the centerpiece. This approach is in contrast to predominantly top-down orientation in which policy or legislative edict drives reform, a situation that is all too familiar in America's educational history (Hargreaves, 1994). A top-down approach is effective in establishing a common framework with legal mandates; however, too often, stakeholders do not believe in such mandates and are passive or reluctant participants in reform initiatives conceived by others. A quality standard of successful reform is when the service providers, the teachers, administrators, support-service personnel, parents, and community leaders can explain the system and how the proposed innovations will lead to improved services for students. When school services are redesigned by the stakeholders, there is heightened ownership and passion for the implementation of that system.

Using this stakeholder-centered approach, Iowan's identified concerns related to how the special education system functioned and areas that were in need of improvement. In the late 1980s in Iowa, a series of meetings were held across the state that involved over 4,000 individuals. The general consensus was that Iowa had a good system, but it could be better. Problems were identified with the existing system, including: (1) Special education had become separated from general education in the process of delivering services to students requiring special education; (2) pull-out programs had been the primary delivery method for providing services to all students with disabilities; (3) the types of programs and services available through special education had been strictly limited to students determined to be "entitled"; (4) the requirements of special education laws and regulations not only severely limited the number of students that could benefit from such services, but also maintained a level of rigidity in the options that are available to those who were eligible; (5) there had been an overemphasis on standardized assessment techniques utilized primarily to determine whether a given student is eligible for special education programs and services; and (6) evaluation of special education activities had too frequently been based upon compliance with minimum legal requirements rather than student outcomes. These perceptions were consistent with the viewpoints and issues being identified across the nation (Epps & Tindal, 1988; Heller, Holtzman, & Messick, 1982; Kavale, 1990; Madden & Slavin, 1983; National Association of School Psychologists and National Coalition of Advocates for Students, 1985; Will, 1986). Within Iowa, these concerns were expressed by parents, educators, professional associations, advocacy groups, and educational agencies. A general consensus emerged in Iowa that it was time to consider a new direction.

Foundation Principles of Reform

Based on this large-scale input, a strategic planning effort set out to identify a set of principles that would form the foundation for improved services. The quest was not for a new set of procedures or innovative practices, including CBM. The direction was to revisit the fundamental purpose of special education, to rethink the conceptual structure that supports the service delivery system, to identify principles to guide change, and then to provide flexibility for school systems to address these principles in a manner meaningful to their constituents.

A statewide committee with diverse membership (e.g., teachers, administrators, university faculty, professional organizations, parents, and others) was established to identify the beliefs and principles related to the reform. This effort required five 1-day meetings within 6 months. From this work came a Request for Proposal (RFP) for schools to develop local plans to apply these principles. In Iowa, the RFPs focused on the Area Education Agencies (AEAs), which are intermediate units, that in turn worked directly with school districts in their region. The entire process took 1 year from the development of principles, submission of RFP, approval, and beginning process of implementation. The unifying factor for the Iowa special education reform effort is the use of principles to guide the effort. From this foundation, procedures and practices were envisioned to emerge from each educational agency's plans.

The guiding principles (e.g., functional assessment, progress monitoring, outcome criterion) were established without a clear picture of how to implement the process. Schools were responsible for designing ways to meaningfully address the principles while responding to the needs of students and other stakeholders in their system. The concepts were organized into three sections: guiding principles, organization of resources, and use of resources (see Table 2.1).

TABLE 2.1. Principles in Iowa's Special Education Reform Initiative

Foundation principles

Integrate the resources of general education, compensatory education, and special education in addressing the needs of students with learning and behavior problems.

Provide *increased flexibility in the use of special education support service personnel* will not be strictly limited to students requiring special education.

The renewed delivery system will create the opportunity to *broaden the range of intervention alternatives* available to students.

The preferred environment for delivery of quality instructional and support services for students with learning and adjustment difficulties shall be the local attendance center which is closest to the home of the student and is age appropriate.

Promote meaningful involvement of parents in the decision-making process and subsequent delivery of programs and services.

Organization of resources

Staff development. Students will benefit when personnel working in education receive needed staff development. This staff development will enable regular and special education personnel to acquire skills needed to implement "best practices" for students with learning and adjustment difficulties.

District/building plan. Students will benefit from better coordination and utilization of current instructional and support service personnel. This can be done in a prescriptive manner through the establishment of local building plans.

Utilization of resources

Functional assessment. Students will benefit by requiring assessments that are functionally oriented and built upon a question-oriented assessment plan that tests hypotheses leading to an understanding of factors directly effecting the individual's learning or behavioral difficulty.

Developing appropriate instructional and support interventions. Students will benefit from a variety of innovative instructional and support interventions which will focus on bringing services to students and not students to the services.

Direct and frequent progress monitoring. Students will benefit by procedures that directly and frequently monitor behaviors that are the focus of interventions. Monitoring procedures permit ongoing decision making and adjustment of interventions when needed, and thereby heightening the probability of helping students acquire new skills, knowledge, or ways of functioning.

Outcome-oriented criterion. Students will benefit by an outcome criterion, focusing on gains in students' skills, when adopted and applied to decisions about programming, placement, and reviews/evaluations.

IMPLEMENTING REFORM: CBM AS A VEHICLE

In the sections that follow, we discuss how CBM procedures were used as one vehicle supporting a system reform initiative. Iowa's foundation principles of special education reform adopted four cornerstones of a Problem-Solving system: (1) functional assessments, (2) expanded range of interventions, (3) monitoring of performance improvement, and (4) evaluation of interventions using an outcome criterion. These principles were the focus of the reform, not adoption of CBM or any other educational innovation. It was, and is, the case that for basic skills measurement, CBM can be used to assist in making a series of important decisions for students within a Problem-Solving service delivery model. CBM was often selected by educational agencies as the best technology available for meeting the purposes established by the system as priorities. We want to be clear about this point: If better technologies become available to meet the same purposes, Iowans would adopt them, thus improving the system. To this point, however, other general outcome measures (Fuchs & Deno, 1991) or dynamic indicators (see Shinn and Bamonto, Chapter 1, this volume) that improve on CBM as basic skills indicators have not been developed.

When adopting CBM as a vehicle for system change, a Problem-Solving assessment framework must be adopted along with the CBM procedures. The Problem-Solving framework provides the structure within which educational decisions are made. In its absence, CBM procedures are just a set of curriculum-linked achievement tests that are useful for formative evaluation and have acceptable technical characteristics (Marston, 1989). The most common case, in our experience, where CBM procedures have been adopted and used in an inappropriate manner is when CBM *procedures* are implemented but the *Problem-Solving system* in which they are embedded is not. A frequent example is where CBM procedures have been used as a substitute for nationally normed, published achievement tests to make eligibility decisions. The problem with this approach is that when used in this way, CBM may not improve significantly on the use of published, norm-referenced instruments and hence does not improve the system. Some nationally normed achievement tests have acceptable technical characteristics and are in fact useful for assisting in entitlement decisions. The problem with these tests in a Problem-Solving system is they typically do not provide useful information for program planning and progress monitoring (Howell, Fox, & Morehead, 1993).

Principle-Based Reform Using CBM

Recall that the foundation principles generated for Iowa's reform initiative (which became known as the Renewed Service Delivery System; RSDS) were established to guide reform efforts to better accomplish the fundamental purposes of special education. Many reasons support using a principle or purpose focus for selecting special education innovations. Most importantly, innovation carried out by replacing old procedures with new procedures often does not result in implementors' understanding *why* the change is occurring. Another reason for a purpose orientation to reform is that focusing on underlying purposes for the innovation allows the system to continually improve as new technologies are developed. Most educational innovations are technologies in one form or another; CBM is not an exception. All technologies must be evaluated in the context of other technologies for accomplishing the same purposes. Thus, a purpose focus allows improvements in practice to be evaluated systematically in the context of a current practice. Moreover, it allows improved practices to be integrated into a developing system when they accomplish a specific educational purpose better than do existing technologies. CBM was developed initially as a method for formatively evaluating basic skill acquisition for students with learning disabilities. Throughout approximately 15 years of research, CBM procedures have been systematically validated for making additional special education decisions (e.g., Deno, 1986; Fuchs, Allinder, Hamlett, & Fuchs, 1990; Fuchs, Fuchs, Hamlett, & Stecker, 1990; Shinn & Habedank, 1992). A final rationale supporting a purpose focus is that it decreases the potential of being caught up by the "bandwagon phenomenon." Rather than focusing on innovations in a sociopolitical context, a purpose focus causes potential system improvements to be objectively evaluated in the context of current practice. The outcomes that are targeted for improvement must be specified and the effects of the innovation measured. Hence, systems can adopt a "Show me" attitude and require clear evidence prior to wide-scale adoption of an innovation.

Educational Decision Making as the Focus: Problem Solving as the Structure

A critical first step in implementing CBM is to clarify why the procedures are being adopted. It is the assumption underlying the current discussion that the purpose of adopting CBM is system improvement in special education decision making, as it was in Iowa. Other purposes are also possible including adopting a measurement system that (1) is more in line with a particular curriculum, (2) improves on how a single educational decision is made (e.g., problem identification, evaluating solutions, etc.), and (3) adds to or augments a current set of assessment practices. Each of these purposes is valid and can be accomplished through a targeted adoption of CBM methodology. Each of these purposes limits, however, the degree to which CBM can be used to improve an overall system.

CBM's links to a Problem-Solving model (Shinn & Hubbard, 1992) are fundamental to using CBM as a vehicle for system change. Adoption of a Problem-Solving model is important for four reasons. First, it provides a structure for systematic reexamination of the current service delivery system. When the Problem-Solving model is considered, it provides a framework for examining current procedures in relation to important special education decisions. Second, a Problem-Solving model provides an important structure for determining which system components might be changed and in what order. Once current procedures are examined within the problem-solving structure, decisions can be made regarding the overall direction of the reform effort. Third, a Problem-Solving model helps communicate the "why" of reform to implementors and recipients of services. Because a Problem-Solving model focuses explicitly on decisions to be made rather than procedures, it provides a useful vehicle for communicating the purpose of the change effort. Fourth, a Problem-Solving model always references its effectiveness in relation to important educational outcomes for students. This principle has been called an *outcomes criterion*. Simply, the outcomes criterion states that "the usefulness and value of human services should be determined by the outcomes produced with the recipients of those services" (Reschly & Tilly, 1993).

In a Problem-Solving assessment system, assessment procedures are subordinate to *assessment questions* that define the purpose for data collection. Thus, the focus of a system change is not on substituting new procedures for old (e.g., CBM vs. published tests). Instead, the issue is what educational decisions are to be made within the system to reach the outcomes criterion, and how shall these decisions be made? In our experience, this distinction is extremely important for potential implementors to make. CBM procedures should be adopted because their use enables better decision making for children. Once this perspective has been communicated, understood, and adopted, a major hurdle has been crossed in moving toward using CBM appropriately as a vehicle for system change. The Problem-Solving model provides a vehicle for reexamining the system; the CBM procedures provide initial answers to questions of "how we might make special education decisions differently and better."

In a Problem-Solving model, a range of educational decisions are made including Problem Identification, Problem Certification, Exploring Solutions, Evaluating Solutions, and Problem Solution (Shinn, 1989). It is important to note that because of the way the Individuals with Disabilities Act (IDEA) is structured, these decisions are made implicitly in all special education service delivery systems, no matter what procedures or models are in place. In many cases, decisions may not be made explicitly, or in a data-based manner, but they are nonetheless made. For example, if a referral for a "comprehensive evaluation" is made and further assessment is pursued, a screening decision has been made that a problem exists warranting further assessment. The fact that this decision is not made in a data-based manner does not equate with its not being made. Alternatively, progress on an IEP goal might be monitored informally using procedures with undocumented effectiveness for that purpose. Again, the Evaluating Solutions purpose is accomplished, but with unknown quality. The same analysis could be made for each of the special education decisions.

A Progression of Implementation Questions

Once a Problem-Solving model to service delivery has been adopted and initial orientation to the approach accomplished, a predictable series of events often occurs. As with most reform initiatives, the rate of progress through the issues, the order in which they are addressed, and the answers to the questions will vary. However, adoption of a Problem-Solving model to service delivery usually causes a systematic reevaluation of decision-making practices in the current system and consideration of alternative procedures. A logical progression of discussions and questions typically follows. In general terms, the progression includes the following issues:

1. *Is it true that our system already makes these decisions?* This discussion causes implementors of a system to examine the decisions that are inherent in both the federal regulations and a Problem-Solving model. It is important to illustrate for participants in these discussions the underlying legal, ethical, and professional-practice reasons that each of the educational decisions is important.

2. *How do we currently make these decisions for different types of problems?* The answer to this questions forces a reevaluation of how different special education decisions are made in the system. For many, it provides the first opportunity for reexamination of existing procedures since 1975, when Public Law 94-142 was passed and, for some, initial insight into the purposes underlying many special education procedures.

3. *Given what has been learned in 20 years (or since the last major revision of procedures), how could our system improve its decision-making practices for a particular special education decision or decisions?* Two components of this question must be specified for a response to be possible. First, which decisions will be the focus of the discussion must be specified. Second, the educational domains that will be the focus of discussion must be identified. For elementary- and middle-school students, this discussion usually leads to the basic skills. A focus on basic skills coupled with any group of special education decisions can lead the discussion naturally to the literature on CBM.

Answering this set of questions provides a grounding in the purposes for which CBM will be adopted and momentum for moving forward.

TEN IMPORTANT WAYS TO SUPPORT
CBM IN SYSTEM CHANGE

Few universals exist in education reform. Successful reform occurs when persons at a local level take responsibility for the change process and the innovations that drive the change process (Tilly, Grimes, & Reschly, 1993). Thus, no two initiatives will look exactly alike, even when the innovations are identical. With regard to CBM, a number of components, in our experience, have been present in systems that have been successful with long-term adoption. Some of these components focus on system structures, some on system processes, and some on individual action. This section provides brief descriptions of some of the most critical components and recommendations regarding how they are implemented in practice.

Plan for the Long Term

When embarking on systemwide change initiatives, planning should be done to address a 3- to 5-year period. Critical outcomes of the initiative must be specified, and a systematic plan for reaching those goals must be constructed. Successful adoptions of CBM in our experience have taken multiple years to accomplish. Initially, implementors often adopt CBM to improve educational decision making in one or two areas. As success for these purposes is experienced during the initial implementation, users become comfortable with using CBM and examine how implementation can be expanded and other uses can be added.

To support this "phase in" approach to adoption, planning discussions must include both content and process variables. A content variable that must be determined first is with which special education decisions CBM will be used to assist. The system needs to be clear as to *why* CBM is being adopted, precisely how it will be used, and what are the anticipated benefits. Once purpose is determined, then specific CBM methodologies can be identified for implementation and methods for increasing practitioner's knowledge and skills can be determined. A timeline for implementation of these procedures should be constructed, and a commitment to its implementation must be secured from agency leadership. It has been our experience that planning time prior to implementation is seldom wasted, and taking the time to establish a shared direction is beneficial over the course of implementation.

Process variables are as critical to successful CBM implementation as content variables. Indeed, most failed CBM implementation efforts in our experience resulted more from problems with process variables than content variables. Process variables fall in two classes: political and structural. Politically, frequent and accurate communication is an imperative for any change initiative. During the planning stage of a CBM adoption, critical constituents of the education system must be identified, engaged, and their support garnered. The amount and type of information that each constituent group needs should be identified, and a schedule for communication should be established and strictly adhered to. Most importantly, communication must include the purpose for adopting CBM, the benefits, the specifics of the implementation, and how effectiveness of the adoption will be gauged. Thus, the implementation can be treated as an experiment, and effectiveness of the implementation can be demonstrated over time in a data-based manner.

A second class of process variables, structural variables, are supports created to maintain the change process over time. As innovation is begun, it is important for a person or persons in leadership positions to become familiar with the process of systemic educational reform. Documentation and analysis of the educational change process has expanded markedly within the past 20 years, and there are important lessons to be learned from this literature (e.g., Fullan, 1991; Hargreaves, 1992; Schmuck & Runkel, 1985).

Know the Whys, Not Just the Whats

When beginning a reform effort using CBM as a vehicle, implementors must understand CBM as completely as possible prior to implementation. Each implementation of CBM looks a bit different, and, as a result, in-depth knowledge of CBM is important so that boundaries of customization can be identified. Implementors must understand which components of CBM are critical and must be adhered to strictly and which components can be modified and to what extent. CBM tests are relatively simple protocols to administer and score, yet the decision-making processes underlying their use is complex. Unless implementors understand these complexities and characteristics of CBM procedures, it is possible to render the procedures ineffective due to inappropriate modification of one or more critical components.

Many strategies are available for acquiring the knowledge and skills necessary for successful implementation of CBM. For example, reading the professional literature regarding CBM and its uses is an important first step (a good starting point is the book *Curriculum-Based Measurement: Assessing Special Children;* Shinn, 1989). This survey of the literature can occur individually, but study groups of professionals reading and discussing the research have proven exceptionally effective. Additionally, a self-study package is available that has been documented to result in significant knowledge gains on the part of inservice professionals (University of Oregon School Psychology Training Program, 1993). Fundamental information to master about CBM includes not only how to do it but also how it improves on current practices.

A second strategy for acquiring knowledge about CBM is to engage the services of an expert consultant. Increasing numbers of persons with extensive experience implementing and researching CBM could be engaged to assist in the programmatic implementation of CBM. Presentations and consultation can be an effective component of an overall staff development effort, but they should not be the only component, and their role in an overall staff development plan must be clarified. One caveat regarding selection of a consultant is to be sure that whoever is selected has extensive experience *implementing* CBM in practice, not just a theoretical background. Conceptual understanding of CBM is important, but consultants skills are often most useful in heading off common implementation errors and troubleshooting implementation problems. Without a broad-based knowledge of different strategies and options available for appropriate CBM implementation, maximum benefit will not be obtained from a consulting relationship.

Use an Adequate Staff Development Model

Perhaps the most fundamental component of innovation adoption and educational change is staff development. Without planful staff development, it can be predicted with near certainty that meaningful systems-level change will not occur. There are a number of staff development models that might be used as a basis for a staff development plan (e.g., Gall & Vojtek, 1994; Showers, 1990; Wood, Killian, Quarrie, & Thompson, 1993). No matter which model is used, however, a number of components are critical. First, programmatic staff development must be considered an ongoing component of a reforming system. The term "reforming" is used intentionally in this context, since systems that adopt a data-based approach to change never really become "reformed." There are always system components that can be improved, and staff development is critical to this task. Staff development in this context must be programmatic in its intent, with later training building on earlier skills development. Indeed, planning for long-term staff development while continuing to provide services is a complex process. One Iowa administrator has described the process as similar to "trying to rewire a house with the electricity on."

A second critical staff development component requires a system's administration to make an overt commitment to providing ongoing professional development. This commitment should include long-term planning (usually 3–5 years in scope) and often requires creating a line item in an agency budget to support training and follow-up over time. For implementations of CBM, costs associated with initial skills training are only a beginning. Costs related to ongoing support and follow-up must be factored in if the intent is systemic implementation and maintenance of the innovation. Specifics of this budgeting process will be unique to the individual implementation. However, discussions with experienced users of CBM can identify realistic estimates of costs of implementing CBM.

A third requirement of staff development systems for system reform is that staff must be trained to a "skills" level of performance, not simply an awareness level. In our experience, this necessity has required rethinking and redesigning of traditional staff development procedures and processes. Drive-by workshops (e.g., 1- or 2-day meetings without follow-up), although they may be informative and entertaining, have not resulted in wide-scale professional behavior change. In-service professionals learn new skills precisely the same way that children do, by performing new skills in controlled circumstances and receiving feedback on their performance. In Iowa, we have found that we can no longer ignore what we know about human learning if we truly expect professional behavior change that will significantly improve our system. Thus, staff development efforts have become slower in their introduction of new skills, require guided practice of new skills with feedback during acquisition phases of learning and massed practice with feedback as implementors build fluency, and require participants to demonstrate some facility with new skills prior to the introduction of new skills.

Engage Leadership

Leadership in this context refers to a role, not a position. Barker's (1992) description of a leader as a person you would follow to a place you wouldn't go yourself applies. In any education system, there are persons whose support can influence CBM implementation positively. These persons likely will include school administrators, teachers, related-service persons, and parents. In any major initiative, it makes sense to commission a steering committee whose role is to provide guidance and direction. Including system leaders as decision makers in a CBM initiative has distinct advantages. First, inclusion of leaders will cause the system to "take CBM seriously" from the beginning and may promote greater levels of implementation early in the project. Second, involving leaders from diverse groups lends credibility and balance to the overall implementation effort. When questions or concerns arise from a constituent, there will be a peer on the leadership team who credibly can address the concerns. Third, including opinion leaders as decision makers for the initiative allows these persons' questions and concerns to be dealt with proactively, directly, and positively, which decreases the possibility of these persons' leadership influencing implementation negatively.

Publicize Success

In every CBM implementation effort, there will be successes and challenges to be overcome. Often, it is possible to build significant support for CBM by publicizing initial successes through sharing results with others. CBM data-collection procedures yield data that can be graphed to depict student performance (a key outcome variable in any educational system), and these graphs can be used to illustrate the benefits of using a Problem-Solving model. With readily available computer software, graphs can be generated quickly to assist making any educational decision where CBM is used. The following illustrations present examples of how CBM data might be summarized to communicate important student performance information to varied constituencies. The reader is encouraged to consider how these types of graphics might be useful in practice.

Figure 2.1 contains a display of CBM normative data for one grade level with a school district. It is used to explain the meaning of a CBM "cover sheet" to parents and educators without the use of statistical jargon. This figure usually is accompanied by an explanation such as "If we randomly selected a hundred children from our school district and lined them up against the wall from lowest performer to highest performer, this box shows how their scores would be distributed." This same type of description can be used for each CBM measure displayed on the cover sheet.

Figure 2.2 illustrates how a CBM normative data "cover sheet" can be used to assist in making Problem Identification (screening) decisions for an individual student. The assessment question in this case is "Is more assessment warranted?" The measurement activities focus on individual performance data in all areas of concern. The evaluation activity requires a determination to be made regarding whether the student's performance is discrepant from typical performance to the extent that further assessment is warranted. In the example, the school district criteria for further assessment was "at or below the 16th percentile." Chad B.'s CBM scores are overlaid on the winter cover sheet for his school district. It is clear from this depiction that Chad's current performance in all basic skills areas does not meet the criteria for further assessment. Note that areas where no box plot is shown do not have sufficient variability in the normative data to create a box plot.

Figure 2.3 illustrates how a CBM normative data "cover sheet" can be used to assist in making Problem Certification (entitlement) decisions.

How to Interpret a Cover Sheet

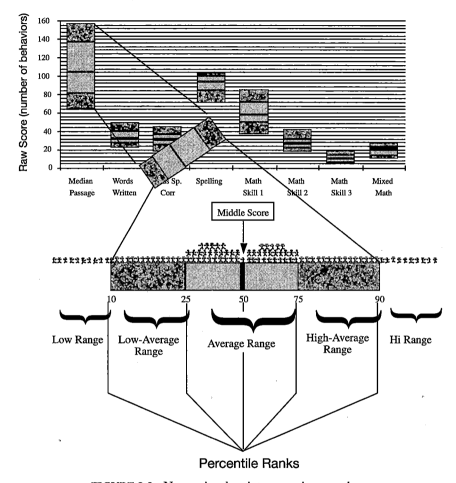

FIGURE 2.1. Normative data interpretation template.

Problem Certification decisions answer the question "Is a problem severe enough to warrant the use of resource beyond general education to resolve the problem?" The measurement activities focus on collecting student performance data in successively lower levels of the curriculum. The evaluation activity requires a determination to be made regarding how far behind the individual's performance is in the school's curriculum. CBM reading passage scores for Karen S. are overlaid on an across-grade reading graph. This graphic depicts typical grade-level performance in grade-level material (e.g., first graders' performance in first-grade materials, sec-

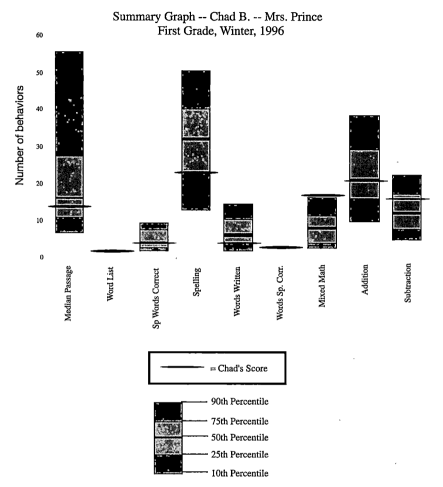

FIGURE 2.2. CBM data summary for an individual student: Norm-referenced peer comparison—screening decision.

ond graders' performance in second-grade material, etc.). It is clear from this depiction that Karen's reading performance compared to fourth graders is far below the 10th percentile. If she were a third grader reading third-grade material, her performance would also place her below the 10th percentile compared to third graders. When Karen reads second- and first-grade materials, her performance appears to more closely approximate typical second- or first-grade performance. Since Karen is a fourth grader, her performance appears to be at least 2 years behind in the curriculum. Hence, these data might be used to support a conclusion that

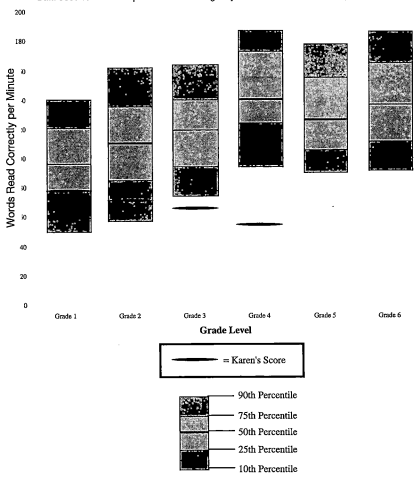

FIGURE 2.3. Survey-level CBM procedure used to identify a student's performance in successively easier levels of the curriculum—eligibility determination decision.

resources not available in general education might be warranted to resolve this problem.

Figure 2.4 illustrates how CBM performance monitoring data can be used to assist in making "Evaluating Solutions" decisions. The assessment question in this case is "Is the reading intervention working?" The measurement activities focus on collecting CBM data frequently and repeatedly across time. The evaluation activity requires a determination to be

Student's Name __Ben M.__   District __Des Moines__   School __Primary__   School Year __9x–9x__   Teacher __Smith__

Goal Statement: __In 32 weeks, when presented with a randomly selected passage from Silver-Burdette–Ginn level 3-2,__
__Ben will read 108 words correct per minute__

Expected Level of Performance: Goal Criterion (#) __108__ Quarterly Objective 1 (#) __58__ Quarterly Objective 2 (#) __74__ Quarterly Objective 3 (#) __91__ Quarterly Objective 4 (#) __(Same as Goal Criterion)__

Service: Primary Provider __Smith (RR Teacher)__   Supporting Provider __Jacobs (3rd grade teacher)__   Supporting Provider __Sally M. (mother)__

Parent Participation: __Parent Conferences: 10-12, 11-2, 2-6, 3-5, notes 10-1, 10-31, 11-1, 12,14,3-17__

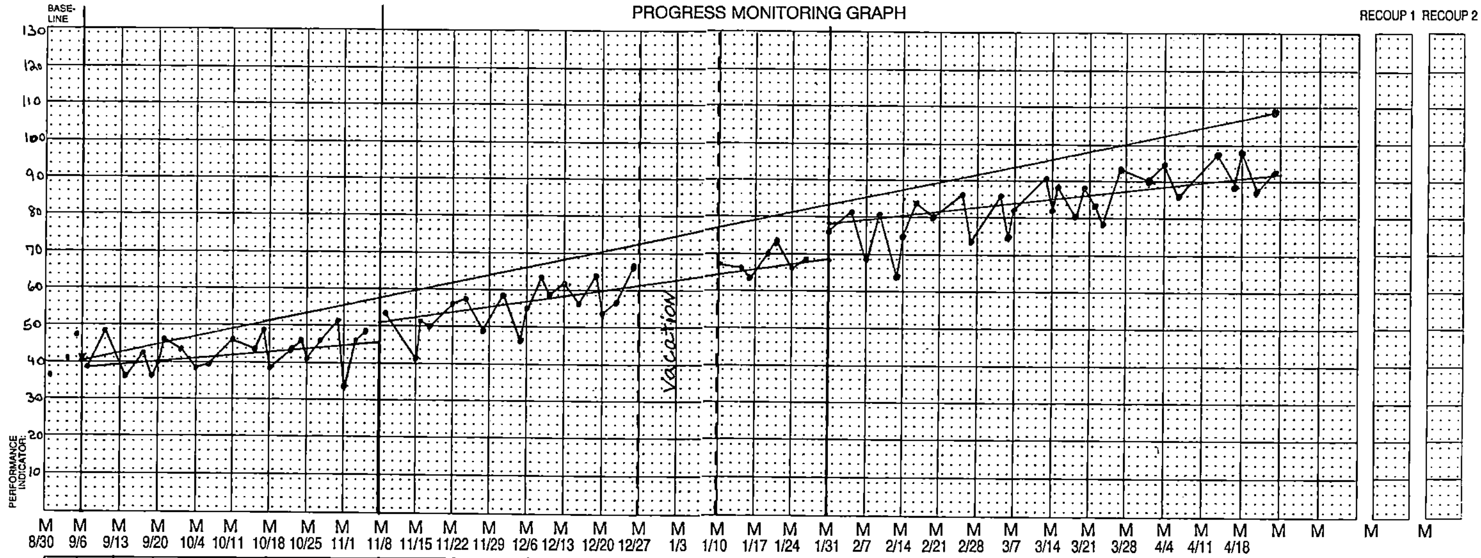

PROGRESS MONITORING GRAPH

FIGURE 2.4. Ben's individual CBM progress monitoring graph.

made regarding whether the student's performance is improving at an acceptable rate (i.e., is the intervention working?). In this case, Ben M's graph illustrates how CBM data can be used to determine when to change the reading intervention program. The chart format used in this example was developed across a 4-year period by a large number of Iowa educators. These educators borrowed liberally from other CBM implementation projects across America and integrated many good ideas into a format that is exceptionally useful for progress monitoring. The graph is printed on 17" by 22" paper and is prepared so that when folded in half, it fits into a typical 8½" by 11" notebook. A copy of this form is available from the first author.

Figures 2.5 and 2.6 depict first-grade students' performance on CBM reading tasks during the fall and spring of the year. Figure 2.5 illustrates the fact that many children enter first grade as very disfluent readers. By the end of first grade (see Figure 2.6), however, many of these students have improved their reading fluency markedly. This type of display can be generated for each grade to illustrate changes in groups of students performance across time.

No matter which decisions are the focus of improvement, CBM data can provide an impressive display that can be shared with important constituent groups. Useful strategies include presenting CBM data at a PTA meeting, working with an administrator on a presentation for the school board, and preparing a graph for each child in the school for sharing at the time of parent–teacher conferences.

Work Smart

It is not often possible to expect persons in school to work any harder. Creating meaningful change in educational delivery systems entails significant work. Adopting CBM is no exception. The only alternative to working harder (which is somewhat unavoidable) is to work strategically to build a reform effort. Components of working smart include starting CBM on a small scale, working with innovation leaders, and letting innovation spread naturally.

An important rule should be adhered to when embarking on a CBM initiative: Don't begin more innovation than can be supported by the system. Systems adopting CBM must examine the capacity of their system to provide follow-up and support to all implementors. The reality is that if CBM cannot be made to work at a small scale, then it will not work on a large scale. Working smart frequently means identifying persons in the system who are interested in early adoption of CBM procedures. Often, these persons are teachers wishing to experiment with the procedures in their classrooms. Working smart also means working directly with these persons early in the implementation of CBM and providing sufficient re-

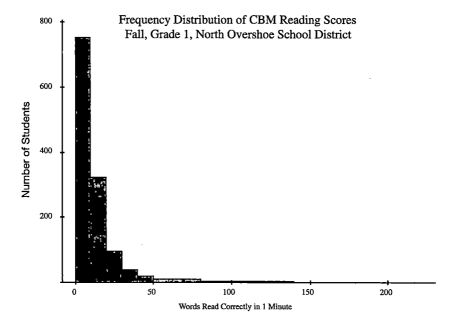

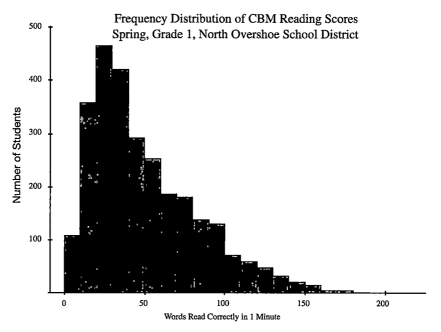

FIGURES 2.5 and 2.6. Frequency distributions of first graders' CBM reading performance during fall and spring—system analysis decision.

sources to ensure their success. These persons often will become advocates of the procedures and can contribute significant energy, based on their experiences, to the start-up of a larger CBM initiative. Finally, it is usually best to begin a CBM initiative on a small scale and allow expansion to occur naturally. A question is sometimes asked, "How do you sell CBM to teachers?" The answer is that it is best not to. CBM improves educational decision-making practices when used appropriately. When educators experience this benefit, they typically share their perceptions with others. Sales are not required.

Let No One Fail Alone

Adoption of CBM procedures often involves risks. Sometimes these risks are unwarranted (e.g., If CBM replaces current procedures, will my skills still be valued?) and sometimes they are realistic (e.g., Will there be enough time to implement CBM in my school with fidelity?). In all cases, the perception of risk on the part of implementors must be discussed and solutions identified. One useful strategy is to "let no one fail alone." To accomplish this task, the responsibility for initial implementation of CBM, even at the individual-teacher level, must be shared by more than a single person. Effective strategies include pairing teachers together who will initially have responsibility for using CBM to monitor a small group of students' progress. Alternatively, a principal, a group of teachers, and a related service person may spearhead a CBM norming project. Or a group of special education teachers may use CBM procedures to examine the potential for reintegration for a small group of special education students. The common feature among all of these implementations is *joint* responsibility for successes or missteps. When CBM is implemented initially by pairs or groups of persons, it has been our experience that a climate of trust and collegiality is established that creates tolerance of mistakes. It is inevitable that initial implementations of CBM will result in implementation errors. The key of this strategy, then, is to assist teams to identify mistakes when they occur, to correct them, and to ensure that the implementation effort continues. Ultimately, when successful results are generated, there is often a shared sense of accomplishment that can support expansion of CBM into use with other educational decisions.

Expect a Dual System

It has been our experience that successful adoption of CBM innovation has not resulted from large-scale abandonment of prevailing procedures prior to significant implementation of CBM. Instead, the educational decisions underlying the adoption of CBM are reexamined, and the adoption of CBM for any specific decision is based on the extent to which CBM improves upon prevailing practices. For many reasons, current educational decision-making procedures are ardently protected when threatened. Many special educators and related-services personnel identify personally with practices that have defined their professional identity for years. Moreover, it is often uncomfortable (and may be unprofessional in some cases) to relinquish an existing set of practices for an unknown alternative, no matter what empirical evidence suggests. Thus, an alternative approach to supplanting less effective decision-making practices is usually warranted.

One effective approach to improving decision making is to continue on with typical practices for making a particular educational decision and then to "add on" CBM procedures. This practice creates what some have called a "dual system," where both current practices and CBM exist in the same system simultaneously. For example, in cases where entitlement assessment practices are targeted for improvement, it is often beneficial to continue using procedures that have always been done, then adding CBM to the database upon which the eligibility decision will rest. Few situations exist where CBM data do not add significant information to the data provided by nationally normed, published, standardized tests. Thus, existing procedures are evaluated in the context of the CBM data and procedures. Over time, as both sets of information are collected repeatedly and consumers begin to experience the benefits of using the CBM database, questions arise. If CBM accomplishes the purposes of current procedures *and* improves significantly on prevailing practices, which procedures should be primary?

This approach to innovation has a number of advantages. First, at the point at which the dual system can no longer be supported and a single set of procedures must be adopted (usually about 2 years into implementation), decisions can be made in an experiential manner. Current practices are not challenged based solely on logical, research-based arguments. Decisions regarding direction are based on *experiences* regarding effective practice and not solely on who can argue most loudly. Second, persons are not asked to abandon practices that have become comfortable simply for the sake of adopting CBM. Instead, they are allowed to experience new procedures, and CBM spreads naturally rather than in a forced or mandated manner. Finally, this approach to implementing CBM begins on everyone's common ground: current practices.

Despite the benefits to the dual-system approach to CBM adoption, there is one potential danger. That danger is the situation where CBM procedures are added on as another source of information, usually to make eligibility decisions, and a Problem-Solving model of service delivery is not adopted. In this case, CBM is used simply to assist with a single decision and is not linked to goal setting, intervention planning, and progress monitoring. When used in this way, CBM does not provide a significant improvement over the previous system and, in fact, becomes an add-on. Hence, adoption of a Problem-Solving model to service delivery is a critical component to adopting CBM as a vehicle for system reform.

Expect Resistance

Any meaningful change will have its vocal detractors, and there may be many reasons underlying the animosity. Indeed, a colleague, after experiencing numerous examples of resistance to change, created a law summarizing the relationship. "Stoner's Law" asserts that "under the best of circumstances, 50 percent of people will be upset by change; in the worst, 95 percent will be angry" (cited in Shinn & Good, 1990). It is axiomatic: Change creates resistance. This resistance typically represents the first stage of the change process (Hord, Rutherford, Huling-Austin, & Hall, 1987). Resistance to change should be planned for and addressed as a part of the change process. Indeed, if resistance is not encountered, implementors should wonder whether meaningful change is occurring.

Dealing with resistance requires understanding, tolerance, creativity, and perseverance. Typically, as communication efforts related to the innovation are effective, large-scale resistance to adoption of potentially effective innovations becomes less problematic. One effective way to deal with resistance head-on is to frame all changes as experiments with clearly specified outcome expectations. The effectiveness of current practices can be used as a baseline against which the effectiveness of innovation can be judged. Results of the experiment will dictate which procedures should be primary. As stated earlier, an expectation of innovation is that the new practices improve upon existing procedures in important and meaningful ways. In this case, use of a data-based approach to adoption does not pose a threat to the ultimate adoption of the innovation. Instead, it provides a responsible structure for implementing innovation, it models the data-based decision-making process that is at the center of CBM adoption, and it provides a safety net for the system. If the new procedures do not attain their promise, they can be abandoned in a data-based way.

Collaborate with Other Implementors

A final component useful for successful CBM implementation is consultation and collaboration with other implementors. Although not imperative, valuable lessons can be learned both from successful and unsuccessful implementors. Indeed, some of the most important lessons can be learned from persons who struggled during initial implementation. Many common implementation errors can be avoided through such visits. Site visits to schools where CBM is institutionalized are seldom a waste of time and can result in the transfer of useful information not available anywhere else.

SUMMARY AND IMPLICATIONS

Introducing new practices into an educational system is a familiar occurrence. Having those practices become valued and sustained within a system across time is a more challenging proposition. Long-term acceptance of new approaches is not a function of the power of the ideas per se, but the extent that the educational system expects, values, and supports professionals in performing these new practices. Generally, for new educational approaches to become incorporated into the overall system requires system change. In this chapter, we have emphasized how CBM has been an important part of an overall change process in Iowa. CBM has served in Iowa as a vehicle to help establish the importance of using a Problem-Solving model for service delivery. In many ways, CBM also was the vanguard technology illustrating that student improvement could be measured dynamically in basic academics and the results communicated in a meaningful way.

When Iowa's administrative rules for special education were revised in 1995, following the years of flexibility, waivers, and experimentation, the overall impact of Iowa's system change became codified. Throughout the rule-revision process, Iowa applied the principle that policy follows practice (Grimes & Tilly, 1996). This principle means that new rules were designed to support practices that had been demonstrated to be feasible, responsible, and desirable. CBM was one of the many forces that influenced the ultimate course of our new rules. Successful experiences with CBM influenced our rules in two major ways. First, the general Problem-Solving model upon which CBM is built has been written into Iowa's new rules of special education. It is now required that prior to referral for special education, a general education intervention is implemented that includes Problem Identification, Problem Analysis, Progress Monitoring, and Program Evaluation decisions. Additionally, Iowa's rules allow intermediate agencies to adopt a Problem-Solving model and Problem-Solving methodologies as their comprehensive structure for providing special education services.

The second way that the concepts underlying CBM influenced our rules was by demonstrating that technically adequate measurement of growth toward meaningful long-term goals is possible. The concept of evaluating the effectiveness of educational services for students has become an explicit expectation of our special education system (see Chapter 41 of Iowa's Administrative Rules). This expectation has led to the creation of a statewide project to examine the extent to which these individual results can be summarized. Thus, aggregated intervention results form a picture of the impact of educational services for students with unique needs. This conceptual framework is illustrated in Figure 2.7.

In this system, individual student growth toward accomplishment of IEP or Individual Family Service Plan (IFSP) goals is a critical indicator of success. Student growth toward goals is the "coin of the realm" in this system, and individual results are used for decision making at two levels of the system. First, at an individual level, they provide a means for reconsidering services provided by the IEP or IFSP. Second, individual results may

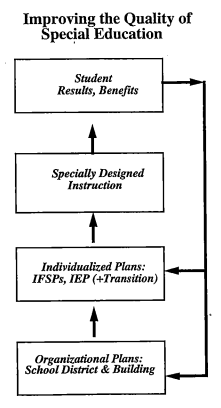

Improving the Quality of Special Education

Student Results, Benefits

Specially Designed Instruction

Individualized Plans: IFSPs, IEP (+Transition)

Organizational Plans: School District & Building

FIGURE 2.7. Illustration of a special education system Improvement Model.

be aggregated across goals and across groups of students to establish a picture of an organization's educational success. The intent of these summaries is ongoing improvement of educational services over time, just as the intent of using CBM formatively is improvement in student performance over time.

The process of improvement in Iowa is not finished. We have embraced an approach in which organizational modification is based on student outcomes and the refinement of the system is viewed as a continuous process. Inherent in such an approach is the challenge of ever-present change. The upside is that services are constantly being adjusted to fit students' emerging educational needs. For this task to be achieved in a reasonable and responsible manner requires data about students outcomes from their educational interventions. Thus, refinements in the educational system will be based upon data just as, within a CBM approach, an individual's educational plan is adjusted to ensure that goal-directed efforts are on course and meeting human needs.

REFERENCES

Barker, J. A. (1992). *Future edge*. New York: Morrow.

Deno, S. L. (1986). Formative evaluation of individual student programs: A new role for school psychologists. *School Psychology Review, 15*, 358–374.

Epps, S., & Tindal, G. (1988). *The effectiveness of differential programming in serving mildly handicapped students: Placement options and instructional programming*. London: Oxford University Press.

Fuchs, L. S., Allinder, R., Hamlett, C. L., & Fuchs, D. (1990). Analysis of spelling curriculum and teachers' skills in identifying phonetic error types. *Remedial and Special Education, 11*(1), 42–53.

Fuchs, L., & Deno, S. L. (1991). Paradigmatic distinctions between instructionally relevant measurement models. *Exceptional Children, 57*, 488–500.

Fuchs, L. S., Fuchs, D., Hamlett, C. L., & Stecker, P. M. (1990). The role of skills analysis to curriculum-based measurement in math. *School Psychology Review, 19*, 6–22.

Fullan, M. (1991). *The new meaning of educational change* (2nd ed.). London: Cassell.

Fullan, M. (1996). Turning systemic thinking on its head. *Phi Delta Kappan, 77*(6), 420–423.

Gall, M. D., & Vojtek, R. O. (1994). *Planning for effective staff development: Six research-based models* (ERIC No. ED372464). ERIC Clearinghouse on Educational Management.

Grimes, J., & Tilly, W. D., III. (1996). Policy and process: Means to lasting educational change. *School Psychology Review, 4*, 464–475.

Hargreaves, A. (1992). *Teacher development and educational change*. London: Falmer Press.

Hargreaves, A. (1994). Restructuring restructuring: Postmodernity and the prospects for educational change. *Journal of Education Policy, 9,* 47–65.

Heller, K. A., Holtzman, W., & Messick, S. (1982). *Placing children in special education: A strategy for equity.* Washington, DC: National Academy Press.

Hord, S. M., Rutherford, W. L., Huling-Austin, L., & Hall, G. E. (1987). *Taking charge of change.* Austin, TX: Southwest Education Development Laboratory.

Howell, K. W., Fox, S. L., & Morehead, M. K. (1993). *Curriculum-based evaluation: Teaching and decision making* (2nd ed.). Pacific Grove, CA: Brooks/Cole.

Kavale, K. (1990). The effectiveness of special education. In T. B. Gutkin & C. R. Reynolds (Eds.), *The handbook of school psychology* (pp. 868–898). New York: Wiley.

Madden, N., & Slavin, R. (1983). Mainstreaming students with mild handicaps: Academic and social outcomes. *Review of Educational Research, 53,* 519–659.

Marston, D. (1989). Curriculum-based measurement: What is it and why do it? In M. R. Shinn (Eds.), *Curriculum-based measurement: Assessing special children* (pp. 18–78). New York: Guilford Press.

National Association of School Psychologists and National Coalition of Advocates for Students (1985). *Position statement: Advocacy for appropriate educational services for all children.* Washington, DC: Author.

Reschly, D. J., & Tilly, W. D. (1993). The why of system reform. *National Association of School Psychologists Communiqué, 22*(1), 1–6.

Shanker, A. (1995). A reflection on twelve studies of educational reform. *Phi Delta Kappan, 77*(1), 81–83.

Schmuck, R. A., & Runkel, P. J. (1985). *The handbook of organization development in schools* (3rd ed.). Palo Alto, CA: Mayfield.

Shinn, M. R. (Ed.). (1989). *Curriculum-based measurement: Assessing special children.* New York: Guilford Press.

Shinn, M. R., & Good, R. H. (Ed.). (1990). *CBA: An assessment of its current status and a prognosis for its future.* Engelwood Cliffs, NJ: Erlbaum.

Shinn, M. R., & Habedank, L. (1992). Curriculum-Based Measurement in special education problem identification and certification decisions. *Preventing School Failure, 36,* 11–15.

Shinn, M. R., & Hubbard, D. D. (1992). Curriculum-Based Measurement and problem-solving assessment: Basic procedures and outcomes. *Focus on Exceptional Children, 24,* 1–20.

Showers, B. (1990). Aiming for superior classroom instruction for all children: A comprehensive staff development model. *Remedial and Special Education, 11,* 35–39.

Sitlington, P. L., Frank, A. R., & Carson, R. (1993). Adult adjustment among high school graduates with mild disabilities. *Exceptional Children, 59,* 221–233.

Tilly, W. D., Grimes, J. P., & Reschly, D. J. (1993). Special education system reform: The Iowa story. *National Association of School Psychologists Communiqué, 22*(1), 1–6.

University of Oregon School Psychology Training Program. (1993). *CBM continuing professional development training package.* Eugene, OR: College of Education, University of Oregon.

Will, M. (1986). *Educating students with learning problems: A shared responsibility.* Washington, DC: U. S. Department of Education.

Wood, F., Killian, J., Quarrie, F., & Thompson, S. (1993). *How to organize a school-based staff development program.* Alexandria, VA: Association for Supervision and Curriculum Development.

CHAPTER 3

◆◆◆

Contemporary Perspectives on Curriculum-Based Measurement Validity

◆

ROLAND H. GOOD III
GRETCHEN JEFFERSON

In the past 10 years, the construct of validity has undergone remarkable evolution and refinement. Past conceptualizations of validity have focused on "whether a test measures what it says it measures" with four types of evidence considered: (1) construct validity, (2) concurrent criterion-related validity, (3) predictive criterion-related validity, and (4) content validity. Although these tried-and-true conceptualizations remain important, there is increasing agreement that they are not enough. The call for an expanded perspective of validity comes from many sources and utilizes a variety of terms. The advocates of special education reform have called for an *outcomes criterion* (Reschly, 1988) in which the quality of assessment procedures depends on whether meaningful student outcomes are enhanced as a result of the measurement activities. From a behavioral assessment perspective comes the idea of *treatment utility*, that assessment ought to contribute demonstrably to the selection of effective interventions (Hayes, Nelson, & Jarrett, 1987). Two common themes have emerged from these discussions of validity.

1. Assessment procedures must also be judged, in part, by their demonstrated contributions to desirable student outcomes.
2. It is also important to evaluate the moral and values implications of assessment in addition to evaluating the psychometric evi-

dence. It is not enough to determine that we *can* measure a construct with a particular test. It also is important to judge whether it is *good, right,* and *appropriate* to measure the construct in that way.

The emerging perspectives of validity are explicated best by Messick (1975, 1986, 1989, 1990, 1995) and are beginning to be used in evaluating assessment (e.g., Gersten, Keating, & Irvin, 1995). Messick describes validity as "an integrated evaluative judgment of the degree to which empirical evidence and theoretical rationales support the adequacy and appropriateness of inferences and actions based on test scores or other modes of assessment" (1989, p. 13). Tightly packed within this definition are four facets of validity: (1) construct validity, (2) values implications, (3) relevance/utility, and (4) social consequences.

The *construct validity* of a test corresponds best to conventional conceptualizations of validity, including the myriad ways of demonstrating that a test measures the construct it says it measures. The *values implications* facet of validity refers to values and moral judgments regarding whether it is good, right, and appropriate to make the inferences the test implies. The *relevance/utility* facet of validity involves evidence that the test results provide an adequate basis for the actions and decisions that are based on the test. Finally, the *social consequences* facet addresses the values and moral implications of taking those actions and making those decisions based on the test. This chapter will be organized around these four facets identified by Messick.

Particularly with respect to the relevance/utility and social consequences facets of validity, it is clear that test validity is evaluated within the context of actions or decisions based on test information. For Curriculum-Based Measurement (CBM), the Problem-Solving model of educational decision making provides an appropriate framework within which to evaluate test-based actions. Thus, five potential actions/decisions will be considered in this chapter: (1) Problem Identification, (2) Problem Certification or Validation, (3) Exploring Solutions, (4) Evaluating Solutions, and (5) Problem Solution.

CONSTRUCT VALIDITY OF CBM

According to Messick, construct validity addresses the adequacy of inferences based on test scores. Whether they realize it or not, educators continually make inferences about students based on test scores. If a student scores low on a reading test, we *infer* that the student has low reading skills; if the student scores high on an intelligence test, we *infer* that he or she is more intelligent. The inferences we draw are directly related to the construct ostensibly measured by the test. The term "construct" is used here to refer to the idea of the thing being assessed. The construct of reading competence, for example, refers to the domain of all reading skills and reading behaviors that conceptually comprise competent reading. Constructs do not have any physical reality. There is nothing that can be held, measured, or weighed that is "intelligence" or "reading competence." We use the term "construct" to distinguish the idea of the thing we are trying to measure from the particular sample of behaviors on a test. Each test is only a sample of behavior, not the construct itself (Salvia & Ysseldyke, 1995). No reading test can measure all of the skills and behaviors that constitute reading competence. A test provides an adequate basis for inferences about the construct if the scores on the test generally correspond to the construct ostensibly measured by the test: in other words, when the test measures what it says it measures.

The problem with construct validity, of course, is that we can never *know* if test scores correspond to the construct, because the construct is not accessible to us. Thus, we need indirect evidence. A common approach referred to as criterion-related validity is to see if the test is correlated with another test (i.e., the criterion) measuring the same construct. The logic of this approach is that if the same construct is responsible for both test scores, then the scores should be correlated. Of course, neither test will be a perfect measure of the construct, and so they cannot be perfectly correlated. This logic is illustrated in Figure 3.1 using CBM reading as an example. If CBM reading and the criterion are correlated, then both are measuring something in common. The "something in common" is presumably the construct of interest. If the two measures are not correlated, or if the magnitude of the correlation is lower than expected, then either the CBM reading measure is not related to the construct, or the criterion is not related to the construct, or both.

One might wonder why it is important that an "alternative" assess-

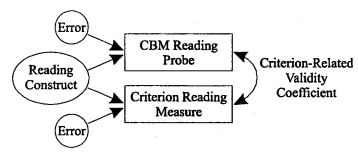

FIGURE 3.1. Logic underlying criterion-related validity as construct validity evidence for a test.

ment procedure such as CBM correlates with conventional measures of achievement. In fact, as discussed by Shinn in Chapter 1, this volume, some critics (e.g., Mehrens & Clarizio, 1993) have accused CBM developers of inconsistency in their arguments. The critics claim that if published achievement tests are "bad," then CBM validation studies should not use them as criterion measures (see Shinn & Bamonto, Chapter 1, this volume, for more detail). The point of this discussion is that the correlation between the CBM reading measure and criterion measures is not important in its own right, but only as evidence that *both* tests are related to the underlying construct of reading competence. Thus, correlations with a *variety* of measures of the same underlying construct, including published achievement tests, strengthen the construct validity of a test. Generally, concurrent, criterion-related validity coefficients in the range .60 to .80 are taken as evidence in support of the validity of a test (Salvia & Ysseldyke, 1995). For example, the Stanford Diagnostic Reading Test reports concurrent validity coefficients of .67 to .88 with the Stanford Achievement Test for the Red Level (Salvia & Ysseldyke, 1995, p. 480).

Concurrent, Criterion-Related Validity of CBM with Other Measures

Many studies have examined the criterion-related validity of CBM probes. Marston (1989) summarized the concurrent validity of CBM probes through 1989. Although exhaustive, Marston's review has three limitations. First, there is so much information on the validity of each type of measure that it is easy to be overwhelmed. Second, additional research has contributed to our understanding of the construct validity of CBM since that review. Third, many of the validity coefficients reported by Marston were computed across grade or age levels. The problem is that across-age or grade correlations generally artificially inflate validity coefficients (Salvia & Ysseldyke, 1995). The validity of a test is supported if the test and the criterion agree in differentiating a third grader with high reading skills (for example) from a third grader with low reading skills. However, calculating a validity coefficient across grades one to six only tells us that the tests agree in differentiating a first grader from a sixth grader, something most of us do not need a test to accomplish accurately.

The purpose of this section is to summarize succinctly the information available about the criterion-related validity of CBM measures. Three criteria were specified for inclusion in this review. First, only within-grade validity coefficients were included. If scores were standardized by grade before calculating the correlation, those validity coefficients also were included. Second, only validity coefficients with publicly available criteria where included. Thus, validity coefficients were included if the criterion was a published, norm-referenced test, a published, criterion-referenced test, or a test from a publisher's basal reader series. Correlations with informal reading measures such as teacher-made tests or experimental measures were not included. Correlations with latent factors (e.g., Shinn, Good, Knutson, Tilly, & Collins, 1992) will be addressed in a subsequent section. Third, to reduce confusion and information overload, the most frequently used and recommended CBM scoring rules and CBM measurement materials were included. Thus, for reading, oral reading fluency on grade-level passages from students' curricula were included, but maze measures were not. For written language, students were asked to write a story based on a story starter, and their stories were scored for the number of correct writing sequences. In math, where consensus on measurement-material rules has not been clearly established, a variety of measurement materials were included in the review.

The median concurrent criterion-related validity coefficients for each measurement area and grade level are reported in Table 3.1. From the

TABLE 3.1. Summary of Concurrent, Criterion-Related Validity for Selected CBM Probes

Grade	Measurement material	Number of validity coefficients	Median validity coefficient
	Reading		
2	Oral reading fluency on passages	3	.69
3	Oral reading fluency on passages	16	.71
4	Oral reading fluency on passages	10	.73
5	Oral reading fluency on passages	13	.62
6	Oral reading fluency on passages	4	.66
	Math		
3	Grade level addition, subtraction, mixed, wide, and narrow probes	12	.32
5	Grade level multiplication, division, mixed, wide, and narrow probes	12	.57
	Written expression		
2	Correct writing sequences with story starters	1	.60
3	Correct writing sequences with story starters	5	.68
4	Correct writing sequences with story starters	1	.58
5	Correct writing sequences with story starters	1	.61
6	Correct writing sequences with story starters	1	.52
8	Correct writing sequences with story starters	1	.56
11	Correct writing sequences with story starters	1	.48

Note. Data from Espin, Deno, Maruyama, and Cohen (1989); Hubbard (1996); Marston (1989); Parker, Tindal, and Hasbrouck (1991); Putnam (1990); and Shinn et al. (1992).

table, it is clear that the most information is available about CBM reading. In CBM reading, multiple validity coefficients are available for each grade level, based on different studies and reading curricula. All CBM reading validity coefficients are in the .60 to .80 range, supporting the construct validity of CBM reading. The construct validity evidence for written language based on number of correct writing sequences was less extensive and lower in magnitude. For most of the grade levels, only one study was identified reporting a within-grade validity coefficient. For elementary grades, most validity coefficients were in the lower end of the .60 to .80 range, providing modest support for the construct validity of CBM for written expression scored with correct writing sequences. In math, information was available only for third and fifth grades (Putnam, 1989), with the magnitude of the validity coefficients providing only modest support for the construct validity of CBM math probes. The consistently lower correlations with published math tests have led some to question the validity of the criterion measures. For example, Marston (1982) found the best correlations with published math tests were a combination of math and reading performance.

Correlations with Latent Constructs

A preferable approach to evaluating the construct validity of CBM measures is illustrated by Shinn et al. (1992). They examined the factor structure of multiple reading measures, including CBM oral reading probes, published, norm-referenced reading measures, and informal measures of reading competence such as reading orally a phonetically regular word list from the Test of Written Language. By using factor-analytic methods, the correlation of each variable with the constructs (e.g., reading competence) shared in common by the measures could be estimated. This approach is superior to the criterion-related validity approach described earlier, because it moves the focus away from correlations between CBM reading probes and specific criterion tests and instead focuses explicitly on the extent to which the CBM reading probes are related to the construct that is shared in common across the set of reading measures. The pattern of correlations with reading constructs from Shinn et al. is illustrated in Table 3.2.

For third-grade students, Shinn et al. (1992) found that the eight reading measures they examined represented one underlying construct that they labeled Reading Competence. The correlations of the reading measures with the Reading Competence construct are summarized in Table 3.2. For third-grade students, CBM oral reading probes correlated .88 and .90 with a latent construct of Reading Competence, higher than any of the other reading measures that were examined. For fifth-grade

TABLE 3.2. Validity Coefficients of CBM Reading Probes with Reading Constructs for Third- and Fifth-Grade Students

Variable	Third-grade Reading Competence	Fifth grade Reading— Decoding	Fifth grade Reading— Comprehension
CBM Reading Probe 1	.88	.90	.75
CBM Reading Probe 2	.90	.89	.74
Phonetically regular words	.76	.77	.64
Nonsense words	.78	.56	.47
Written retell	.69	.43	.51
Cloze exact matches	.85	.71	.86
SDRT Literal Comprehension	.71	.62	.75
SDRT Inferential Comprehension	.72	.60	.73

Note. SDRT, Stanford Diagnostic Reading Test. Adapted from Shinn, Good, Knutson, Tilly, and Collins (1992, pp. 470, 474). Copyright 1992 by the National Association of School Psychologists. Adapted by permission of the author.

students, Shinn et al. found that two reading constructs were required to explain the intercorrelations among the eight reading measures, which they labeled Decoding and Comprehension. The CBM reading probes were correlated most strongly with Decoding, but they also were correlated about .75 with Comprehension, comparable with or greater than other measures of reading comprehension. As a caveat to these findings, it is possible that the constructs of Decoding and Comprehension in Shinn et al. may have been artifacts of the measurement materials. The Decoding construct included only measures where the students read aloud. The Comprehension construct included measures where the student read silently and answered in writing.

In summary, the construct validity of CBM oral reading probes has been demonstrated persuasively. Clearly, CBM reading probes are as valid or more valid indicators of reading competence as other available reading measures. The construct validity of written expression and math also is supported, although less evidence is available, and the magnitude of the validity coefficients is less than CBM reading. Within-grade validity coefficients for spelling were not available.

RELEVANCE AND UTILITY OF CBM

From a contemporary perspective, criterion-related validity is desirable *but not sufficient* for determining the validity of any measure. The *relevance* and *utility* of any measure also must be considered when establishing the validity of that measure. The goal of assessment is to gather information about a student's performance to make decisions about interventions that directly contribute to the *remediation* of problems. Evaluations of the validity of CBM in the Problem-Solving model also must include an examination of the relevance and utility of CBM in resolving academic problems.

Relevance

The *relevance* of a test refers to the directness of the linkage between the assessment measure or method and the proposed purpose of the assessment (Messick, 1995). If the selected assessment measure or method provides information that *directly* addresses or answers the questions posed in the assessment process, that measure or method is more relevant to the purpose of the assessment than one that provides information that requires interpretation or inference. A direct link is established if the information collected during the problem-solving process contributes to *resolution* of the referral problem. Key to problem resolution is an adequate sample of the academic skills that permit an analysis of a student's strengths and weaknesses, educational *goal setting*, and *instructional planning*.

For example, the most frequent validity evidence provided by published, norm-referenced reading tests (PNRTs) is criterion-related validity evidence (Salvia & Ysseldyke, 1995). Criterion-related validity evidence supports the use of the test to determine whether students' reading skills are low compared to other students. If students referred for poor reading performance obtain low scores compared to students their age/grade, we may conclude that the students have low reading skills, because the test has demonstrated construct validity for the assessment of reading. Thus, PNRTs could be used for Problem Identification and Certification decisions.

However, few PNRTs provide *evidence* to support their use in setting educational goals or planning educational programs. Providing evidence for the use of PNRTs in educational goal setting or instructional planning is a separate issue from *claiming* they can be used for these purposes. Educators who claim that PNRTs are useful in setting goals and planning instruction base their claims on scant evidence. In fact, there are good reasons to expect that PNRTs will generally not be helpful for setting goals or planning instruction. First, they generally report performance with scores of relative standing (e.g., standard scores, percentiles, or grade equivalents) that prohibit meaningful comparisons between students' current performance with their past or their expected performance. Second, PNRTs are not sensitive to gradual, but important, improvements in student performance. It is not possible, for example, to determine whether the student has improved in performance from week to week. A third reason why

PNRTs are not helpful for planning instruction is that the behavior samples are limited, typically with at best one or two items at any particular skill level. Distributing item difficulties from far too easy to far too difficult allows the test to differentiate between students with high and low skills, but does not offer a good sample of an individual student's skills for planning instruction (see Carver, 1974, and Howell, Fox, & Moorehead, 1993, among others, for more information on this topic).

Thus, both the current empirical evidence and theoretical rationales do not support the use of PNRT results for Exploring Solutions and Evaluating Solutions decisions within the Problem-Solving model. Although we can use PNRT results to establish the existence and severity of a reading problem, PNRT information does not provide a direct linkage from assessment to problem resolution. The *relevance* of CBM in the Problem-Solving model can be demonstrated with evidence that CBM can be used to make all of the decisions necessary to link assessment information directly to problem resolution.

Utility

The utility of an assessment measure or procedure refers to the *benefits* of assessment relative to its *costs* (Messick, 1995). If an assessment measure or procedure has high utility, educational decisions based on that assessment should result in *greater student achievement* than decisions based on a competing assessment approach (Messick, 1989). Utility, as described by Messick (1995), is similar to the concept of treatment utility proposed by Hayes et al. (1987). Treatment utility refers to "the extent to which assessment is shown to contribute to beneficial treatment outcomes" (p. 196). Treatment utility is directly affected by the relevance of assessment information for planning interventions (Hayes, Nelson, & Jarrett, 1989). The treatment utility of a measure is demonstrated when a direct linkage is shown between assessment and the development of an effective intervention plan. Therefore, in order to evaluate the treatment utility of CBM in a Problem-Solving model, its direct contribution to enhanced student achievement must be examined.

Fundamental to demonstrations of the relevance/utility of assessment is *empirical evidence* of the effectiveness of instructional goals and plans derived from the assessment. Linking assessment to goal setting and instructional planning is necessary, but not sufficient, to establish the relevance/utility of the measure or method. Although assessment might establish educational goals and even be relevant to instructional planning, the relevance/utility of the assessment would be unsatisfactory if the goals are not sufficiently ambitious or the instructional plan is not effective. Evidence of student progress toward educational goals that represent problem resolution is necessary. Thus, examinations of student progress provide an empirical basis for evaluating the relevance/utility of CBM in a Problem-Solving model as the degree to which CBM assessment results provide information that leads *directly* to the development of *effective* intervention plans. The relevance and utility of CBM will be discussed with respect to each phase of the Problem-Solving model: (1) Problem Identification, (2) Problem Certification, (3) Exploring Solutions, (4) Evaluating Solutions, and (5) Problem Solution.

Problem Identification and Certification

Problem Identification and Certification are the first two phases in the Problem-Solving model. During the Problem Identification phase, educators must determine if a problem exists that warrants further assessment. In the Problem Certification phase, the educator decides if an identified problem is sufficiently severe to warrant a special program, which may or may not require special education. Both phases require the comparison of the referred student's academic skills with expected performance. The key issue in evaluating the relevance and utility of CBM in both the Problem Identification and Certification phases of the Problem-Solving model is whether CBM can distinguish between students with and without severe educational problems. Evidence that CBM can be used to make Problem Identification and Certification decisions is provided by studies that examine whether (1) groups with different educational needs (e.g., special education and general education) differ on CBM, and (2) CBM discrimination of groups is similar to other bases for distinguishing groups (e.g., teacher referral or PNRTs).

A series of studies have examined the extent to which CBM can distinguish between groups with different educational needs. If CBM can be used to decide which students should be targeted for special education services, students with special needs should be distinguishable from students who do not have special needs. Students who are referred by their teachers for academic concerns and nonreferred students are significantly different on CBM measures of reading in first through sixth grades and on CBM measures of spelling, math, and written expression in fourth through sixth grades (Shinn & Marston, 1985; Shinn, Tindal, Spira, & Marston, 1987a; Shinn, Tindal, & Spira, 1987b). For example, referred students' reading performance on CBM measures is consistently well below the performance of their nonreferred, same-grade peers (Shinn et al., 1987b).

In addition, students receiving special education services and students in general education are significantly different on CBM measures of spelling, math, and written expression in fourth through sixth grades and on CBM measures of reading for first through sixth grades (Shinn &

Marston, 1985; Shinn et al., 1987a; Shinn, Ysseldyke, Deno, & Tindal, 1986). For example, first-grade students receiving special education services in the learning-disabled (LD) category can be differentiated from their peers in general education on the basis of CBM reading performance (Shinn et al., 1987a). Finally, low-achieving students can be distinguished from students in special education on CBM measures of math, written expression, and spelling measures in fourth through sixth grades (Shinn & Marston, 1985; Shinn et al., 1986). For example, students receiving remedial reading services who generally are characterized by low reading achievement can be distinguished from students receiving mildly handicapped special education services using CBM reading, spelling, math, and written expression measures in sixth grade (Shinn & Marston, 1985).

In addition to the evidence that CBM can distinguish between students with different educational needs, evidence also supports the ability of CBM to make those decisions as well or better than teacher judgment and PNRTs (Marston, Mirkin, & Deno, 1984). For example, Marston et al. (1984) examined the accuracy of referral decisions based on CBM reading, spelling, and written expression for elementary students in third through sixth grades. Students identified as eligible for special education using CBM also demonstrated low performance on PNRTs of aptitude and achievement consistent with special education eligibility. Indeed, more accurate classifications of students as needing special education services were made using the CBM measures than were made using teacher judgment.

Taken together, these studies indicate that CBM *can* be used to identify the presence of educational problems and establish their severity. CBM provides a direct measure of students' educational needs that forms an accurate basis for Problem Identification and Problem Certification decisions in the Problem-Solving model. Educators may rely on student CBM performance to determine if special education services are needed to reduce the discrepancy between actual and expected student performance.

Exploring Solutions

Within the Exploring Solutions phase of the Problem-Solving model, educators use assessment information to: (1) develop annual goals for students, (2) design an instructional plan for obtaining these goals, and (3) select instructional methods to accomplish the plan. The CBM information obtained in previous phases of the Problem-Solving model is used in this phase, providing a direct linkage between assessment and intervention and supporting the relevance of CBM for problem resolution. In both the Problem Identification and Certification phases of the Problem-Solving model, educators obtain samples of the students' basic academic skills. These samples are analyzed in the Exploring Solutions phase to determine which skills should be targeted for instruction and to document current levels of performance. In addition, information on the local normative context obtained in the Problem Identification and Problem Certification phases is used to establish goals for intervention. The student's current performance, progress, and goal for resolving the problem provide a basis for evaluating the effectiveness of interventions within the Evaluating Solutions phase of the Problem-Solving model.

Setting annual student goals may be one of the most critical tasks educators perform in the Exploring Solutions phase of the Problem-Solving model. In developing annual goals, educators must consider both the *structure* and *content* of these goals. Goals may be structured as *long-term* or *short-term* goals and as *dynamic* or *static*. Long-term goals represent desired achievement of more general skills (e.g., reading), whereas short-term goals specify subskills that must be acquired to promote achievement of long-term goals (e.g., word attack skills). Dynamic goal setting involves modification of educational goals when student progress is sufficiently discrepant from the expected rate of progress. Static goal setting refers to maintaining educational goals regardless of student progress or lack of progress.

Using CBM to develop long-term annual goals within a dynamic goal-setting process has been demonstrated to promote greater student achievement on general measures of achievement (Fuchs & Fuchs, 1986a; Fuchs, Fuchs, & Hamlett, 1989b; Fuchs, Fuchs, Hamlett, & Ferguson, 1992). For example, students whose teachers used CBM in a long-term, dynamic goal-setting approach achieved an average of +0.52 standard deviations above a control group, whereas students whose teachers used a static goal-setting approach did not demonstrate similar gains (Fuchs et al., 1989b). A meta-analysis of 18 studies supports a +0.10 effect size advantage on global achievement measures when progress is regularly measured toward long-term goals (effect size of 0.51 over control condition) compared to short-term goals (effect size of 0.41 over control; Fuchs & Fuchs, 1986a). Thus, constructing long-term goals on the basis of CBM assessment contributes to student achievement gains.

In addition to goal setting, instructional planning decisions occur in the Exploring Solutions phase. In general, assessment information that allows more specific instructional plans is more relevant to instructional planning, and assessment that results in more effective instructional plans has greater utility. Using CBM to design instructional programs results in greater specificity in instructional plans and higher student achievement in math, spelling, and reading (Fuchs, Fuchs, & Hamlett, 1989c; Fuchs, Fuchs, Hamlett, & Allinder, 1991a; Fuchs, Fuchs, Hamlett, & Stecker,

1990). For example, teachers who used CBM for both progress monitoring and skills analysis incorporated significantly more specific skills in their intervention plans than teachers who used CBM for progress monitoring only, or who used standard Individualized Education Plan (IEP) forms and teacher-made tests (Fuchs et al., 1990). In addition, students performed better (about +0.12 effect size) when instructional programs were designed using a CBM-based skills analysis.

The selection of instructional methods is based on the linkage of Exploring Solutions and Evaluating Solutions phases of the Problem-Solving model. Initially, instructional methods that are generally effective for most children are implemented. Based on individual, case-by-case evaluations of student progress using CBM in the Evaluating Solutions phase, effective instructional methods are maintained and instructional methods that are not resulting in adequate student progress are modified.

Evaluating Solutions

The Evaluating Solutions phase follows the implementation of instructional interventions. The educator must determine whether the selected intervention is sufficiently effective or whether it must be modified to increase effectiveness. The referred student's performance is monitored throughout the intervention. Students' actual rate of progress is compared to their expected rate of progress as specified in the students' annual goal to determine intervention effectiveness. A relevant assessment measure is sensitive to changes in student performance over short periods of time and reflects progress toward annual goals. Assessment with high utility enhances student achievement outcomes. Using CBM in the Evaluating Solutions phase of the Problem-Solving model is a vital part of the linkage of assessment information to problem resolution. Indeed, the relevance and utility of CBM in the Problem-Solving model is perhaps *most evident* within the Evaluating Solutions phase, where positive effects on student achievement have been demonstrated (Fuchs & Fuchs, 1986b; Fuchs, Fuchs, & Hamlett, 1989a; Fuchs et al., 1989c; Fuchs, Fuchs, & Hamlett, 1989d; Fuchs et al., 1992; Shinn & Hubbard, 1992). Evidence for the relevance and utility of CBM for Evaluating Solutions decisions derives from two sources: (1) generic effects of monitoring progress with direct and frequent measures on student achievement, and (2) effects of CBM progress monitoring on student achievement.

When the generic effects of systematic evaluation, of which CBM is one exemplar, on student achievement are examined, important benefits are identified. For example, in a meta-analysis of 21 studies, students whose progress toward their educational goals was systematically monitored earned achievement measure scores +0.7 standard deviations higher than those students whose progress was not systematically monitored (Fuchs & Fuchs, 1986b). These effects were further enhanced when progress was evaluated according to specific data-utilization rules and when progress was displayed graphically (Fuchs & Fuchs, 1986b). Because CBM in a Problem-Solving model entails systematic progress monitoring with specific decision rules and graphic display of data, similar effects would be expected.

As expected, the use of CBM in Evaluating Solutions decisions has resulted in enhanced student achievement (Fuchs & Deno, 1994; Fuchs et al., 1991a; Fuchs et al., 1992; Fuchs et al., 1990; Shinn & Hubbard, 1992). For example, Fuchs, Fuchs, Hamlett, and Ferguson (1991b) demonstrated that student performance on oral-reading fluency and maze-reading tasks was significantly greater for students whose teachers used CBM for progress monitoring than for those students whose teachers relied on criterion-referenced tests for evaluating progress. In addition, Shinn and Hubbard (1992) summarized the results of nine studies that investigated the use of CBM measures to monitor student achievement. They found that individuals whose progress is monitored using CBM over time could be expected to perform +0.36 standard deviations higher, on average, than students whose progress is monitored using traditional methods. Thus, using CBM for Evaluating Solutions decisions within a Problem-Solving model has clearly established relevance and utility for resolving problems.

Problem Solution

The final phase of the Problem-Solving model is Problem Solution, which completes the direct linkage of assessment to problem resolution. Following implementation of an effective instructional intervention, the educator must determine if the student's problem has been resolved and special educational services should be terminated. In this phase of the Problem-Solving model, CBM is used to determine if students' skills remain significantly discrepant from the skills of their general education peers. If students' skills are consistent with their general education peers, the educational problem has been resolved, and it is likely that the student will fit instructionally in the general education classroom. At this time, the student may be a candidate for reintegration into the general education classroom for instruction. Although Problem Solution decisions appear to be made infrequently in practice (Shinn, 1986) a substantial number of children in special education appear to be potential candidates for reintegration (e.g., Shinn, Habedank, Rodden-Nord, & Knutson, 1993). The relevance and utility of CBM for Problem Solution decisions is supported by evidence that (1) CBM can be used to identify potential candidates for reintegration, (2) the CBM information affects the willingness of teachers and parents to reintegrate the student, and (3) students who are reintegrated on the basis of CBM in Problem Solution decisions can be successful receiving general education instruction.

First, CBM can be used to determine whether a student is an appropriate candidate for reintegration into the general education classroom (Rodden-Nord, Shinn, & Good, 1992; Shinn et al., 1993). For example, Shinn et al. (1993) found that 44% of 85 special education students (most receiving services under the LD category) were identified using CBM reading as having skills within the range of students in the low reading group.

Second, the information provided by CBM in Problem Solution decisions appears to be relevant to teachers and thereby parents in deciding whether to attempt a trial reintegration (Rodden-Nord et al., 1992; Shinn, Powell-Smith, & Good, 1996). For example, after general education teachers were shown how reintegration candidates performed on CBM reading measures, their attitudes toward reintegration of the student changed significantly (Rodden-Nord et al., 1992).

Finally, students who are reintegrated based on CBM Problem Solution information can be successful receiving general education instruction, and CBM can be used to evaluate the success of the trial reintegration (Shinn et al., 1996; Shinn, Powell-Smith, Good, & Baker, in press). For example, Shinn et al. (in press) examined the reading progress of students reintegrated into general education low reading groups on the basis of CBM information compared to the reading progress of general education students in the low reading group. The academic gains of the reintegrated students were evaluated using CBM reading measures administered on an ongoing basis after reintegration. The reintegrated students made, on average, academic gains comparable to their general education low reading peers.

The evidence summarized here supports the relevance and utility of CBM reading measures for identifying students whose educational problems have been resolved and who are potential candidates for reintegration into general education reading instruction. However, even with evidence for the construct validity of CBM measures, evidence for the relevance and utility of CBM in a Problem-Solving model is not sufficient to evaluate the validity of CBM. Also necessary is consideration of whether it is *appropriate* to use CBM to infer student characteristics (values implications facet of validity) and make educational decisions (social consequences facet of validity).

VALUES IMPLICATIONS

Evidence for the relevance/utility of CBM in a Problem-Solving model is desirable, but, like criterion-related validity, it is not sufficient to conclude that CBM is "valid." The value implications facet of validity addresses the *appropriateness* of inferences and interpretations based on test results. In this discussion, the important distinction is between the *adequacy* of inferences, which refers to evidence that the test *can* measure what it says it measures (i.e., construct validity) and the *appropriateness* of inferences, which refers to whether we *should* make the inferences implied by test results. In other words, the values implications facet of validity goes beyond objective, scientific evidence and extends the validity discussions to the moral and ethical consequences of the inferences we make based on test results. Unfortunately, perhaps, there are no correlations, coefficients, or statistics that quantify the appropriateness of test-based inferences with respect to absolute standards. Instead, discussions of the values implications of test-based inferences are based on comparisons of competing approaches using rational, philosophical argument, more akin to ethical argument or moral philosophy (Messick, 1995). Our approach, then, will be to compare the values implications of CBM inferences with the values implications of inferences based on competing measurement approaches.

When comparing the values implications of CBM and competing measurement approaches, the *unintended implications* of test-based inferences are of particular interest. Generally, test inferences are intended to have positive implications for consumers, and so the intended implications are less effective in differentiating the values implications of tests. In contrast, the unintended implications seldom are subjected to overt examination and comparison. Thus, an evaluation and comparison of the unintended implications of test-based inferences provides the most information on the values implications of a test. We pose this discussion as the beginnings of argument or discussion. Unlike the evidential basis of validity (construct validity and relevance/utility) which is supported through scientific consensus, the consequential basis of test inferences (values implications) may be clarified best by argument (Messick, 1989, p. 63). First we will propose some guidelines for evaluating the values implications of CBM, and then compare CBM inferences with inferences based on competing measurement approaches with respect to the guidelines.

Guidelines for Evaluating the Values Implications of CBM

Clearly, some guidelines or principles are needed to form a basis of comparison when evaluating the values implications of CBM in a Problem-Solving model. Five interrelated factors to consider when evaluating the values implications of test constructs and theories are proposed in Table 3.3. These factors affect the likelihood of unintended negative values implications of test-based inferences about a student. For example, broad in-

TABLE 3.3. Factors Affecting the Likelihood of Unintended Negative Effects of Test-Based Inferences

Area	Consideration
1. Valence	The extent to which the inferred attributes are *valenced* as socially desirable or undesirable. Constructs that carry a higher social valence are more likely to have unintended value implications.
2. Judgmental	The extent to which inferred attributes are *judgmental* or value laden as opposed to *descriptive*. More judgmental inferences are more likely to have unintended value implications.
3. Breadth of the construct	Constructs that are too broad carry needless and potentially harmful baggage, while constructs that are too narrow are not helpful, referring only to specific behaviors. "The broader the construct, the more likely it is that hidden value implications will flourish unheeded" (Messick, 1989, p. 60).
4. Personological versus situational constructs	Personological inferences characterize an inherent aspect of the person; situational inferences characterize the situation, circumstances, or conditions. Negative attributions that are believed to characterize the person are more likely to be generalized to new settings than those that emphasize a person's response to a situation.
5. Amenable or resistant to intervention	Inferring a negative attribute that is believed to be amenable to intervention or education invites the investment of resources and effort. Inferring a negative attribute that is believed to be resistant to intervention invites the withdrawal of resources and effort.

ferences about personological constructs that are judgmental, socially valenced, and thought to be resistant to intervention are most likely to have unintended values implications.

Evaluating CBM Using the Values Implications Guidelines

The values implications facet of validity will be evaluated for CBM in a Problem-Solving model by comparing the values implications of inferences based on CBM with the values implications of a competing measurement approach, a severe discrepancy between intelligence test and achievement. A reading problem for a student could be identified by CBM reading measures in a Problem-Solving model, or by a discrepancy between published, norm-referenced tests of intelligence (e.g., Wechsler Intelligence Scale for Children—III [WISC-III]) and reading achievement (e.g., Woodcock–Johnson Psycho-Educational Battery, Broad Reading Cluster). Using CBM, the inference is that the student has "severe low reading skills." Based on the discrepancy between intelligence and achievement, the inference is that the student has a "learning disability in reading."

These inferences differ in terms of the five guidelines identified previously. First, although both inferences are negatively valenced (i.e., few would voluntarily elect either condition), an inference of "a learning disability in reading" carries a stronger social stigma. Generally, ability to learn is a core value of our society. Second, inferences of a deficit in such a core value will likely carry more stigma and be more judgmental of the individual. Third, "low reading skills" is a narrower construct than a "learning disability in reading." An inference of "low reading skills" conveys sufficient information to be helpful while minimizing needless and potentially harmful baggage. In contrast, a "learning disability in reading" is widely believed (in the absence of evidence) to be theoretically linked to other constructs, such as perceptual difficulties and need for unique, specialized instruction. More than one teacher, for example, has maintained that a child should be removed from their classroom because he or she believed specialized "learning disability instruction" was needed. Fourth, an inference of "low reading skills" is situational: "Low reading skills" might be due to lack of instruction, poor quality instruction, or inadequate curriculum. An inference of a "reading learning disability" is more personological, attributing a characteristic to the person instead of the situation or condition. If the reading problem is inferred to be a within-person attribute, educators may be less likely to examine instructional solutions. Instead, the descriptor becomes the explanation: The student has low reading skills because they have a reading learning disability; and we know they have a reading learning disability because of their low reading skills. Fifth, an inference of a "reading learning disability" that implies resistance to intervention is more likely to affect a student adversely by reducing ameliorative effort. There may be an implication that the student's low reading skills are acceptable or understandable because of the learning disability.

In general, CBM-based inferences in reading, math, spelling, and written language are *narrow* inferences focusing on *descriptions* of performance in basic academic skill areas that are comparatively *neutral* in valence. When used in a Problem-Solving model, a problem is defined *situationally* as a discrepancy between observed and expected behavior (see Shinn and Bamonto, Chapter 1, this volume, or Deno, 1989, for more information). In addition, the inferences based on CBM in a Problem-Solving model emphasize the linkages to interventions. Compared to competing assessment procedures, the validity of CBM in a Problem-Solving model with respect to the values implications facet is supported. However, like the other facets of validity, the values implications facet does not, in itself, provide a sufficient basis for test use.

SOCIAL CONSEQUENCES

The social consequences facet of validity addresses the *appropriateness* of *actions* taken on the basis of test results. Evaluating the social consequences of test actions parallels the evaluation of test values implications; that is, evaluating social consequences entails (1) a rational, philosophical discussion of the values and worth of test consequences; (2) a comparison of actions based on the test or measurement procedure to actions based on competing procedures, including not testing at all; and (3) a focus on unintended as well as intended effects. The social consequences facet differs from the values implications facet in that the focus is on test-based *actions or decisions* rather than inferences and interpretations. The social consequences facet also differs from the relevance/utility facet. Although the relevance/utility facet of validity incorporates evidence that the test *can* be used as a basis for action, the social consequences facet of validity examines whether the test *should* be used as a basis for action. Thus, although CBM can be used to make Problem Certification decisions, the question in the social consequences facet of validity is whether it should.

Evaluating the social consequences of test use need not be bounded by current legal definitions or standard operating procedures. Instead, the social consequences of test use involve what *ought* to be (Messick, 1989). Only by clarifying what ought to be can we establish the direction that laws and procedures should take. If we are not clear on the direction that laws and procedures *should* be moving, we are doomed to have laws and procedures imposed on us by lawyers and bureaucrats. Ideally, good practice should drive the laws which, in turn, should support and codify good practice. Periodic reexamination of laws with respect to good practice is necessary to avoid rigid application of procedures that are no longer the best practice.

As stated earlier, examinations of social consequences are based on a rational comparison of competing tests or measurement procedures for making decisions or taking action. Of the actions or decisions in the Problem-Solving model, Problem Certification decisions carry the greatest social consequences and will be examined in depth. Problem Certification decisions are based on evidence that the student needs a "special" (i.e., beyond the norm provided by general education) intervention to reduce the discrepancy between observed and expected behavior (Deno, 1989). In practice, Problem Certification decisions typically correspond to special education eligibility decisions. The consequential validity of CBM in a Problem-Solving model will be evaluated by comparing three test-bases for special education eligibility decisions: (1) severe low achievement on CBM, (2) severe low intelligence on an intelligence test (mental retardation), and (3) severe discrepancy between intelligence and achievement (learning disability).

Context for Comparing Social Consequences Validity

To evaluate the social consequences validity of CBM for Problem Certification decisions, the consequences of the three test bases for children will be compared with respect to a reading problem. The distribution of performance that would be found on a measure of intelligence and a measure of reading achievement such as CBM reading or a published, norm-referenced reading achievement test is illustrated in Figure 3.2, which is very like one obtained by Shaywitz, Fletcher, Holahan, and Shaywitz (1992) for the Wechsler Intelligence Scale for Children—Revised (WISC-R) and the Woodcock–Johnson Psycho-Educational Battery, Broad Reading Cluster in their Connecticut Longitudinal Study. A similar distribution would be expected for any combination of achievement and intelligence tests, which generally are correlated in the range .60 to .80. Thus, this same figure could generically represent the distribution of the WISC-III and CBM reading performance, for example.

Using Figure 3.2, the social consequences of using CBM to make

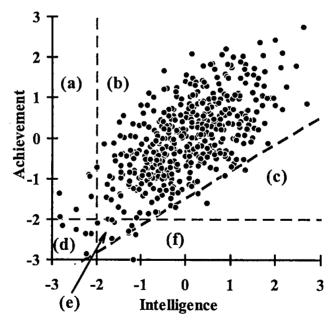

FIGURE 3.2. Individuals identified as eligible for special education services using extremely low academic skills (areas d, e, and f); extremely low intelligence (areas a and d); and an extreme discrepancy between intelligence and achievement (areas c and f).

Problem Certification decisions can be compared to (1) using severe low intelligence on an intelligence test, or (2) using a severe discrepancy between intelligence and achievement test. Using CBM in a Problem-Solving model, students could be considered eligible based on their extremely low reading scores alone. Using CBM to make Problem Certification decisions would correspond to areas (d), (e), and (f) in Figure 3.2. Students scoring in these areas all displayed extremely low reading skills, below −2 standard deviations from the mean, regardless of their score on the intelligence test. Determining eligibility on the basis of severe low intelligence on an intelligence test (below −2 standard deviations from the mean) would correspond to students in areas (a) and (d). Finally, basing eligibility on a severe discrepancy between an intelligence test and an achievement test would identify students in areas (c) and (f) as eligible.

In evaluating the social consequences of Problem Certification decisions based on CBM compared to severe low intelligence and a severe discrepancy between intelligence and achievement, three interrelated consequences will be considered: (1) increased likelihood that selected children with severe educational needs will be served, (2) reduced likelihood that selected children who do *not* have severe educational needs will be identified as mentally retarded or learning disabled, and (3) a shift in the focus of the problem away from within-child variables to instructional and curricular variables. One of the most important social issues for the United States today is the patterns of social, economic, and educational inequality between White and minority individuals (Sternberg, 1995). Because minority students, especially Hispanics and African Americans, tend to score below Whites on measures of intelligence, the social consequences of test use bear directly on issues of racial inequality.

Social Consequences for Children with Severe Educational Needs

The consequences of using CBM in a Problem-Solving model are substantial for children who have severe educational needs but do not display severe low intelligence or a severe discrepancy between intelligence and achievement. The children in area (e) of Figure 3.2 all share extremely low academic skills (below −2 standard deviations from the mean). Without remediation, they are likely to experience severe social consequences such as illiteracy and reduced employment opportunity (Adams, 1990; Anderson, Hiebert, Scott, & Wilkinson, 1984). Using CBM procedures for Problem Certification, students with the severe low reading skills, area (e), *would* be eligible for special educational services.

The social consequences of the denial of services to children with severe educational needs may be even more severe for some groups of students, such as children from minority backgrounds. Because all of the children in area (e) scored below the mean on intelligence (most between −1 and −2 standard deviations below the mean), minority children can be expected to be overrepresented in this group (Kaufman, Harrison, & Ittenbach, 1990). Thus, one advantage of CBM in a Problem-Solving model with respect to the social consequence of test use is increased likelihood of providing remediation to students with severe educational needs. A social consequence of using severe low intelligence or a severe discrepancy between intelligence and achievement is decreased likelihood of providing services to students with severe educational needs, who are more likely to be students from minority backgrounds.

Social Consequences for Children Who Do Not Have Severe Educational Needs

In addition to providing services to children with severe educational needs, using CBM in a Problem-Solving model reduces the number of children with "average" reading skills who would be eligible for special education services. The children in area (a) of Figure 3.2 have academic skills that are not severely low and may be in the average range compared to other children their age. In reading, they may read like many other students, no better and no worse. However, their score on the intelligence test is extremely low and consistent with identification as mentally retarded. In a sense, these children represent errors of prediction. Their reading skills are not as low as would be predicted based on the intelligence test. It may seem somewhat preposterous to consider identifying these children as needing special education services. After all, why would one pay more attention to the predictor than to the criterion? Indeed, this illustrates the indirect nature of intelligence tests as a basis for decision making, an issue of "the relevance of the test to the particular applied purpose" (Messick, 1995, p. 744). In general, more *direct* bases for action are preferable.

One might object that these children are rare or do not exist. Indeed, they may be seldom seen in a referral population, in part because referrals typically are consistent with very low academic skills (Shinn et al., 1987b). However, a recent random sample of schoolchildren (as opposed to a referral population) yields a distribution with many children with low intelligence test scores whose reading skills are average (Shaywitz et al., 1992). One also might argue that even if the children in area (a) are not displaying severe low reading skills, they most likely would display severe low achievement in other academic areas. Of course, this *may* be correct. However, there are more direct measures of academic skills in those other areas as well. The best way to determine if a child's skills are low in an academic area is to measure the skills directly.

The children in area (c) of Figure 3.2 also represent errors of prediction. They have higher intelligence test scores than other children with reading difficulty, most of which are *above* the mean. Although their reading skills are severely discrepant from their intelligence test scores, their reading skills are not severely low and may be average (i.e., no better and no worse than other children their age). With average reading skills, it is difficult to argue that they experience severe educational need in reading. Although the children in area (c) may not have severe educational needs, certification as learning disabled may have positive social consequences, as when students seek identification as learning disabled to gain entrance to college (e.g., Ackerman, 1987; Meyers, 1985) or extended time for the Graduate Record Examination.

The social consequences of the errors of prediction for children without severe educational needs may also adversely impact minority children. Because children from minority backgrounds are more likely to score below the mean on intelligence tests, they would tend to be overrepresented in area (a) and underrepresented in area (c) of Figure 3.2. The most problematic aspect of this over- and underrepresentation is that the group differences in the adverse consequences of test use are the result of "construct irrelevant variance" (Messick, 1995, p. 742). In other words, because *neither* group is displaying severe low reading skills, both groups represent errors of prediction resulting from indirect measures of educational need. Thus, direct measures of educational need using CBM in a Problem-Solving model also have advantages with respect to the social consequences for children without severe educational needs.

Social Consequences for Instruction

Finally, the children in areas (d) and (f) of Figure 3.2 all share severe low reading skills. Because these children may be identified as eligible for special education services using either CBM in a Problem-Solving model or severe low intelligence, or a severe discrepancy between intelligence and achievement, it might at first appear as if the comparison of methods is equivalent—the same children are identified. However, important social consequences derive from the *way* the children are identified. First, providing services on the basis of mental retardation (severe low intelligence) or a learning disability (severe discrepancy between intelligence and achievement) attributes the *cause* of the problem to variables solely within the child. Attributing the focus of the problem within the child may have the unintended effect of effectively absolving the school (or home, or community) from responsibility (Shinn & Good, 1993). If the assumption is that the child is mentally retarded or has a learning disability, then it is perceived as reasonable that he or she has severe low academic skills. After all, the argument goes, we should expect lower skills because they are mentally retarded or learning disabled. Thus, the frequent response may be to reduce expectations for progress and perhaps even reduce effort, services, and resources for instruction. In contrast, using CBM in a Problem-Solving model to make Problem Certification decisions shifts the focus to instructional variables. The first question asked should be: Can the student's low skills be explained by poor or inadequate instruction or opportunities to learn? Indeed, we have the skills and the instructional technology to ensure that the vast majority of children with mild disabilities successfully master basic academic skills (e.g., Adams, 1990; Kameenui & Simmons, 1990). The barrier to effective instruction is more frequently one of implementation of effective instruction than that our best instruction is not effective.

Thus, the values implications of the constructs ostensibly assessed and the theoretical framework of assessment (need vs. disability) have social consequences in terms of the likelihood of effective intervention: CBM in a Problem-Solving model is more likely to lead to effective intervention, because the focus is on instructional variables with documented effectiveness. Identification as mentally retarded or learning disabled is less likely to lead to effective intervention, because the focus is on within-child characteristics with no documented treatment utility.

In summary, the social consequences facet of validity for use of CBM in a Problem-Solving model can be evaluated by means of a rational, philosophical discussion of the values and worth of test consequences. The appropriateness of test use for Problem Certification decisions in reading was examined as an example because the decisions entail clear differences in social consequences. The social consequences of CBM in a Problem-Solving model to identify need were contrasted with competing assessment procedures based on intelligence tests and intelligence–achievement discrepancies. Substantial differences in the social consequences favoring CBM and its use in a Problem-Solving model were identified, including (1) increased likelihood of serving selected children with severe educational needs, (2) reduced likelihood of identifying selected children who do not have severe educational needs as learning disabled or mentally retarded, and (3) increased focus on instructional variables with documented effectiveness. However, even consideration of the social consequences of assessment in isolation is not sufficient to establish the validity of CBM in a Problem-Solving model.

SUMMARY

According to Messick, validity is "an integrated evaluative judgment of the degree to which empirical evidence and theoretical rationales support the adequacy and appropriateness of inferences and actions based on test scores or other modes of assessment" (Messick, 1989, p. 13). Key to this definition of validity is the importance of an *overall judgment* based on consideration of *all* of the evidence, *all* of the rational discussion, and *all* of the theoretical justification. Construct validity, relevance/utility, values implications, and social consequences are not separate, distinct "validities." Professionally, we need to go beyond mere examinations of criterion-related validity. Throughout this chapter we have adopted the perspective that "both meaning and values, as well as both test interpretation and test use, are intertwined in the validation process. Thus, validity and values are one imperative, not two, and test validation implicates both the science and the ethics of assessment, which is why validity has force as a social value" (Messick, 1995, p. 749). From the evidence reviewed here, and the rational comparisons with existing decision-making practices, CBM within a Problem-Solving model provides a valid basis for test interpretation and use with students in the basic academic skills areas.

REFERENCES

Ackerman, P. T. (1987). A profile of male and female applicants for a special college program for learning-disabled students. *Journal of Clinical Psychology, 43,* 67–78.

Adams, M. J. (1990). *Beginning to read: Thinking and learning about print.* Cambridge, MA: MIT Press.

Anderson, R. C., Hiebert, E. H., Scott, J. A., & Wilkinson, I. A. G. (1984). *Becoming a nation of readers: The report of the Commission on Reading.* Washington, DC: National Institute of Education.

Carver, R. P. (1974). Two dimensions of tests: Psychometric and edumetric. *American Psychologist, 29,* 512–518.

Deno, S. L. (1989). Curriculum-Based Measurement and special education services: A fundamental and direct relationship. In M. R. Shinn (Ed.), *Curriculum-Based Measurement: Assessing special children* (pp. 1–17). New York: Guilford Press.

Espin, C., Deno, S. L., Maruyama, G., & Cohen, C. (1989, March). *The Basic Academic Skills Samples (BASS): An instrument for the screening and identification of children at risk for failure in regular education classrooms.* Paper presented at the 70th Annual Meeting of the American Educational Research Association, San Francisco.

Fuchs, L. S., & Deno, S. (1994). Must instructionally useful performance assessment be based in the curriculum? *Exceptional Children, 61,* 15–24.

Fuchs, L. S., & Fuchs, D. (1986a). Curriculum-Based Assessment of progress toward long-term and short-term goals. *Journal of Special Education, 20,* 69–82.

Fuchs, L. S., & Fuchs, D. (1986b). Effects of systematic formative evaluation: A meta-analysis. *Exceptional Children, 53,* 199–208.

Fuchs, L. S., Fuchs, D., & Hamlett, C. L. (1989a). Computers and Curriculum-Based Measurement: Effects of teacher feedback systems. *School Psychology Review, 18,* 112–125.

Fuchs, L. S., Fuchs, D., & Hamlett, C. L. (1989b). Effects of alternative goal structures within Curriculum-Based Measurement. *Exceptional Children, 55,* 429–438.

Fuchs, L. S., Fuchs, D., & Hamlett, C. L. (1989c). Effects of instrumental use of Curriculum-Based Measurement to enhance instructional programs. *Remedial and Special Education, 10*(2), 43–52.

Fuchs, L. S., Fuchs, D., & Hamlett, C. L. (1989d). Monitoring reading growth using student recalls: Effects of two teacher feedback systems. *Journal of Educational Research, 83,* 103–110.

Fuchs, L. S., Fuchs, D., Hamlett, C. L., & Allinder, R. M. (1991a). The contribution of skills analysis to Curriculum-Based Measurement in spelling. *Exceptional Children, 57,* 443–452.

Fuchs, L. S., Fuchs, D., Hamlett, C. L., & Ferguson, C. (1991b). Effects of expert system advice within Curriculum-Based Measurement using a reading maze task. *Exceptional Children, 20,* 49–66.

Fuchs, L. S., Fuchs, D., Hamlett, C. L., & Ferguson, C. (1992). Effects of expert system consultation within Curriculum-Based Measurement using a reading maze task. *Exceptional Children, 58,* 436–450.

Fuchs, L. S., Fuchs, D., Hamlett, C. L., & Stecker, P. M. (1990). The role of skills analysis in Curriculum-Based Measurement in math. *School Psychology Review, 19,* 6–22.

Gersten, R., Keating, T., & Irvin, L. (1995). The burden of proof: Validity as improvement of instructional practice. *Exceptional Children, 61,* 510–519.

Hayes, S. C., Nelson, R. O., & Jarrett, R. B. (1987). The treatment utility of assessment: A functional approach to evaluating assessment quality. *American Psychologist, 42,* 963–974.

Hayes, S. C., Nelson, R. O., & Jarrett, R. B. (1989). The applicability of treatment utility. *American Psychologist, 44,* 1242–1243.

Howell, K. W., Fox, S. L., & Moorehead, M. K. (1993). *Curriculum-based evaluation: Teaching and decision making.* Pacific Grove, CA: Brooks/Cole.

Hubbard, D. (1996). *Technical adequacy of formative monitoring systems: A comparison of three curriculum-based indices of written expression.* Unpublished doctoral dissertation, University of Oregon, Eugene.

Kameenui, E. J., & Simmons, D. C. (1990). *Designing instructional strategies: The prevention of academic learning problems.* Columbus, OH: Merrill.

Kaufman, A. S., Harrison, P. L., & Ittenbach, R. F. (1990). Intelligence testing in the schools. In T. B. Gutkin & C. R. Reynolds (Eds.), *The handbook of school psychology* (2nd ed., pp. 289–327). New York: Wiley.

Marston, D. B. (1982). *The technical adequacy of direct repeated measurement of academic skills in low-achieving elementary students.* Unpublished doctoral dissertation, University of Minnesota, Minneapolis.

Marston, D. B. (1989). A curriculum-based measurement approach to assessing academic performance: What it is and why do it. In M. R. Shinn (Ed.), *Cur-*

riculum-based measurement: Assessing special children (pp. 18–78). New York: Guilford Press.

Marston, D. B., Mirkin, P., & Deno, S. (1984). Curriculum-based measurement: An alternative to traditional screening, referral, and identification. *Journal of Special Education, 18*, 109–117.

Mehrens, W. A., & Clarizio, H. F. (1993). Curriculum-Based Measurement: Conceptual and psychometric considerations. *Psychology in the Schools, 30*, 241–254.

Messick, S. (1975). The standard problem: Meaning and values in measurement and evaluation. *American Psychologist*, 955–966.

Messick, S. (1986). *The once and future issues of validity: Assessing the meaning and consequences of measurement* (Research Rep.). Princeton, NJ: Educational Testing Service.

Messick, S. (1989). Validity. In R. L. Linn (Ed.), *Educational measurement* (3rd ed., pp. 13–103). New York: Macmillan.

Messick, S. (1990). Test validity and the ethics of assessment. *American Psychologist, 35*, 1012–1027.

Messick, S. (1995). Validity of psychological assessment: Validation of inferences from persons' responses and performances as scientific inquiry into score meaning. *American Psychologist, 50*, 741–749.

Meyers, M. J. (1985). The LD college student: A case study. *Academic Therapy, 20*, 453–461.

Parker, R., Tindal, G., & Hasbrouck, G. (1991). Countable indices of writing quality: Their suitability for screening-eligibility decisions. *Exceptionality, 2*, 1–17.

Putnam, D. (1989). *The criterion-related validity of CBM measures of math.* Unpublished master's thesis, University of Oregon, Eugene.

Putnam, D. (1990). *Reliability of CBM Math.* Unpublished doctoral dissertation, University of Oregon, Eugene.

Reschly, D. J. (1988). Special education reform: School psychology revolution. *School Psychology Review, 17*, 459–475.

Rodden-Nord, K., Shinn, M. R., & Good, R. H. (1992). Effects of classroom performance data on general education teachers' attitudes towards reintegrating students with learning disabilities. *School Psychology Review, 21*, 138–154.

Salvia, J., & Ysseldyke, J. E. (1995). *Assessment* (6th ed.). Boston: Houghton Mifflin.

Shaywitz, B. A., Fletcher, J. M., Holahan, J. M., & Shaywitz, S. E. (1992). Discrepancy compared to low achievement definitions of reading disability: Results from the Connecticut Longitudinal Study. *Journal of Learning Disabilities, 25*, 639–648.

Shinn, M. R. (1986). Does anyone really care what happens after the refer–test–place sequence: The systematic evaluation of special education program effectiveness. *School Psychology Review, 15*, 49–58.

Shinn, M. R., & Good, R. H. (1993). CBA: An assessment of its current status and prognosis for its future. In J. J. Kramer (Ed.), *Curriculum-Based Measurement* (pp. 139–178). Lincoln, NE: Buros Institute of Mental Measurements.

Shinn, M. R., Good, R. H., Knutson, N., Tilly, W. D., & Collins, V. L. (1992).

Curriculum-based measurement reading fluency: A confirmatory analysis of its relation to reading. *School Psychology Review, 21,* 459–479.

Shinn, M. R., Habedank, L., Rodden-Nord, K., & Knutson, N. (1993). Using Curriculum-Based Measurement to identify potential candidates for reintegration into general education. *Journal of Special Education, 27,* 202–221.

Shinn, M. R., & Hubbard, D. D. (1992). Curriculum-based measurement and problem-solving assessment: Basic procedures and outcomes. *Focus on Exceptional Children, 24*(5), 1–20.

Shinn, M. R., & Marston, D. (1985). Differentiating mildly handicapped, low-achieving, and regular education students: A curriculum-based approach. *Remedial and Special Education, 6*(2), 31–38.

Shinn, M. R., Powell-Smith, K. A., & Good, R. H. (1996). Evaluating the effects of responsible reintegration into general education for students with mild disabilities on a case-by-case basis. *School Psychology Review, 4,* 519–539.

Shinn, M. R., Powell-Smith, K. A., Good, R. H., & Baker, S. (in press). The effects of reintegration into general education reading instruction for students with mild disabilities. *Exceptional Children.*

Shinn, M. R., Tindal, G., Spira, D., & Marston, D. (1987a). Practice of learning disabilities as social policy. *Learning Disability Quarterly, 10,* 17–28.

Shinn, M. R., Tindal, G. A., & Spira, D. A. (1987b). Special education referrals as an index of teacher tolerance: Are teachers imperfect tests? *Exceptional Children, 54,* 32–40.

Shinn, M. R., Ysseldyke, J., Deno, S., & Tindal, G. (1986). A comparison of differences between students labeled learning disabled and low achieving on measures of classroom performance. *Journal of Learning Disabilities, 19,* 542–552.

Sternberg, R. J. (1995). For whom the bell curve tolls: A review of *The Bell Curve. Psychological Science, 6,* 257–261.

CHAPTER 4

♦♦♦

Computer Applications to Address Implementation Difficulties Associated with Curriculum-Based Measurement

♦

LYNN S. FUCHS

In developing Curriculum-Based Measurement (CBM), Deno and colleagues (see Deno, 1985) sought to establish a measurement system that (1) teachers could use efficiently; (2) would produce accurate, meaningful information with which to index student improvement over time; (3) could answer questions about the effectiveness of programs in producing academic growth; and (4) would provide information that helped teachers plan better instructional programs. Toward that end, Deno and colleagues undertook a program of research to describe the technical features of CBM and to develop a set of methods for connecting the assessment database to instructional planning in an effective, meaningful manner (see Fuchs, 1995 for an summary of that research).

This research on teachers' use of CBM for instructional planning indicates that this assessment system can help teachers plan better programs and effect superior academic growth among students with disabilities and other nondisabled pupils (e.g., Fuchs, Deno, & Mirkin, 1984; Fuchs, Fuchs, Hamlett, & Ferguson, 1992b; Fuchs, Fuchs, Hamlett, & Stecker, 1991c; Jones & Krouse, 1988; Wesson, 1991). With CBM, the special educator plans an initial instructional program that, based on research, has a good probability of helping the student learn. Given the student's history of academic failure, however, the teacher does not assume that the planned instructional program will in fact be successful for that child.

Rather, while implementing the planned program, the teacher conducts routine assessments to monitor the extent to which the student is actually learning. The teacher uses this ongoing assessment database to tailor an instructional program over time that does, in fact, produce superior learning for a given student. In response to a mounting database supporting efficacy, CBM is cited frequently as a potential method for enhancing the quality of services for students with disabilities and other low-performing, nondisabled children (e.g., Christenson, Ysseldyke, & Thurlow, 1989; Gersten, Carnine, & Woodward, 1987; Reisberg & Wolf, 1988; Will, 1986; Zigmond & Miller, 1986).

Unfortunately, despite support for the efficacy of CBM as well as calls for its implementation, teachers frequently do not choose to use CBM. At least two reasons explain teachers' reluctance (see Fuchs, Fuchs, Hasselbring, & Hamlett, 1987a; Wesson, King, & Deno, 1984). First, substantial time is necessary to collect and manage ongoing assessment information, a practice that requires teachers to prepare materials for testing, administer and score tests, and graph and analyze scores. Second, teachers often find it difficult to translate systematic assessment information into meaningful instructional changes that can be implemented feasibly within their programs, which often serve large numbers of students.

Given the demonstrated promise of CBM to enhance the quality of services provided to individuals with disabilities and other chronically low-achieving students, my colleagues and I undertook a program of research in 1985 to explore how computers can be used to surmount these difficulties in the areas of reading, spelling, and mathematics. In this chapter, I describe the chronology and purposes of this research program and synthesize findings. Then, I draw implications for the fields of special and general education, technology, and assessment.

RESEARCH PROGRAM ON COMPUTER APPLICATIONS TO CBM

Data Management and Data Collection

Electronic Management of Data That Have Been Collected by Hand

Early discussions (Hasselbring & Hamlett, 1985; Walton, 1986) about the potential for computers to solve the problems associated with ongoing assessment systems focused on computer applications to manage data: software to store, graph, and analyze data (i.e., draw lines of best fit through graphed scores, draw goal lines, and formulate decisions about the need to modify programs to improve progress or raise goals when actual progress exceeds anticipated progress) that teachers had collected and scored. The initial step in the research program, therefore, was in response to these discussions: My colleagues and I sought to develop and evaluate this type of data-management technology.

During 1985 and 1986, we created and examined the use of data-management software among 20 special educators, each of whom conducted CBM with two pupils in reading, spelling, and mathematics. All teachers were required to prepare, administer, and score the CBM tests by hand. Teachers were assigned randomly to a condition in which they used computers to manage the data or to one in which they managed the data by hand.

Despite earlier speculation (see Hasselbring & Hamlett, 1985; Walton, 1986) that computerized data-management systems would improve the efficiency of routine measurement, findings revealed that this type of software application significantly *reduced* teacher efficiency. The data-management software actually required teachers to complete extra steps: After administering and scoring tests by hand, teachers still needed to go to a computer, load software, identify pupils and academic areas to the computer, enter measurement dates and scores, save data, and view or print graphs. By contrast, the noncomputer teachers simply located graphs and placed symbols at appropriate places on those graphs (Fuchs et al., 1987a).

Interestingly, however, although the use of data-management software required additional teacher time, teachers were more satisfied with CBM in the computerized data-management condition (Fuchs et al., 1987a). Moreover, with the addition of a tutorial routine in the software, which explained the rationale for the program-changing and goal-raising decisions formulated by the computer, teachers in the computerized data-management condition understood the CBM data analysis better and complied better with CBM decisions (Fuchs, Fuchs, & Hamlett, 1988). Consequently, although the data-management software failed to improve CBM feasibility, this work began to shed light of the capability of computers to supplement and enhance CBM methods that relied on humans to collect and manage the assessment database. In subsequent years of our research program, we began to take increasing advantage of those capabilities.

Automatic Data Collection

Initial work with data-management software highlighted the need to use computers in more dramatic ways than simply managing information that teachers had already collected. In the next phase of this research program, my colleagues and I therefore investigated the use of computers to generate, administer, and score CBM tests. In 1986 and 1987, we (Fuchs, Hamlett, Fuchs, Stecker, & Ferguson, 1988) developed and evaluated software that automatically generated CBM tests, administered those tests to students at the computer, scored the tests, provided test feedback to students, and saved the data for storage and analysis by the data-management software. Twenty special educators implemented CBM, each with two pupils in reading, spelling, and mathematics for 15 weeks. Ten teachers collected data by hand but used the data-management software; the other half used the data-collection software that automatically saved scores for the data-management program.

Direct observations of data-collection and evaluation activities indicated that teachers spent reliably and substantially less time in measurement and evaluation when CBM data were automatically collected by computers. Most teachers, in fact, spent *no* time in administering, scoring, or analyzing assessments. In addition, teacher satisfaction with CBM was greater with the data-collection software, and the ease with which teachers could be trained in CBM was greatly facilitated: We could quickly ensure that teachers understood their students' assessment profiles, while avoiding spending large amounts of time training them to criterion in how to administer, score, or analyze the data accurately and reliably.

Increasing Teachers' Capacity to Analyze the Database to Improve Instructional Decision Making

The combination of data-collection and data-management software greatly reduced the amount of time and number of mechanical tasks required of teachers to implement CBM. Nevertheless, a second, persistent implementation problem remained—teachers' difficulty in translating assessment information into meaningful instructional decisions that could be implemented within the context of the large class size frequently found today in special and general education. In our research program on computer applications to CBM, we have addressed this problem in three stages: through computerized skills analysis, through expert systems, and through classwide data analysis and instructional recommendations.

Skills Analysis

With every CBM administered throughout the year, student performance is sampled on all the skills embedded in the year's curriculum (see Fuchs & Deno, 1991, for a related discussion). Consequently, two types of CBM information are always available: (1) the total test score, which represents a student's overall proficiency on the year's curriculum; and (2) an analysis of a student's performance on each of the specific skills contained in that curriculum. For example, in mathematics, a student's total CBM test score may be 53 digits (or 16 problems). However, one can also analyze a student's performance on an item-by-item basis across several recent tests to determine which skills the student can and cannot do well. Unfortunately, this type of item-by-item analysis is extremely time consuming for humans to complete; even with great time expenditures, this analysis cannot be done by hand in an accurate, reliable manner. By contrast, computers are ideal for completing a laborious, intricate, item-by-item analysis quickly and accurately.

Therefore, to enhance teachers' use of assessment information for instructional decision making, we began by developing computerized skills analysis to complement the CBM total scores. In 1987 and 1988, we developed software that could complete item-by-item skills analyses in reading, spelling, and mathematics. In math, for example, in addition to receiving a graph showing a student's total scores over time, the teacher also received a skills analysis (see Figure 4.1 for sample graph and skills analysis in the area of mathematics computations and applications). The skills analysis describes the student's performance for each half-month interval on 10 clusters of skills represented in the annual curriculum. Each skill cluster is placed in one of five mastery categories: mastered, probably mastered, partially mastered, not mastered, or not attempted. The rows represent the different skill clusters; the columns represent half-month intervals. A black box represented mastery; a black box with a dot, probably mastered; a checkered box, partially mastered; a striped box, not mastered; and an empty box, not attempted. Consequently, increasingly darker boxes signify increasing mastery. The type and format of the skills analysis differed by academic area (see Fuchs, Fuchs, & Hamlett, 1989, for more information about reading, and Fuchs, Fuchs, Hamlett, & Allinder, 1991b, for more information about spelling).

We ran three experiments (one in each academic area) in which special educators were assigned randomly to a control group or to one of two experimental groups: CBM with computerized data collection and management (but no skills analysis) or CBM with computerized data collection, management, and skills analysis. Our findings were robust: Regardless of academic area, teachers who planned students' programs with skills analyses designed more specific program adjustments to assist students who were demonstrating inadequate overall progress (as shown in their CBM total scores). These teachers who had automatic skills analysis feedback also effected reliably greater achievement among their students (Fuchs et al., 1989, 1991b; Fuchs, Fuchs, Hamlett, & Stecker, 1990).

Elizabeth Smith

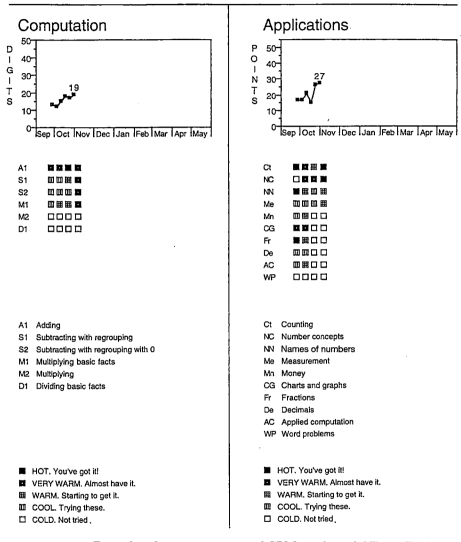

FIGURE 4.1. Examples of computer-generated CBM graphs and skills profiles in mathematics computations and applications.

Andy Farr

Computation

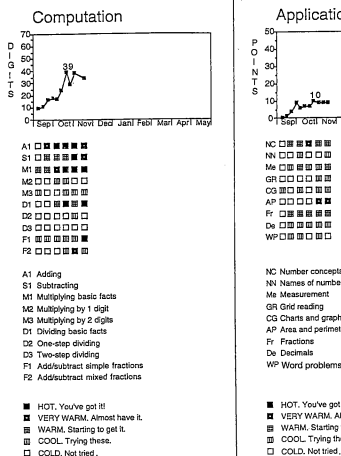

A1 Adding
S1 Subtracting
M1 Multiplying basic facts
M2 Multiplying by 1 digit
M3 Multiplying by 2 digits
D1 Dividing basic facts
D2 One-step dividing
D3 Two-step dividing
F1 Add/subtract simple fractions
F2 Add/subtract mixed fractions

■ HOT. You've got it!
◪ VERY WARM. Almost have it.
▦ WARM. Starting to get it.
▥ COOL. Trying these.
□ COLD. Not tried.

Applications

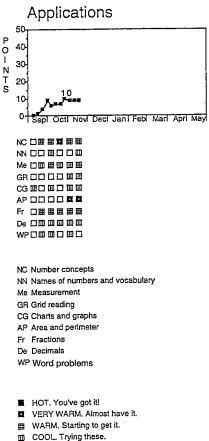

NC Number concepts
NN Names of numbers and vocabulary
Me Measurement
GR Grid reading
CG Charts and graphs
AP Area and perimeter
Fr Fractions
De Decimals
WP Word problems

■ HOT. You've got it!
◪ VERY WARM. Almost have it.
▦ WARM. Starting to get it.
▥ COOL. Trying these.
□ COLD. Not tried.

FIGURE 4.1. *cont.*

Expert Systems

Use of skills analysis helped teachers plan more specific adjustments to their students' instructional programs, which also enhanced program success. This increased "specificity" occurred in teachers more clearly referencing the skills they were targeting for remediation (i.e., a better description of *what* they would teach.)

A persistent problem in the manner in which teachers design instructional adaptations for students who are experiencing failure, however, is an inadequate focus on *how* they will teach. When a student has failed to learn a skill, many teachers will reteach that skill using the original instructional method (see Fuchs, Fuchs, & Bishop, 1992a; Putnam, 1987). Although recycling students through the same instructional procedure may work in some cases, a higher level of adaptation occurs when teachers not only modify what they teach students, but also use a different strategy to provide an alternative route for the student's learning (see Corno & Snow, 1986).

Unfortunately, teachers frequently are knowledgeable and comfortable with only one or two instructional methods and, after a student has experienced failure with these methods, teachers often have difficulty identifying an additional instructional strategy to address the same content. Consequently, although the skills analysis addressed teachers' difficulties in pinpointing which skills to reteach, the computerized skills analysis did not help teachers identify alternative strategies for reteaching that material.

In the next phase of our research program, therefore, we developed and evaluated the use of expert systems to address teachers' difficulty in identifying how to teach students who were experiencing difficulty with the content teachers already had taught. In 1988 and 1989, we developed expert systems in reading, spelling, and mathematics, which provided recommendations for *what* and *how* to teach students whose CBM data indicated that their academic progress was inadequate. Each participating teacher was assigned to a control group or to a CBM experimental group. For each academic area, half of the CBM-participating teachers used expert systems to help determine how to adjust instructional programs; the other half formulated instructional adjustments on their own, using their own judgment. In math, for example, the expert system entered into dialogue with the teacher, requesting information about a student's graphed CBM performance, the student's CBM skills analysis, the student's work habits, the teacher's previous instructional program and the teacher's curricular priorities. The expert system identified which skills should be taught, instructional strategies for teaching those skills to acquisition, methods for retaining already mastered material, as well as motivational strategies.

The extent to which these expert systems helped teachers plan better programs and effect greater achievement varied as a function of content area. In mathematics (Fuchs et al., 1991c), effects supporting the expert system were impressive. Teachers who used the expert system designed better instructional programs that incorporated attention to a more diverse set of skills and relied on a more varied set of instructional design features. Additionally, students in the expert system CBM experimental group achieved significantly and dramatically better than students in the nonexpert system CBM group, and better than the control, non-CBM group.

In reading (Fuchs et al., 1992b), effects differed for instructional planning and achievement. Teachers in the expert system CBM group planned instructional programs that incorporated more reading skills and utilized more instructional methods. With respect to achievement, students in the expert system group achieved reliably better than nonexpert system CBM pupils and control students on outcomes measures involving written retells—an outcome measure that mirrored expert system teachers' greater use of written story grammar instructional activities. On other reading outcome measures (i.e., oral reading fluency and maze), however, both CBM groups achieved comparably well and did better than control group students.

Results in the area of spelling (Fuchs, Fuchs, Hamlett, & Allinder, 1991a) were least supportive of the expert system. Nonexpert and expert system CBM teachers both effected reliably better achievement outcomes than the control teachers. The achievement of the two CBM groups was not, however, reliably different. Our analysis of teachers' instructional plans indicated that teachers in the expert system relied on practice routines recommended by the expert system to a great extent but utilized the expert system's teacher-directed instructional recommendations less frequently. Consequently, the expert system advice did not substantially add to or improve decisions formulated by the teachers on their own.

Although findings differed across the three academic subjects, we identified two important generalizations across content areas. First, without the assistance of the expert systems, teachers found it difficult to generate important instructional adaptations that differed in meaningful ways from their standard instructional routines. This finding corroborated previous CBM work.

Our findings also contributed to the CBM research base in a more novel way. We found that, without the assistance of expert systems, teachers tended to design instructional adaptations that mirrored the measurement system closely. For example, in reading, the nonexpert-system teachers implemented a relatively large number of instructional changes that involved a cloze technique—when the CBM reading measurement task was a closely related maze technique (i.e., multiple-choice cloze). In spelling and math, teachers' instructional adjustments tended to involve reteaching problematic skills—as identified in the skills analysis—but using the same instructional strategy that previously had proved unsuccessful for the student. Consequently, across academic areas, expert systems tended to help teachers move beyond their standard instructional routines and to identify alternative teaching procedures that might assist students in learning the content with which they were experiencing difficulty.

Nevertheless, even with technology that could help teachers identify alternative, potentially effective instructional strategies, an important feasibility problem with meaningful CBM implementation remained: Given CBM's focus on the individual learner, teachers frequently needed to adjust different students' instructional programs in different ways at different times. Given the large numbers of students with whom many special and general educators work, such an individual focus is problematic. Therefore, the next step in our research program was to develop technology for helping teachers integrate CBM information and instructional recommendations across learners.

Classwide Analysis

In a series of research and development stages beginning in 1990, we have developed classwide CBM analyses. As shown in the sample mathematics class report in Figure 4.2, a classwide CBM analysis covers one half-month interval and contains four types of *descriptive* information about class performance. First, at the top of the Class Summary in Figure 4.2, classwide graphs show students' overall progress in mathematics computation and applications, with three paths of CBM scores over time: a path for the 25th percentile scores in this teacher's class, a path for the 50th percentile scores in the class, and one for the 75th percentile scores in the class. Below this graph, the names of students who are performing below the 25th percentile in that class are listed, with advice to the teacher to "watch" these students. The second type of descriptive information is shown in the middle of the Class Summary, where the report identifies the skills on which the class has improved over the past month.

The third type of descriptive information appears in the Class Skills Profile—Computation in Figure 4.2, with a classwide skills analysis that shows every student's mastery status on each skill cluster for the current half-month interval. The students are listed in rows; the skills are represented in columns; the boxes are coded the same way as the individual student's skills analysis—with black boxes representing mastery (or hot), black boxes with dots representing probable mastery (very warm), checkered boxes representing partial mastery (warm), striped boxes represent-

<u>CLASS SUMMARY</u>
Teacher: Mrs. Stephens
Report through 11/8

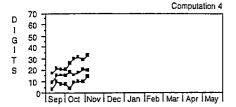

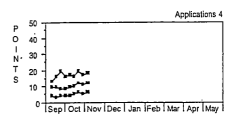

<u>Students to Watch</u>

Lewis Campbell
Omar Faruk
Sylvia Montegro
Diane Fernandez
Luis Castro

<u>Most Improved</u>

Sylvia Montegro
Diane Fernandez
LaShonda Aron
Long Thu
Matthew Stone

<u>Areas of Improvement: Computation</u>

A1   Adding
M2   Multiplying by 1 digit
D1   Dividing basic facts
S1   Subtracting

<u>Areas of Improvement: Applications</u>

Fr   Fractions

<u>Whole Group Instruction: Computation</u>

M2 Multiplying by 1 digit

57% of your students are either COLD or
COOL on this skill.

<u>Whole Group Instruction: Applications</u>

NN Names of numbers and vocabulary

79% of your students are either COLD or
COOL on this skill.

<u>Small Group Instruction: Computation</u>

A1 Adding

Annie Hernandez
Diane Fernandez
Matthew Stone
Steven Smith

<u>Small Group Instruction: Applications</u>

NC Number concepts

Annie Hernandez
Diane Fernandez
Omar Faruk
Sylvia Montegro

(*continued*)

FIGURE 4.2. Example of a computer-generated CBM classwide report in math.

CLASS SKILLS PROFILE - Computation

Teacher: Mrs. Stephens
Report through 11/8

Name	A1	S1	M1	M2	M3	D1	D2	D3	F1	F2
Adam Quave	■	□	⊞	Ⅲ	Ⅲ	⊞	Ⅲ	⊞	Ⅲ	Ⅲ
Annie Hernandez	Ⅲ	Ⅲ	⊞	Ⅲ	Ⅲ	⊞	□	□	Ⅲ	Ⅲ
Anthony Hodges	Ⅲ	Ⅲ	◪	Ⅲ	Ⅲ	⊞	Ⅲ	□	Ⅲ	□
Carlos Gonzalez	⊞	Ⅲ	◪	Ⅲ	Ⅲ	Ⅲ	Ⅲ	Ⅲ	Ⅲ	Ⅲ
Damien Allen	■	⊞	Ⅲ	⊞	Ⅲ	Ⅲ	□	□	Ⅲ	□
Daniel Shinh	■	■	■	⊞	Ⅲ	◪	Ⅲ	⊞	□	□
David Anderson	■	Ⅲ	⊞	◪	Ⅲ	◪	Ⅲ	Ⅲ	◪	■
Diane Fernandez	Ⅲ	□	Ⅲ	□	Ⅲ	◪	□	□	□	□
Gwendolyn Evans	■	Ⅲ	■	◪	Ⅲ	■	□	Ⅲ	◪	□
Kathy Thompson	■	■	■	■	Ⅲ	■	Ⅲ	⊞	□	□
Kendra Lois	■	⊞	⊞	Ⅲ	Ⅲ	⊞	□	□	□	□
Kevin LaBounty	Ⅲ	Ⅲ	Ⅲ	⊞	Ⅲ	□	□	□	□	Ⅲ
LaShonda Aron	■	■	◪	◪	Ⅲ	Ⅲ	□	□	⊞	□
Lewis Campbell	Ⅲ	⊞	Ⅲ	□	Ⅲ	Ⅲ	Ⅲ	Ⅲ	□	□
Lisa Summerall	■	□	◪	□	Ⅲ	Ⅲ	Ⅲ	Ⅲ	Ⅲ	Ⅲ
Long Thu	■	■	■	□	Ⅲ	⊞	Ⅲ	□	Ⅲ	◪
Luis Castro	□	□	□	□	□	□	□	□	Ⅲ	□
Matthew Stone	Ⅲ	Ⅲ	Ⅲ	Ⅲ	Ⅲ	⊞	□	□	□	□
Meagan McGarver	■	◪	◪	■	Ⅲ	⊞	□	Ⅲ	Ⅲ	Ⅲ
Melinda O'Grady	■	⊞	⊞	◪	Ⅲ	◪	□	□	◪	□
Michael Patterson	■	⊞	◪	■	Ⅲ	◪	Ⅲ	□	□	□
Michael Stevens	■	Ⅲ	◪	Ⅲ	Ⅲ	Ⅲ	Ⅲ	Ⅲ	Ⅲ	Ⅲ
Omar Faruk	◪	⊞	◪	□	Ⅲ	Ⅲ	□	□	□	□
Rehanii Nirji	■	⊞	Ⅲ	Ⅲ	Ⅲ	◪	□	□	□	□
Steven Smith	Ⅲ	⊞	■	■	Ⅲ	■	□	Ⅲ	□	□
Sylvia Montegro	⊞	⊞	⊞	□	Ⅲ	Ⅲ	Ⅲ	Ⅲ	Ⅲ	Ⅲ
Tiffany Miller	■	◪	⊞	□	Ⅲ	⊞	□	□	Ⅲ	□
Uri Gurgais	■	◪	■	⊞	⊞	◪	□	□	□	□

		A1	S1	M1	M2	M3	D1	D2	D3	F1	F2
□	COLD. Not tried	1	4	1	8	1	2	16	16	12	18
Ⅲ	COOL. Trying these.	7	8	6	8	26	8	12	10	12	8
⊞	WARM. Starting to get it.	2	9	7	4	1	8	0	2	1	0
◪	VERY WARM. Almost have it.	1	3	8	4	0	7	0	0	3	1
■	HOT. You've got it!	17	4	6	4	0	3	0	0	0	1

FIGURE 4.2. *cont.*

CLASS SKILLS PROFILE - Applications

Teacher: Mrs. Stephens
Report through 11/8

Name	NC	NN	Me	GR	CG	AP	Fr	De	WP
Adam Quave	▦	▥	▦	▥	▥	☐	■	▥	▦
Annie Hernandez	▥	▦	▥	▥	▥	▥	▥	▥	☐
Anthony Hodges	▦	▥	▦	◪	▥	▥	▥	▥	▥
Carlos Gonzalez	▦	▥	◪	☐	▥	◪	▥	▥	▥
Damien Allen	▦	▦	▥	▥	▥	▥	▦	▥	▥
Daniel Shinh	■	▥	▦	■	☐	▥	■	▥	▦
David Anderson	▦	▦	▦	◪	▦	▥	▦	▥	▥
Diane Fernandez	▥	▥	▥	☐	☐	▥	▥	▥	▥
Gwendolyn Evans	▦	▥	▥	▥	▦	▦	▥	▥	▦
Kathy Thompson	▦	▥	▦	◪	▦	▥	■	▥	▦
Kendra Lois	▥	▦	▦	▥	▦	▥	■	▥	▦
Kevin LaBounty	▥	▥	▥	☐	▥	▥	■	▥	▥
LaShonda Aron	▥	▥	▥	☐	▥	▥	▥	▥	▥
Lewis Campbell	▥	▥	▥	☐	▥	▥	◪	▥	▥
Lisa Summerall	▦	▥	▥	☐	▥	▥	■	▥	▥
Long Thu	▦	☐	▥	▥	▥	◪	▦	▥	▥
Luis Castro	▥	▦	▥	▥	▦	☐	☐	☐	☐
Matthew Stone	▦	▥	▥	◪	▥	▥	◪	▥	▥
Meagan McGarver	▥	▥	▥	■	▥	▥	▥	▥	▥
Melinda O'Grady	▦	▥	▦	▥	▥	▥	▦	▥	▥
Michael Patterson	◪	▥	▥	◪	▦	◪	■	▥	▦
Michael Stevens	▦	▥	▦	▥	▦	▦	▦	▥	▦
Omar Faruk	▥	▦	▥	▥	☐	▥	▦	▥	☐
Rehanii Nirji	▦	▥	▦	☐	▥	▥	▦	▥	▥
Steven Smith	▦	▥	▦	☐	▥	☐	▦	▥	▦
Sylvia Montegro	▥	▥	▥	☐	▥	▥	▥	▥	☐
Tiffany Miller	▥	▥	▥	▥	▦	▥	■	▥	▥
Uri Gurgais	▥	☐	▥	▥	▥	◪	▦	▥	▥

		NC	NN	Me	GR	CG	AP	Fr	De	WP
☐	COLD. Not tried.	0	2	0	9	3	3	1	1	4
▥	COOL. Trying these.	12	20	17	12	17	19	8	27	16
▦	WARM. Starting to get it.	14	6	10	0	8	2	9	0	8
◪	VERY WARM. Almost have it.	0	0	1	5	0	4	1	0	0
■	HOT. You've got it!	2	0	0	2	0	0	9	0	0

(*continued*)

FIGURE 4.2. *cont.*

RANKED SCORES - Computation

Teacher: Mrs. Stephens
Report through 11/8

Name	Score	Growth
Kathy Thompson	38	+2.65
Long Thu	33	+3.71
Steven Smith	30	+2.01
Daniel Shinh	30	+2.20
Gwendolyn Evans	29	+2.26
Uri Gurgais	27	+1.87
LaShonda Aron	27	+1.39
Michael Patterson	26	+0.89
Melinda O'Grady	26	+2.57
David Anderson	26	+2.13
Michael Stevens	25	+0.12
Meagan McGarver	24	+2.08
Rehanii Nirji	20	+1.32
Tiffany Miller	19	+1.27
Kendra Lois	18	+0.53
Damien Allen	18	+1.26
Carlos Gonzalez	18	+1.74
Adam Quave	18	+0.88
Lisa Summerall	16	+0.60
Anthony Hodges	16	....
Sylvia Montegro	13	....
Omar Faruk	13	+0.66
Lewis Campbell	13	+1.14
Annie Hernandez	12	+0.67
Kevin LaBounty	11	+0.11
Matthew Stone	10	+0.61
Diane Fernandez	9	+0.67
Luis Castro	0	....

FIGURE 4.2. *cont.*

RANKED SCORES - Applications

Teacher: Mrs. Stephens

Report through 11/8

Name	Score	Growth
Michael Patterson	20	+0.36
Michael Stevens	18	+0.40
Kathy Thompson	17	+0.13
Kendra Lois	16	+1.32
Daniel Shinh	16	+0.70
Adam Quave	16	+1.27
David Anderson	15	+0.40
Damien Allen	15	+1.09
Gwendolyn Evans	14	-0.14
Carlos Gonzalez	14	+0.41
Melinda O'Grady	13	+0.59
Matthew Stone	13	+1.12
Kevin LaBounty	12	+0.57
Steven Smith	11	+0.49
Anthony Hodges	11	....
Lisa Summerall	10	-0.06
Annie Hernandez	10	+1.15
Uri Gurgais	9	+0.90
Tiffany Miller	9	+0.43
Rehanii Nirji	9	-0.06
Long Thu	9	+1.12
Meagan McGarver	8	-0.56
Luis Castro	8	....
Lewis Campbell	7	+0.42
LaShonda Aron	6	+0.02
Omar Faruk	5	+0.31
Diane Fernandez	5	-0.55
Sylvia Montegro	4	....

(*continued*)

FIGURE 4.2. *cont.*

PEER　TUTORING　ASSIGNMENTS

Teacher: Mrs. Stephens
Report through 11/8

S1 Subtracting	First Coach	Second Coach
	▪ Kathy Thompson	☐ Luis Castro
	⊞ Michael Patterson	☐ Diane Fernandez
	⊞ Michael Stevens	⊞ Carlos Gonzalez
	⊞ Rehanii Nirji	⊞ Gwendolyn Evans
	⊞ Steven Smith	⊞ Anthony Hodges
	⊞ David Anderson	☐ Lisa Summerall
	⊞ Melinda O'Grady	⊞ Matthew Stone
	◼ Uri Gurgais	⊞ Kevin LaBounty
	⊞ Kendra Lois	⊞ Annie Hernandez
	⊞ Lewis Campbell	☐ Adam Quave

Fr Fractions	First Coach	Second Coach
	▪ Daniel Shinh	⊞ Meagan McGarver
	▪ Tiffany Miller	⊞ Long Thu
	⊞ Omar Faruk	⊞ LaShonda Aron
	⊞ Damien Allen	⊞ Sylvia Montegro

CLASS STATISTICS

Teacher: Mrs. Stephens
Report through 11/8

Score

Average score	33.9
Standard deviation	10.3
Discrepancy criterion	23.6

Slope

Average slope	+1.91
Standard deviation	1.01
Discrepancy criterion	+0.90

Students identified with dual-discrepancy

	Score	Slope
Diane Fernandez	14.0	+0.12
Kevin LaBounty	23.5	+0.68

FIGURE 4.2. *cont.*

ing nonmastery (cool), and empty boxes representing nonattempts (cold). The teacher can look across any row to determine how any individual student in the class is doing on the multiple skills embedded in the year's curriculum. The teacher can also look down any column to determine how the class is doing on a particular skill. At the bottom of each column, a frequency count shows the numbers of students in each mastery status.

The fourth type of descriptive information appears in the Ranked Scores—Applications in Figure 4.2. This summary rank-orders the students in the class from the highest to the lowest CBM median score over the past half-month. It also provides a slope of improvement over time for each student, which indicates the average number of digits correct gain per week.

The group analysis also provides *instructional recommendations*. For example, the bottom of the Class Summary in Figure 4.2, identifies skills to teach in large- and small-group arrangements and, for small groups, indicates which students should be included for each skill. In the Peer-Tutoring Assignments in Figure 4.2, the computer reports peer-tutoring recommendations it has formulated. Skills for remediation during peer tutoring are listed. Under each skill, the report lists students who have the requisite skills to serve as first coaches (i.e., tutors for the first half of each session, who model the skills); other students who require remediation are listed as second coaches (i.e., who serve tutors for the second half of each session). The computer-assisted instruction and peer-tutoring recommendations allow teachers to use the CBM information flexibly to adapt their instruction to meet individual needs, using routines that can be feasibly integrated into existing classroom structures. (We have also developed classwide peer-tutoring methods that teachers can use to structure the process by which classwide peer tutoring occurs. For additional information on these classwide peer-tutoring methods, see Fuchs et al., 1997).

During 1991 and 1992, we conducted an experiment to examine the utility of classwide CBM reports and instructional recommendations within general education classrooms that incorporated mainstreamed students with learning disabilities for instruction on a daily basis (Fuchs, Fuchs, Hamlett, Bishop, & Bentz, 1994). Results indicated that teachers who employed classwide CBM with instructional recommendations on the CBM mathematics-operations curriculum planned more responsively to individual student needs and effected substantially and significantly better mathematics operations achievement than teachers who did not use CBM. These effects held across learning-disabled, low-achieving nondisabled, and average-achieving students. Additionally, and importantly, the general educators found the CBM process, which included both measurement and instructional decision making as deliberate emphases of the intervention, to be feasible to implement and enjoyable for them and for their students. In subsequent work, we have corroborated findings on the mathematics-applications curriculum with learning-disabled, low-achieving nondisabled, average-achieving, and high-achieving students (Fuchs et al., 1997).

ADDITIONAL DIRECTIONS FOR COMPUTER APPLICATIONS

Although most of our work has focused on helping teachers connect CBM to their instructional decision making in meaningful, effective, and feasible ways, we recently have developed and investigated how CBM software might be used to provide ongoing, technically strong information relevant to special education referral and placement decisions. Our computerized programs to assist teachers in making sound prereferral and referral decisions rely on portions of an innovative CBM identification model, which capitalizes on CBM's capacity to focus explicitly on questions about student learning (i.e., change over time). (For an extended description of this alternative CBM identification model and discussion of the conceptual and technical basis for proposing an alternative CBM identification model, see Fuchs, 1995.)

One central feature of this alternative CBM referral and identification model is that before a student can be considered for prereferral intervention, he or she must demonstrate sizable discrepancies *from other students in his or her classroom* on CBM performance *level* and CBM *rate of improvement* over time (i.e., growth rate or slope). The first key dimension is reliance on the student's own classmates for the normative comparison. The rationale for this focus is as follows: To determine whether a student manifests a serious learning problem that requires special intervention, it is necessary to interpret that problem relative to students who are receiving the same instruction. The need for this situational interpretation is illustrated in work by Fuchs (1995), showing that the effectiveness of regular classroom instructional settings can vary dramatically. Even within the same school at the same grade, effect sizes comparing the CBM growth rates of most effective and least effective teachers (difference between mean CBM slopes, computed on the basis of 30 weekly, classwide CBM assessments, divided by the pooled standard deviation) were between 0.62 and 1.82 standard deviations, for mathematics computations; between 1.10 and 1.50 standard deviations, for mathematics applications.

These data, demonstrating the differential efficacy of regular classroom instructional settings, illustrate how a student's responsiveness to instruction cannot be judged in absolute terms. In a classroom environment where the instruction is relatively ineffective (and slopes are generally low), a child with a CBM mathematics growth rate of 0.30 digits per week might represent the typical level of responsiveness to the instruction provided by that teacher. Consequently, a growth rate of 0.30 would not suggest the presence of a learning problem (although one might target the *classroom* for intervention in an attempt to improve the overall level of effectiveness). By contrast, a growth rate of 0.30 digits per week in an effective teacher's classroom, where the mean growth rate is perhaps 0.80 digits per week, might place a child one or more standard deviations below the class mean—suggesting a lack of responsiveness to this effective learning environment and indicating the potential presence of a learning problem. Because lack of responsiveness and learning problems must therefore be judged situationally, a CBM database that generates general education classwide growth rates is helpful in interpreting individual students' potential difficulties.

The second key dimension of the innovative CBM referral/identification process is that in determining whether a student's learning problem warrants special consideration, analysis focuses simultaneously on a student's CBM *level* of performance and his or her *rate of improvement* over time. A student whose CBM level score is one or more standard deviations below the mean CBM level of the class demonstrates a poor learning history. Nevertheless, despite a history of difficulties, that child may be responding well to the current instructional environment—as shown in a respectable CBM slope. Such a child, who is substantially below the level of his or her class, but who is nonetheless demonstrating good learning in this classroom, should not be identified for special intervention. On the other hand, a student who is already a proficient reader, with a high CBM level of performance, but who is no longer demonstrating a strong rate of improvement, also presents a profile that does not warrant special intervention. Alternatively, we argue for the identification of students who present a dual set of CBM discrepancies—showing a poor learning history (as demonstrated in CBM performance level) as well as poor responsiveness to the current instructional environment (as demonstrated in CBM slope or rate of growth).

To begin to address this question, we studied the appropriateness of groups of students identified with *dual* discrepancy criteria by (1) comparing them to the pools that would have been identified on the basis of a single discrepancy on CBM performance level, (2) contrasting the percentages of identified students to national prevalence estimates, and (3) estimating decision-consistency reliability with respect to students with school-identified mild/moderate disabilities labels (see Fuchs, 1995).

As might be expected, use of these dual-discrepancy criteria frequently identified a pool of students whose performance levels were lowest
in the class—similar, but identical, to the pool that would be identified on
the basis of a single discrepancy on performance level. Use of the dual-
discrepancy criteria did, however, contribute important additional information beyond a sole focus on CBM performance level: Between 29%
and 71% of students who demonstrated discrepancies in performance level equal to or greater than 1.5 standard deviations were eliminated from
consideration because their growth rates were acceptable. For example, in
one classroom, the lowest-performing student (whose performance level
was 2.55 standard deviations below the class mean) had a slope of 0.73
digits per week, placing him only 0.88 standard deviations below the mean
on growth. Similarly, in another class, the lowest-performing student,
whose performance level was 2.47 standard deviations below the class
mean, had a slope of 0.55 digits, placing him only 0.68 standard deviations below the mean on growth. Neither of these two students was selected by any of the dual-discrepancy criteria we applied.

To explore further the decision validity of the dual-discrepancy criteria, we compared the percentage of students identified for further assessment to national prevalence estimates. Different dual-discrepancy criteria
that required students to be 1 standard deviations below the class mean on
CBM level and growth rate identified between 9.4% of the sample of 469
students. As an initial phase in a multistep process, where false negatives
are highly undesirable because additional children will be eliminated from
the special education eligibility pool at subsequent stages, a dual criterion
of 1st standard deviation on level and 1st standard duration on slope
seemed appropriate.

Finally, we explored the consistency of decisions with respect to
school-identified mild/moderate disability status. The dual discrepancy
criteria of 1/1 generated, among a pool of 469 students, between 20
(6.2%) and 30 (6.3%) false positives. Again, this rate seemed appropriate
within a multistage identification process, where false positives will be reduced throughout subsequent stages. These analyses lend tentative empirical support for use of a dual-discrepancy model, in relation to classroom
norms, for initial identification in a first stage of a multiphase eligibility assessment procedure.

Over the past 2 years, we developed software that automatically conducts these dual-discrepancy analyses and piloted a special education
identification process within one school, which relies on dual CBM discrepancies in level and growth, using the classroom as the normative
framework. The computerized analyses are shown in the Class Summary
portion of the classwide CBM report (see Figure 4.2). Our pilot work
demonstrates consistency in decision making and promise for the use of

dual discrepancies within a multistage special education identification process.

IMPLICATIONS

This 10-year research program on computer applications to CBM permits several conclusions about special education, general education, technology, and assessment. First, technology can be used to reduce dramatically the need for teachers to conduct the mechanical tasks associated with assessment, such as test construction and administration, scoring, graphing, and data analysis. Although data-management software, alone, does not increase teacher efficiency in measurement, data-generation/collection software (used in combination with data-management software) totally eliminates most teachers' time in such tasks. Computers are ideally suited for the completion of this type of repetitive, routine work, and related computer applications for other types of assessment procedures should be developed to help reduce the need for teachers to engage in unchallenging work and to increase their availability for the more critical instructional responsibilities.

Second, in addition to completing the mechanical, repetitive aspects of measurement, computers can be used to complete work that human beings would not ordinarily be capable of performing accurately (even with great expenditures of time). For example, the computer-generated skills analyses provide a useful supplement to the traditional CBM total test score indicators of overall proficiency, allowing teachers to plan more specific instructional programs and to effect greater achievement for their students. Without the use of technology, such skills analyses are not possible. Another example of information that computers can easily generate, which teachers would not be capable of producing reliably even with time expenditures, is the group reports. These reports aggregate information about many students and automatically organize instructional recommendations. Our research again indicates that these group reports increase teachers' capacity to plan responsive instructional programs, even in the context of large groups of students, and to effect better achievement outcomes. Researchers and developers should continue to consider how technology can be used not only to save teachers time but also to *enhance* the quality and effects of teachers' efforts by providing information and completing work that humans would otherwise not be capable of generating.

Third, our work with expert systems and other instructional recommendation systems indicates their value in helping teachers plan more sound, effective instruction. Nevertheless, our research also suggests that caution is in order: Use of our expert systems produced differing, depending on instructional area. Clearly, the availability of computer-generated instructional recommendations alone is insufficient to increase teachers' capacity to plan better programs. The nature of the advice and the conditions under which that advice is offered are critical to efficacy. As electronic information and communication systems are developed to increase teachers' access to information, researchers and developers need to consider carefully the quality and nature of the available information and the conditions under which that information is offered. In addition, the efficacy of such electronic information and communication systems needs to be evaluated rigorously before we can assume beneficial outcomes for students or teachers.

ACKNOWLEDGMENTS

Research described in this chapter was supported in part by Grant Nos. H180E20004, H023E90020, H023A10010, G008730087, and G008530198 from the U.S. Department of Education, Office of Special Education, to Vanderbilt University. Statements should not, however, be interpreted as official policy of the agencies.

REFERENCES

Bishop, N., Fuchs, L. S., Fuchs, D., & Hamlett, C. L. (1992). *Adaptive peer tutoring: Framework and procedures.* Unpublished manuscript.

Christenson, S. L., Ysseldyke, J. E., & Thurlow, M. E. (1989). Critical instructional factors for students with mild handicaps: An integrative review. *Remedial and Special Education, 10*(5), 21–31.

Corno, L., & Snow, R. E. (1986). Adapting teaching to individual differences among learners. In M. Wittrock (Ed.), *Third handbook of research on teaching* (pp. 605–629). New York: Macmillan.

Deno, S. L. (1985). Curriculum-based measurement: The emerging alternative. *Exceptional Children, 52,* 219–232.

Fuchs, L. S. (1995, May). *Incorporating curriculum-based measurement into the eligibility decision-making process: A focus on treatment validity and student growth.* Paper presented at the 2nd Workshop on IQ Testing, National Research Council, Washington, DC.

Fuchs, L. S., & Deno, S. L. (1991). Paradigmatic distinctions between instructionally relevant measurement models. *Exceptional Children, 57,* 488–501.

Fuchs, L. S., Deno, S. L., & Mirkin, P. K. (1984). The effects of frequent curriculum-based measurement and evaluation on pedagogy, student achievement, and student awareness of learning. *American Educational Research Journal, 21,* 449–460.

Fuchs, L. S., Fuchs, D., & Bishop, N. (1992a). Teacher planning for students with learning disabilities: Differences between general and special educators. *Learning Disabilities Research and Practice, 7,* 120–129.

Fuchs, L. S., Fuchs, D., & Hamlett, C. L. (1988). Effects of computer-managed instruction on teachers' implementation of systematic monitoring programs and student achievement. *Journal of Educational Research, 81,* 294–304.

Fuchs, L. S., Fuchs, D., & Hamlett, C. L. (1989). Monitoring reading growth using student recalls: Effects of two teacher feedback systems. *Journal of Educational Research, 83,* 103–111.

Fuchs, L. S., Fuchs, D., Hamlett, C. L., & Allinder, R. M. (1991a). Effects of expert system advice within curriculum-based measurement on teachers planning and student achievement in spelling. *School Psychology Review, 20,* 49–66.

Fuchs, L. S., Fuchs, D., Hamlett, C. L., & Allinder, R. M. (1991b). The contribution of skills analysis to curriculum-based measurement in spelling. *Exceptional Children, 57,* 443–452.

Fuchs, L. S., Fuchs, D., Hamlett, C. L., Bishop, N., & Bentz, J. (1994). Classwide curriculum-based measurement: Helping teachers meet the challenge of student diversity. *Exceptional Children, 60,* 15–24.

Fuchs, L. S., Fuchs, D., Hamlett, C. L., & Ferguson, C. (1992b). Effects of expert system consultation within curriculum-based measurement using a reading maze task. *Exceptional Children, 58,* 436–450.

Fuchs, L. S., Fuchs, D., Hamlett, C. L., & Stecker, P. M. (1990). The role of skills analysis in curriculum-based measurement in math. *School Psychology Review, 19,* 6–22.

Fuchs, L. S., Fuchs, D., Hamlett, C. L., & Stecker, P. M. (1991c). Effects of curriculum-based measurement and consultation on teacher planning and student achievement in mathematics operations. *American Educational Research Journal, 28,* 617–641.

Fuchs, L. S., Fuchs, D., Hasselbring, T., & Hamlett, C. L. (1987a). Using computers with curriculum-based progress monitoring: Effects on teacher efficiency and satisfaction. *Journal of Special Education Technology, 8*(4), 14–27.

Fuchs, L. S., Fuchs, D., Phillips, N. B., Hamlett, C. L., Karns, K., & Dutka, S. (1997). Enhancing students' helping behavior during peer-mediated instruction with conceptual mathematical explanations. *Elementary School Journal, 97,* 223–250.

Fuchs, L. S., Hamlett, C. L., Fuchs, D., Stecker, P. M., & Ferguson, C. (1988). Conducting curriculum-based measurement with computerized data collection: Effects on efficiency and teacher satisfaction. *Journal of Special Education Technology, 9*(2), 73–86.

Gersten, R., Carnine, D., & Woodward, J. (1987). Direct instruction research: The third decade. *Remedial and Special Education, 8*(6), 48–56.

Haynes, M. C., & Jenkins, J. R. (1986). Reading instruction in special education resource rooms. *American Educational Research Journal, 23,* 161–190.

Jones, E. D., & Krouse, J. P. (1988). The effectiveness of data-based instruction by student teachers in classrooms for pupils with mild handicaps. *Teacher Education and Special Education, 11*(1), 9–19.

Putnam, R. T. (1987). Structuring and adjusting content for students: A study of live and simulated tutoring of addition. *American Educational Research Journal, 24,* 13–48.

Reisberg, L., & Wolf, R. (1988). Instructional strategies for special education consultants. *Remedial and Special Education, 9*(6), 29–40.

Shinn, M. R. (Ed.). (1989). *Curriculum-based measurement: Assessing special children.* New York: Guilford Press.

Walton, W. T. (1986). Educators' response to methods of collecting, storing, and analyzing behavioral data. *Journal of Special Education Technology, 7,* 50–55.

Wesson, C. L. (1991). Curriculum-based measurement and two models of follow-up consultation. *Exceptional Children, 57,* 246–257.

Wesson, C. L., King, R. P., & Deno, S. L. (1984). Direct and frequent measurement: If it's so good for us, why don't we use it? *Learning Disability Quarterly, 7*(1), 45–48.

Will, M. (1986). Educating children with learning problems: A shared responsibility. *Exceptional Children, 52,* 411–415.

Zigmond, N., & Miller, S.E. (1986). Assessment for instructional planning. *Exceptional Children, 52,* 501–509.

CHAPTER 5

◆◆◆

Assessing Early Literacy Skills in a Problem-Solving Model: Dynamic Indicators of Basic Early Literacy Skills

◆

RUTH A. KAMINSKI
ROLAND H. GOOD III

Reading is a cultural imperative in today's information-based society. Reading competence will certainly become increasingly important as an avenue to rewards and success. And yet, many children experience significant difficulty learning to read that will impact their success throughout school and beyond. Children from families with low socioeconomic status (SES) are particularly at risk (Bowey, 1995). However, identifying children with reading problems and providing intervention is generally not sufficient to remediate reading problems. For example, Johnston and Allington, in their review of remedial reading interventions, concluded that "remedial reading is generally not very effective at making children more literate" (1991, p. 1001). Instead, a more efficacious approach is to *prevent* reading problems by ensuring that children have the necessary early literacy skills for successful reading instruction. "One irrepressible interpretation is that the likelihood that a child will succeed in the first grade depends most of all on how much she or he has already learned about reading before getting there" (Adams, 1990, p. 82).

Effective early intervention to prevent reading problems has been hampered by two factors. First, until recently, it has been unclear *what* early literacy skills should be taught (see, e.g., Masland & Masland, 1988). For kindergarten and preschool teachers, uncertainty about what to teach is especially problematic, because the outcome of instruction (reading competence) will not be evident until later. Second, even when the efficacy of teaching early literacy skills has been supported by research (e.g., Byrne & Fielding-Barnsley, 1993, 1995), effects have been demonstrated only for *groups* of children. Although children provided with an effective intervention might read better *as a group* than children given a competing intervention, the intervention may not be effective for each individual child (Deno, 1990).

In the absence of clear evidence regarding what to teach and the effectiveness of instruction for each individual student, teachers must use a "teach-and-hope" approach to early literacy skills instruction based primarily on *beliefs* about reading acquisition and *beliefs* about what will work to assist children in learning to read. However, belief-driven intervention is hamstrung by the time lag between the intervention and outcome, and by the lack of accurate feedback on effectiveness for individual children. Important advances in *intervention* regarding what to teach and advances in *assessment* regarding the evaluation of outcomes for individual students are beginning to empower educators to effect improved literacy outcomes.

ADVANCES IN INTERVENTION

We now understand better than ever *what* early literacy skills to teach to assist children in successful reading instruction and to prevent reading difficulty (Adams, 1990). Adams presents a summary of the research on early reading acquisition commissioned by the U.S. Department of Education. She notes that the probability of success in learning to read is the result primarily of the early literacy skills that children bring to early reading instruction. The three most crucial early literacy skills noted by Adams are (1) phonological awareness skills, (2) language skills, and (3) awareness of print. In particular, phonological awareness skills appear to be an important key to the development of the alphabetic principal and subsequent literacy for children. Although the importance of phonological awareness skills is clear, teacher training programs have not done an adequate job of training teachers to instruct phonological awareness (Moats, 1995). In addition, early reading curricula generally have not addressed phonological awareness skills adequately (Simmons et al., 1995).

Phonological awareness refers to the explicit awareness of the *sound structure* of language, including the ability to manipulate sound units smaller than words. For example, the word "cat" is composed of the sounds /k/ /a/ /t/, where the slashes indicate the sound of the letter rather than the name of the letter. Phonological awareness includes a range of skills including rhyming, blending, segmentation, and deletion. Phonological awareness includes tasks requiring knowledge of the smallest sound unit of the language (phonemic awareness) and larger sound units such as onsets (initial consonant or consonant sounds) and rimes (vowel and any final consonant sounds). Phonological or phonemic awareness is not the same as phonics: *Phonics* refers to the pattern of letter–sound correspondences in *written* language, whereas phonological awareness refers to the component sounds of *spoken* language. Phonological awareness may be an essential preskill for phonics-based reading instruction to make sense, however. "Faced with an alphabetic script, the child's level of phonemic awareness on entering school may be the single most powerful determinant of the success she or he will experience in learning to read and of the likelihood that she or he will fail" (Adams, 1990, p. 304).

The steps in the logic linking phonological awareness to successful reading instruction have been demonstrated. Phonological awareness skills can be taught (e.g., Byrne & Fielding-Barnsley, 1995; Koehler, 1996; O'Connor, Jenkins, Leicester, & Slocum, 1993). When children learn phonological awareness skills, they experience greater success in learning to read (Iverson & Tunmer, 1993; Lundberg, Frost, & Petersen, 1988). In addition, explicit instruction on phonological awareness skills may mediate SES differences in reading success (Bowey, 1995). The possibilities for important social outcomes are staggering. By ensuring that *all* children have adequate phonological awareness skills when they enter first grade, we may be able to mitigate the effects of many differences in the initial skills required for successful reading instruction and prevent many cases of reading failure.

However, knowing that an early literacy skills intervention is effective in general is not sufficient for a teacher working with a specific child. Although phonological awareness interventions have been developed with documented effectiveness (e.g., Byrne & Fielding-Barnsley, 1991; Torgesen & Bryant, 1994), their effectiveness is for *groups* of students. Even investigations of effective interventions have identified individual children who did not respond to the intervention, or at least who had not yet responded at termination of the study (e.g., Blachman, 1994; Byrne & Fielding-Barnsley, 1995; Torgesen, Wagner, & Rashotte, 1994). For example, Byrne and Fielding-Barnsley (1995) examined the effects of the Sound Foundations phonological awareness training program (Byrne & Fielding-Barnsley, 1991). They found that the experimental group receiving the Sound Foundations program scored significantly better than the control group on "pseudowords" (e.g., neb, lim) in first and second grade. However, 3 of the 63 children in the experimental group failed the phoneme identity posttest. Similarly, Torgesen et al. (1994) found that "about 30% of our at-risk sample showed no measurable growth in phonological awareness following an 8-week training program that produced significant growth in awareness in the majority of children" (p. 284). Thus, even generally effective interventions are not necessarily effective for all students. A methodology is needed to identify and evaluate the effectiveness of interventions for *individual* students in a timely manner, so that the intervention can be modified on a timely basis.

ADVANCES IN ASSESSMENT

In addition to the significant contribution of phonological awareness instruction to enhancing reading outcomes, advances in assessment and educational decision making can enhance achievement outcomes. These advances in assessment and decision making are epitomized by the use of Curriculum-Based Measurement (CBM) in a Problem-Solving model. Development and refinement of the Problem-Solving model provides a set of decision-making procedures that are grounded in a theoretical model (e.g., Deno, 1989; Shinn & Hubbard, 1992). In the Problem-Solving model, five linked decisions are made: (1) Problem Identification, (2) Problem Validation or Certification, (3) Exploring Solutions, (4) Evaluating Solutions, and (5) Problem Solution (Deno, 1989). CBM provides a measurement technology to operationalize the decisions represented by the Problem-Solving model.

By continuously assessing the progress of individual students using CBM reading in a Problem-Solving model, educators can evaluate the effectiveness of their intervention within weeks instead of waiting until the end of the year (or even the following year) to tell if their interventions are working (Deno, 1986). The use of this *formative* evaluation strategy to evaluate the effectiveness of interventions for individual students has a positive effect on reading achievement (Fuchs & Fuchs, 1986). In their meta-analysis of the effects of systematic progress monitoring on student's reading skills, Fuchs and Fuchs found that formative evaluation, with progress toward an ambitious goal graphed on an ongoing basis, reinforcement for progress, and data-based decision rules for modifying intervention, resulted in an effect size of +0.70 for reading outcomes.

APPLYING THE PROBLEM-SOLVING MODEL
TO EARLY LITERACY SKILLS

It seems reasonable to combine effective interventions targeting the acquisition of early literacy skills (including phonological awareness) with a Problem-Solving model of assessment to further enhance learning outcomes for children at risk of difficulty learning to read. Dynamic Indicators of Basic Early Literacy Skills (DIBELS) were developed to make educational decisions in a Problem-Solving model regarding (1) *which children* require early literacy skills interventions beyond the general "curriculum"; (2) *which interventions* are effective in resolving the early literacy skills problem on an individual, case-by-case basis; and (3) *when interventions have successfully reduced the risk* of reading failure by remediating early literacy skills. The steps of the Problem-Solving model and the type of data the DIBELS measures are intended to provide for each decision step are detailed in Table 5.1.

Development of the DIBELS measures followed a review of the literature on the importance and contribution of different early literacy skills. The criteria used to develop and evaluate the DIBELS measures in a

TABLE 5.1. Using DIBELS in a Problem-Solving Model for Kindergarten Students

Phase	Decision	Data-based comparison
1. Problem Identification	• Which children are potentially at risk of difficulty learning to read because of low early literacy skills?	• Compare individual student's performance to local normative context or expected performance to evaluate discrepancy.
2. Problem Validation	• Are the child's low early literacy skills of sufficient severity and persistence that intervention is warranted?	• Compare individual student performance to local normative context or expected performance to evaluate discrepancy. • Compare child's performance to past performance to evaluate trend.
3. Exploring Solutions	• What skills should we teach and how should we teach them? • What are the goals of instruction?	• Error analysis of performance on DIBELS measures to identify low skills and location on the continuum of skill development. • Normative expectations of performance.
4. Evaluate Solutions	• Is the intervention effective in improving the child's early literacy skills?	• Monitor child's progress during intervention (compare to past performance) to evaluate trend and projected performance.
5. Problem Solution	• Is the child no longer at risk for difficulty learning to read because of low early literacy skills?	• Compare individual student performance to local normative context or expected performance to evaluate discrepancy.

Problem-Solving model were drawn from the criteria used for CBM measures (see Deno, 1985; Marston, 1989), including that the measures be

1. Reliable and valid measures of early literacy skills.
2. Simple and efficient to administer.
3. Easily understood by teachers, parents, and students.
4. Inexpensive to produce in terms of time and resources.
5. Vital signs of growth in basic skills and student educational health, not exhaustive measures of every early literacy skill.
6. Sensitive to improvement in student's skills over time.
7. Sensitive to effects of intervention and short-term growth on an individual, case-by-case basis.
8. Relevant to the content of instruction.
9. Available in multiple forms of short duration to facilitate frequent administration by teachers/educators.
10. Based on production-type responses, so that student skills can be observed rather than inferred.
11. Relevant across a range of educational decisions.

Following the review of literature and establishment of criteria, trial measures were developed and field-tested. The measures that best met the criteria of reliability and validity were examined further, with ongoing research examining the sensitivity of the measures to the effects of interventions. Three DIBELS measures have initial evidence for reliability, validity, and utility within a Problem-Solving model: (1) Phonemic Segmentation Fluency, (2) Onset Recognition Fluency, and (3) Letter-Naming Fluency. The behavior sampled and technical adequacy of each measure is summarized in Table 5.2. All measures use a fluency metric for scoring, with the score being the number of segments, onsets, or letters named correctly per minute. Phonemic Segmentation Fluency is a measure of phonological awareness appropriate for most children from the middle of kindergarten through the middle of first grade. Onset Recognition Fluency is also a measure of phonological awareness that is appropriate for most children from late preschool through the middle of kindergarten. Letter-Naming Fluency is a measure of alphabetic knowledge and fluency that appears to be appropriate for most children from fall of kindergarten through the middle of first grade.

DIFFERENCES BETWEEN CBM AND DIBELS
IN A PROBLEM-SOLVING MODEL

Although DIBELS and CBM share common development criteria and a common linkage to the Problem-Solving model, there are some key differ-

TABLE 5.2. Behavior Sampled, Reliability, and Validity of DIBELS Measures for Kindergarten Students

Measure	Behavior sampled	Reliability and validity
Phonemic Segmentation Fluency	The child is asked to segment a spoken word into component sounds. For example, if the stimulus is "fish" the child would say /f/ /i/ /sh/.	Reliability of 1 probe: .88 Reliability of 3 probes[a]: .96 Validity[b]: .73–.91
Onset Recognition Fluency	The child is presented with four pictures and asked to identify the one that begins with a verbally presented onset. For example, "Which picture begins with /b/?" The child is asked to produce the onset for a verbally presented word accompanied by a picture of the object. For example, "What sound does 'hat' begin with?"	Reliability of 1 probe: .65 Reliability of 5 probes[a]: .90 Validity[c]: .44–.60
Letter-Naming Fluency	The child is presented with random sequence of upper- and lower-case letters and asked to name the letters in order. For example, "When I say 'start' begin here, go across the page and tell me as many letters as you can. Try to name each letter."	Reliability of 1 probe: .93 Reliability of 3 probes: .98 Validity[b]: .72–.98

Note. Reliability and validity summarized from Kaminski and Good (1996) and Otterstedt (1993).
[a]Based on Spearman–Brown prophecy formula.
[b]One-year predictive validity with reading criterion measures.
[c]Concurrent validity with Phonemic Segmentation Fluency.

ences between using CBM for basic academic skills and using DIBELS for early literacy skills. Differences between DIBELS and CBM in a Problem-Solving model include (1) the rationale and definition of a problem, (2) the consequences of decision errors, (3) the nature of skills development and performance, (4) the selection of measurement material, (5) the duration of measured skills, and (6) the relation of measured skills to tool-outcome skills.

Rationale

A first difference between DIBELS and CBM regards the rationale for problem solving and the definition of a problem. CBM in a Problem-Solving model generally is used to *remediate* severe academic problems. In contrast, the goal of DIBELS in a Problem-Solving model is to *prevent* severe academic problems. In both cases, a problem is defined as a discrepancy between observed and expected behavior. For CBM in basic academic skills areas, the *social importance* of the problem is clear. For example, reading competence is an explicit goal of elementary education that is a cultural imperative. A cultural imperative is "the implicit or explicit standards of conduct or performance imposed on all who would be members of a culture" (Deno, 1989, p. 8). Students whose reading skills are discrepant from cultural and normative expectations are readily judged as displaying a socially important problem (for a discussion of the social importance of reading, see Anderson, Hiebert, Scott, & Wilkinson, 1984). Thus, informal teacher referrals or nominations are fairly accurate indices of a reading problem (e.g., Shinn, Tindal, & Spira, 1987).

In contrast to reading skills, early literacy skills, especially phonological awareness, seldom are considered social imperatives. Consequently, attainment of phonological awareness may not be an explicit educational goal, and teachers may not be explicitly aware of their students phonological awareness skills (e.g., Moats, 1995). For DIBELS, in a Problem-Solving model, a problem is defined as the discrepancy between current early literacy skills and the level of early literacy skills necessary for later reading success. However, because early literacy skills problems may not be explicitly included in the curriculum and may be less obvious to teachers, teacher referrals or nominations of early literacy skills problems may be less accurate than for reading skills. Since reliance on teacher referrals to initiate the Problem-Solving model may miss children with phonological awareness skills problems, an active screening procedure may be necessary.

Consequences of Decision Errors

Because the emphasis of DIBELS in a Problem-Solving model is prevention instead of remediation, the corresponding intervention strategies involve *low-stakes* testing. In contrast, when the emphasis is on remediation of severe problems, the stakes are high. High-stakes tests are "those whose results are seen—rightly or wrongly—by students, teachers, administrators, parents, or the general public as being used to make important decisions that immediately and directly affect them" (Madaus, 1988, cited in Meisels, 1989). For example, using a test to certify a child as eligible for special education services is high-stakes testing with severe consequences of decision errors, and the test should meet rigorous standards of reliability and validity. Using a test to identify children who are low on early literacy skills and to evaluate the effectiveness of general education interventions on the early literacy skills entails much less serious consequences of decision errors (i.e., lower stakes).

One advantage of making lower stakes decisions is that a less rigorous standard of reliability and validity is appropriate, because the cost of a decision error is relatively low. If a child were removed from class and placed in special education by mistake, his or her parents might rightfully be concerned. If a child were mistakenly provided with additional instruction, modeling, and practice on phonological awareness skills in the regular class, his or her parents would most likely be unconcerned.

Early Development

A third important difference between DIBELS and CBM regards developmental differences between the children of the respective target ages. The target ages for the DIBELS measures include older preschool, kindergarten, and early-first-grade children. Young children, in particular, are characterized by variability in performance, rapid changes in skills, and malleability.

Although variability in performance is characteristic of all people, and especially children, young children can be extremely variable in performance depending on sleep, food, interest, emotional state, and the context. This variability has important consequences for assessment. First, it is important to avoid high-stakes decisions as much as possible. When high-stakes decisions are unavoidable, they should be based on information obtained on multiple days, in multiple contexts, with multiple sets of stimulus materials. By considering information gathered under multiple conditions, young children's variability in performance can be considered, in addition to their *level* of skills. Thus, when using DIBELS in a Problem-Solving model, more variability in performance is expected than when using CBM with older children. More data points may be needed to obtain the same amount of confidence in a performance estimate.

In addition to variability in performance, young children's performance is characterized by malleability, with rapid changes and growth possible. For young children, changes in rate of growth are even more pronounced than for elementary-school children. Young children enter school and learning settings from an extremely varied range of previous learning environments. When exposed to or instructed in new information or skills, they may respond rapidly. Consequently, for young children, current performance on the DIBELS measures is not as predictive of future performance as the prediction of future performance based on current CBM performance for elementary-school-aged children.

For example, the reading skills of children even as early as the end of first grade are extremely predictive of their later reading skills. Juel (1988) found that a poor reader in first grade has a .88 probability of remaining a poor reader in fourth grade. Others also have found that relative standing in reading skills is remarkably stable for children in elementary school (e.g., Clay, 1979; Jorm, Share, Maclean, & Matthews, 1986). With younger preschool and kindergarten children, rapid changes in response to instruction are likely. For example, Good and Kaminski (1996) described the rapid progress and response to instruction of a kindergarten child who had low phonological awareness skills in the middle of the kindergarten year but responded favorably to phonological awareness instruction. Indeed, it is in the kindergarten and early first grades that teachers have the best opportunity to establish an adequate trajectory of growth on academic skills.

Material Selection

A fourth difference between DIBELS and CBM regards the selection of measurement material. For CBM, the selection of measurement material is determined by the current general education curriculum (Shinn, 1989). Curriculum materials are used to establish expected levels of performance when determining whether there is a problem warranting intervention. In addition, curriculum is the vehicle by which school boards and communities establish the cultural imperatives for schooling and the best approximation of the tool-outcome skills that children will need for success in their society beyond school. As stated in *Becoming a Nation of Readers* (Anderson et al., 1984), "Reading is a basic life skill. It is a cornerstone for a child's success in school and, indeed, throughout life. Without the ability to read well, opportunities for personal fulfillment and job success inevitably will be lost" (p. 1).

In contrast, when using DIBELS, early literacy skills (e.g., phonological awareness), in and of themselves, generally are not a cultural imperative like reading. However, regardless of whether there is a phonological awareness curriculum (Moats, 1995), or whether the phonological awareness curriculum is adequate (Simmons et al., 1995), phonological awareness is an essential early literacy skill to measure because of its contribution to future reading competence (e.g., Yopp, 1995). Because the selection of measurement materials is driven by their linkage to later literacy success, linkage to the specific kindergarten curriculum is less important. In fact, if the kindergarten curriculum does not address skills linked to literacy, the kindergarten curriculum should be evaluated to determine whether it should be changed.

Duration of Measurement Materials

A fifth fundamental difference between DIBELS and CBM regards the *duration* of skills assessed. CBM measurement materials generally have a *long duration,* meaning they may be used over an entire school year or even across years. In CBM reading, for example, a third-grade reading passage may be reliable and valid for students in first through sixth grade (Fuchs & Deno, 1992). In contrast, the duration of DIBELS measurement materials is shorter. For example, the Phonemic Segmentation Fluency test appears to have a floor effect for children beginning kindergarten, with many children receiving a score of 0. From winter of kindergarten through fall of first grade, most children score above 0 on Phonemic Segmentation Fluency probes. By the middle of first grade, however, the performance of typical children on Phonemic Segmentation Fluency is asymptotic (i.e., most children receive close to the maximum score), with fewer meaningful differences between children. To monitor a child's attainment of early literacy skills, it is necessary to change the measurement material more frequently to more difficult material or to activities measuring higher level skills.

Necessary But Not Sufficient Skills

Finally, DIBELS and CBM differ in that the skills targeted by DIBELS are necessary but not sufficient for important life outcomes, whereas CBM skills are direct measures of important life outcomes. One implication of this difference is that when skills increase when testing on CBM reading over time, for example, it is clear that the student is *reading* better. DIBELS progress monitoring, in contrast, is one step removed from important outcome variables. Early literacy skills such as phonological awareness, print awareness, and letter naming generally are not important tool skills in their own right. Instead, they are transitory, *enabling* skills that facilitate the acquisition of reading, an important tool skill. Early literacy skills appear to be necessary but not sufficient for success in learning to read (Otterstedt, 1993). Even if all early literacy skills have been mastered at an adequate level, literacy need not necessarily follow. Opportunity to learn and effective instruction also are needed. Thus, the use of DIBELS in a Problem-Solving model must be combined with effective reading instruction across grades in order for important reading outcomes to be attained.

In summary, the DIBELS measures were developed to extend the Problem-Solving model to enable educational decisions regarding the acquisition of early literacy skills, with the goal of preventing later reading failure. In developing measurement procedures to operationalize the Problem-Solving model, DIBELS employed many of the same criteria as CBM. However, key differences between DIBELS and CBM necessitate some alterations in procedures for implementing DIBELS using a Problem-Solving model.

DECISION MAKING WITH DIBELS

DIBELS are used much the same way in the Problem-Solving model as other CBM measures. The five decisions to be made are (1) Problem Identification, (2) Problem Certification or Validation, (3) Exploring Solutions, (4) Evaluating Solutions, and (5) Problem Solution. Because of the differences between CBM and DIBELS in rationale, skills development, materials selection, duration of skills, and relationship to outcomes described earlier, there are some important distinctions in how DIBELS are used in each of the Problem-Solving phases.

Establishing Local Norms

In Problem Identification, Problem Certification, and Problem Solution phases of the Problem-Solving model, comparisons to a local normative context are indicated. In Problem Identification and Problem Certification decisions, the question is whether the student's early literacy skills are substantially below expected level of early literacy skills based on a local normative comparison. In Problem Solution decisions, the question is whether students' skills deficits have been resolved, and their skills are consistent with local normative expectations. In all of these decisions, information is needed on the relative standing of the target student compared to other students in their classroom, school, or district.

Size and Frequency of Norms

The first decision in the establishment of local norms is the size of the unit upon which to base the norms: individual classroom, school building, or school district. In general, it is preferable to establish local norms at the largest unit that is logically defensible and logistically attainable. However, educationally important information is provided with individual classroom norms if that is the only attainable level. Thus, if the school district is supportive of district-level norms, and the district is relatively homogeneous in terms of educational needs and resources, district-level norms are most appropriate. If there are wide disparities in educational needs, resources, or context for specific buildings or clusters of buildings within the district, it may be most appropriate to establish building-level norms.

A second decision to make in the establishment of local norms is the frequency of the norms. Consistent with the recommendation to repeat the Problem Identification phase of the Problem-Solving model three times over the school year, local norms are recommended in the fall, winter, and spring. The final decision in establishing local norms regards the measurement materials to be used. The general guideline is to select materials in which most students will experience some success, but in which most students will have room for improvement. If the measurement materials are so difficult that most students receive a score close to 0, then the local norms will not assist in Problem Identification or Problem Certification decisions. On the other hand, if most students are close to the measure's maximum score, then local norms will not be useful in establishing goals for intervention and evaluating progress. Although the specific choice of measurement materials depends on the local educational context, Table 5.3 provides recommended measures for initial consideration. In general, Onset Recognition Fluency is appropriate in late preschool and the fall and winter of kindergarten, while Phonemic Segmentation Fluency is generally appropriate material for norms established in winter and spring of kindergarten, as well as fall and winter of first grade. However, if the measures are too difficult or easy for a particular setting, an alternative schedule should be developed.

The materials used to monitor a student's progress may not be the same as the measurement materials used to make local normative comparisons. Thus, Onset Recognition Fluency may be most appropriate for monitoring the progress of a student with low phonological awareness skills in spring of kindergarten, but Phonemic Segmentation Fluency may be most appropriate for making normative comparisons.

Local Norming Procedures

The first step in establishing local norms is to assess all of the children in the local normative unit (individual classroom, school building, or school district) using the procedures describe in the Problem Identification data-collection section. For larger normative units such as a school building

TABLE 5.3. Recommended Measures and Times for Establishing Local Norms

Grade	Fall	Winter	Spring
Kindergarten	Onset Recognition Fluency	Phonemic Segmentation Fluency	Phonemic Segmentation Fluency
	Letter-Naming Fluency	Onset Recognition Fluency	Letter-Naming Fluency
		Letter-Naming Fluency	
First grade	Phonemic Segmentation Fluency	Phonemic Segmentation Fluency	Curriculum-Based Measurement Reading
	Letter-Naming Fluency	Curriculum-Based Measurement Reading	

with multiple classrooms or a school district, it is efficacious to enter the scores in a spreadsheet such as Excel. The *sort* function of the spreadsheet can be used to arrange scores in order from largest to smallest. The students with the lowest scores can readily be identified and targeted for intervention. Alternatively, the spreadsheet functions can be used to assign percentile ranks to the scores. An example of the use of the PERCENTRANK( ) function in Excel is illustrated in Figure 5.1. The formula would be entered as typed in Cell C2, then Cell C2 would be copied and pasted to the cells in the C column corresponding to all student scores. A percentile rank of 14, for example, means that the student performed as well or better than 14% of the children in the local normative group. Students performing at the 25th percentile or below might be identified as low performing within the local context.

For smaller normative units such as an individual classroom, entering the scores in a spreadsheet such as Excel is probably overkill. An alterna-

	A	B	C
1	Name	Score	Percentile
2	Gerry	58	= 100*PERCENTRANK(B:B,b2,2)
3	Fitzgerald	58	92
4	Hubert	56	85
5	Alfred	55	78
6	Edwin	53	71
7	Carmen	52	64
8	Oswald	49	57
9	Monica	45	50
10	Ken	43	42
11	Dilbert	29	35
12	Jack	24	28
13	Ned	17	21
14	Betty	14	14
15	Izzy	13	7
16	Laura	12	0

FIGURE 5.1. Example using Excel and the built in PERCENTRANK( ) function to obtain percentile ranks for local norms.

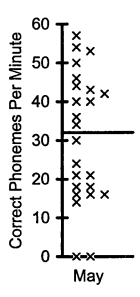

FIGURE 5.2. Example using a paper-and-pencil graph to obtain local normative information.

tive procedure using paper and pencil is illustrated in Figure 5.2. A sheet of graph paper is marked with a scale from 0 to 60 for Phonemic Segmentation Fluency or Onset Recognition Fluency (0 to 90 for Letter-Naming Fluency). An "×" is marked for each student's score, and a line is drawn for the median (middle) score. Using this visual display of the scores, the students whose skills are of concern can be identified. For example, in Figure 5.2, the two students with a score of 0 are discrepant from the expected performance of 32 Correct Segments Per Minute in their classroom.

Problem Identification

For children in kindergarten and first grade, the purpose of Problem Identification with DIBELS is to determine which children differ substantially from their peers in the acquisition of early literacy skills and thus are potentially at risk for difficulty in learning to read. Problem Identification in this context corresponds to the *screening* step in early intervention, a process whereby brief assessment procedures are administered to large numbers of children to identify those who should undergo further, more intensive assessment (Meisels, 1985). The use of DIBELS in a systematic and thorough "screening" process differs from the typical use of CBM in Problem Identification. In CBM, children usually are referred for Problem Identification by teachers. However, because teacher referrals or nominations of early literacy skills problems may be less accurate for phonological awareness skills than for early reading skills, reliance on teachers to initiate referrals may miss children who are at risk for reading problems. By the time teachers have concerns about academic performance and initiate a referral, a serious reading problem may already exist. The focus of intervention then becomes remediation of the existing problem. By screening all children in kindergarten and first grade, those children who are at risk for future reading problems may be identified early, and interventions can focus on *prevention* rather than remediation of problems.

Data Collection

As recommended by Meisels and Provence (1989), the process of early identification should occur on a *recurring* and *periodic* basis. As with screening in early intervention, a one-time measurement using DIBELS provides only a snapshot of the child's early literacy development. By engaging in Problem Identification through ongoing screening, the likelihood of identifying those children who need additional help with early literacy skills is maximized. Therefore, DIBELS should be utilized for Problem Identification by systematically screening all children in kindergarten and first grade at least three times per year (e.g., fall, winter, and spring). During each screening period, kindergarten and first-grade children are administered the DIBELS appropriate for that norming period, as depicted in Table 5.3. For example, during Problem Identification in the fall of kindergarten, children would receive Onset Recognition Fluency and Letter-Naming Fluency probes. During the Winter of first grade, children would receive Letter-Naming Fluency and Phonemic Segmentation Fluency probes. Results of research conducted by Kaminski and Good (1996) indicate that DIBELS administered at a single point in time demonstrate adequate reliability and validity to be used for screening purposes. Thus, a single probe of each measure is sufficient and provides for efficient screening of large groups of children.

DIBELS are individually administered by classroom teachers, teaching assistants/aids, school volunteers, school psychologists, and/or other related services personnel (e.g., speech/language pathologists). Thus, data collection is similar to the collection of CBM reading data. Data collection for Problem Identification is accomplished in a variety of ways, depending on the school and classroom schedules and resources. The screening of a class of 25 kindergarten or first-grade children can be accomplished by a single data collector in approximately 1 ½ hours. Data collection for Problem Identification can be done in one session on a single day or in multiple sessions over the course of a week. If several volunteers are available, data collection for Problem Identification can be accomplished in as little as a half-hour on a single day. As with CBM, training of all data collectors in standardized administration and scoring procedures is essential.

Data Summarization and Decision Making

After the Problem Identification information is collected and organized, those students whose scores are low enough to warrant further assessment are identified. The simplest way to make the decision regarding which students are at risk for reading failure is to use the information collected on the other children as a normative base. As described in the section on local norms, scores for each Problem Identification period are organized by grade level and summarized in tabular and/or graphic form. Based on the normative data and resources available, a cutoff score is established for determining which students to further assess.

As with CBM, cutoff scores can be derived based on percentile rank (Shinn, 1989b). Percentile rank scores are generally easy to understand, are comparable across ages and measures, and can be determined and adjusted based on available data and resources in any given school building or district. For example, in Figure 5.3 the performance of three children on Phonemic Segmentation Fluency in the winter of kindergarten is compared to the average range (25th to 75th percentile) of scores of the nor-

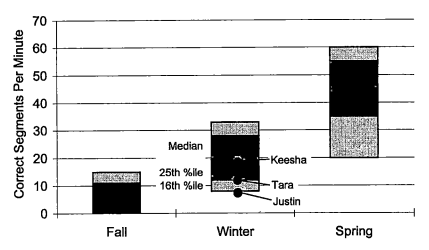

FIGURE 5.3. A comparison of three children's Problem Identification scores to kindergarten winter norms on Phoneme Segmentation Fluency.

mative group. In this figure, the average range of performance on phoneme segmentation in the winter of kindergarten is from 12 to 28 correct segments per minute. For Problem Identification purposes using a normative cutoff, a decision may be made that any child who falls outside the average range (i.e., below the 25th percentile) would be targeted for further assessment. Using this cutoff criterion, both Justin and Tara would be targeted for further assessment. If fewer instructional resources are available, a decision could be made to identify fewer children. For example, all children whose scores fall below the 16th percentile might be identified. If this criterion were used, only Justin would receive further assessment.

Problem Certification/Validation

In a Problem-Solving model, further assessment is conducted to determine if the problem is severe enough to warrant a "special" intervention program. For students in second through sixth grades, this decision frequently entails determining eligibility for special education. With young children in kindergarten and first grade, identifying a "special" program targeting more intensive instruction in early literacy skills is not necessarily a special education decision. In fact, we argue that in most cases the decision should *not* be a special education eligibility decision. In the Problem Certification/Validation phase, the decision to be made is whether a child's performance is sufficiently discrepant from expectations to warrant a modification in the instructional strategies and/or arrangements in the general education classroom.

Data Collection

In contrast to the Problem Identification phase, which utilizes a *single* sample of data from one point in time for screening purposes, Problem Validation decisions are based on *repeated* samples of child performance over time to obtain stable estimates of skills. During Problem Validation, multiple DIBELS probes are administered over a 5- to 10-day period. Alternate forms of the DIBELS measures that are appropriate for the time of the school year (fall, winter, or spring of kindergarten or first grade) are used. Because measures are repeated over the 5- to 10-day period, the child's Problem Identification and Problem Validation scores are recorded and graphed relative to the appropriate norming sample cutoff score. This use of repeated measures allows for (1) a very reliable estimate of level of performance, (2) an estimate of variability of performance, and (3) an initial indication of the current *slope* of acquisition of early literacy skills.

Data Summarization and Decision Making

A normative context based on local norms again is used to determine when additional services or changes in instruction should be considered. In addition, through visual inspection of the graphed data, an initial indication of slope of progress may be obtained. For example, Problem Identification and Problem Validation data on Phonemic Segmentation Fluency for two children are depicted in Figure 5.4. Both Anna and Jeremy performed below the screening cutoff during Problem Identification, and a decision was made to assess further in a Problem Validation phase. Anna's performance over the 2-week Problem Validation phase indicates a level of performance that is above the cutoff, and some indication that the slope of her progress in Phonemic Segmentation Fluency is positive. Because of her performance, a decision was made not to target Anna for special intervention. In contrast, Jeremy's performance over the 2-week Problem Validation period indicates performance below the cutoff and some indication of lack of adequate progress. For Jeremy, a decision to provide special intervention on phonological awareness skills would be appropriate.

Exploring Solutions

The purpose of Exploring Solutions is to determine goals and instructional strategies that will be utilized for those children targeted for intervention during the Problem Validation phase of the Problem-Solving model. The specific questions to be answered are as follows:

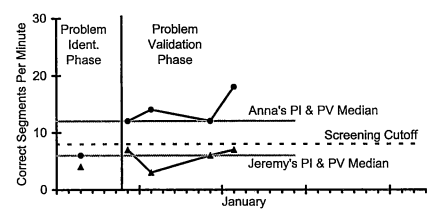

FIGURE 5.4. A comparison of Problem Validation information to cutoff scores for Phonemic Segmentation Fluency.

1. What is the goal of intervention?
2. What is the focus of intervention (i.e., What skills will be taught/learned?)
3. What instructional strategies/arrangements will be used for the intervention?

Intervention Goals

When using CBM in the Problem-Solving model to make special education decisions, the Exploring Solutions phase generally involves the development of long-term statements focused on the ultimate outcome behavior. For example, in reading, this may be a statement of the level of oral reading fluency in the general education reading curriculum in which the child is expected to be reading at the end of 1 year. In contrast, DIBELS goals are shorter term in duration and more directly linked to the ongoing intervention. Goals change periodically throughout the academic year as children master certain skills and move on to higher skills. For example, in the area of phonological awareness, it is expected that Onset Recognition Fluency would be an appropriate goal prior to the middle of kindergarten, and proficiency on Phonemic Segmentation Fluency would be an appropriate goal from the middle of kindergarten to the middle of first grade. After the middle of first grade, oral reading fluency (i.e., CBM) would be the appropriate goal for most children.

Because of the rapid changes in young children's skills and the different goal material used throughout the year, it is recommended that quarterly or biannual goals be developed rather than annual goals. Because limited information exists to suggest appropriate criteria for goals, local normative data may be used as a reference. For example, local normative data might indicate that the typical performance on Phonemic Segmentation Fluency in the spring of kindergarten is 35 phonemes per minute. If a teacher decided that typical kindergarten performance was a reasonable and realistic outcome for a particular child, then 35 phonemes per minute would be the goal for spring of kindergarten.

As always, when developing intervention goals, it is important to balance goal ambitiousness with pragmatic considerations. Although a substantial body of research suggests that ambitious goals relate to greater achievement (Fuchs, Fuchs, & Deno, 1985), it is important that goals not be so difficult as to be unrealistic. Discussing criteria for goals, Fuchs and Shinn (1989) conclude that, with the exception of radically difficult or easy goals, the specific criteria may not be critical as long as systematic measurement is conducted and evaluated with respect to a goal.

Focus of Intervention

With the use of both CBM and DIBELS, it sometimes is necessary to conduct further assessment activities to determine the focus of intervention. Because instructional material can be different from the long-term goal material in CBM, Survey-Level Assessment (SLA) procedures are used to determine the appropriate level of the curriculum for instructional purposes (Howell, 1993; Shinn, Nolet, & Knutson, 1990). In SLA, a student's reading is assessed by having the student read aloud at successively lower levels of the curriculum. The level at which the student should receive instruction is estimated based on instructional placement guidelines (Fuchs & Deno, 1981). See Fuchs and Shinn (1989) for more information. Similar procedures may be used with DIBELS to determine the most appropriate focus of intervention. For example, if a child performs poorly on the Phonemic Segmentation Fluency task, it may be necessary to assess the child's skill in prerequisite phonological awareness skills, such as segmentation of words and syllables or phoneme blending, to determine what phonological awareness skills to teach first.

In CBM, error analysis also may be conducted to determine the appropriate focus of reading interventions. If an error analysis of a child's oral reading indicates consistent errors in specific grapheme/phoneme correspondences, for example, one focus of intervention may be on those specific grapheme/phoneme correspondences. Similarly, if a child performs poorly on phonemic segmentation, error analysis may indicate that the child can segment the initial sounds in words but not the medial or final sounds. The initial focus of intervention then may be on segmentation of final sounds in words. Alternatively, error analysis might indicate that a child can segment single consonants but not blends, in which case the focus of intervention may be on segmenting blends. In either case, error analysis may provide useful information regarding the focus of intervention.

Intervention Strategies/Arrangements

Because DIBELS are used within a problem-prevention model, the interventions considered in kindergarten and first grade are, at least initially, those that may be implemented within the general education classroom. Interventions may be considered as falling along a continuum ranging from broad-based, low-intensity interventions designed to impact the skills of many or all children in the class to high-intensity, individual interventions. The use of low-intensity interventions might include generic modifications of the whole class curriculum. An example of a low-intensity in-

TABLE 5.4. Intervention Options for Early Literacy Skills Ranging from Least Intensive/Intrusive to Most Intensive/Intrusive

	Environmental arrangements	Activity-based intervention	Direct teaching	Individual instruction
Focus	Add Learning Center focused on ELS.	Embed training on ELS within daily teaching activities.	Include instruction of ELS.	Individual instruction on ELS.
Instructional strategies	Increase opportunities throughout day for children to engage in EL activities.	Embed training on ELS within daily teaching activities.	Modify presentation of tasks, prompts, cues, pacing, opportunities to respond, opportunities for practice, error correction procedures.	Modify presentation of tasks, prompts, cues, pacing, opportunities to respond, opportunities for practice, error correction procedures.
Materials	Provide materials for children to engage in EL activities (pictures, flashcards, audiotapes, computers, puppets, games, published materials).	Use materials during daily teaching activities that can facilitate ELS (pictures, flashcards, audiotapes, computers, puppets, games, published materials).	Modify materials used in direct instruction of ELS (pictures, flashcards, audiotapes, computers, puppets, games, published materials).	Modify materials used in individual instruction of ELS (pictures, flashcards, audiotapes, computers, puppets, games, published materials).
Arrangement and setting	Arrange environment to promote ELS (e.g., add bulletin board focused on ELS).	Arrange environment to facilitate teach ELS within daily routine activities.	Modify size of group, composition of group, location.	Modify location, seating arrangements (e.g., floor vs. desk).
Time	Increase/decrease amount of time devoted to ELS.	Increase amount of time devoted to ELS by embedding training on ELS within daily teaching activities.	Increase amount of time, change distribution of time, or change time of day devoted to direct instruction of ELS.	Increase amount of time, change distribution of time, or change time of day devoted to individual instruction of ELS.
Motivational strategies	Modify materials, time, reinforcers, arrangements/settings.	Embed training on ELS within daily teaching activities.	Modify instructional strategies, materials, arrangements/settings, time, reinforcers.	Modify instructional strategies, materials, arrangements/settings, time, reinforcers.

tervention could be as simple as expanding the instructional time for phonological awareness for all children by 10 minutes per day or including a learning center that incorporates phonological awareness games. High-intensity interventions might include small-group or individual, direct teaching of phonological awareness skills using published curricula (e.g., Sound Foundations Program; Byrne & Fielding-Barnsley, 1991).

A list of intervention options along the continuum from least to most intensive/intrusive are depicted in Table 5.4. Ecological arrangements and activity-based interventions are designed to be child centered and nonintrusive with respect to daily routines of children and teachers at school. Direct teaching and individualized instruction provide explicit instruction of specific skills to individuals or small groups of children and are more intrusive. Recommendations for general guidelines to be followed when selecting interventions are adapted from Bailey and Wolery (1992):

1. If child benefit in terms of learning is equal, then less restrictive and less intrusive strategies should be employed.
2. If child benefit in terms of learning is equal, then more child-directed strategies and arrangements are preferred.
3. If child benefit in terms of learning is equal, then parsimonious (simpler/simplest) strategies and arrangements are preferred.
4. The effectiveness (whether children learn) and efficiency (how rapidly and broadly children learn) of instructional procedures and arrangements are more important than their naturalness, their intrusiveness, or their restrictiveness.

It is critical that instructional strategies and arrangements be designed to achieve the desired outcomes, and teachers must repeatedly *evaluate* whether learning of the skills is occurring. Thus, the phases of Exploring Solutions and Evaluating Solutions go hand-in-hand, with decisions made in each phase guiding the procedures implemented in the other.

Evaluating Solutions

A key feature of the Problem-Solving model is that the *outcomes of instruction* drive decision making. In the Evaluating Solutions phase, the primary question is whether the selected interventions are effective in increasing the child's early literacy skills and reducing the discrepancy from expected skills. In the Evaluating Solutions phase, repeated measurements over time are used to monitor the progress of targeted children. When children's progress is adequate, interventions are continued. However, when measurement indicates that child progress in acquisition of early literacy skills is not adequate to meet goals, instructional strategies and arrangements are modified.

Data Collection

In an effort to balance technical and practical considerations, we recommend that DIBELS be administered to at-risk children receiving specialized instruction twice weekly for a period of at least 1 month. Collection of DIBELS data two times per week allows for the collection of approximately 7–9 data points in 1 month. Thus, sufficient time is allowed to evaluate effects of instruction as well as to make further modifications in instruction when necessary. With a longer time frame, teachers run the risk of maintaining ineffective interventions.

Data Summarization and Decision Making

According to Fuchs and Fuchs (1986), use of graphs and data-evaluation rules are related to positive gains in student achievement. We recommend the following procedures be followed for data summarization and decision making with DIBELS:

1. Set an aimline indicating current performance and criteria for success.
2. Establish decision rules for when and how to modify interventions.
3. Graph student scores on an ongoing basis.
4. Use data and decision rules to evaluate effectiveness of interventions.

An aimline is a line on a graph denoting a projected rate of change given intervention based on the child's current performance and goals established during Exploring Solutions. An example of an aimline is depicted in Figure 5.5. In this case, data collected during Problem Identification and Problem Validation provide a baseline, and the goal for the end of kindergarten is 40 segments per minute on Phonemic Segmentation Fluency. An aimline is established by drawing a line connecting the median baseline score (6 correct segments per minute) to the goal of 40 correct segments per minute in June. Student scores are graphed, and performance then can be compared to the aimline to evaluate the effectiveness of the intervention.

Decision rules are used to enable teachers to make decisions about a child's progress toward the goal. When a child's performance falls below the expected rate of progress, changes may be made in the intervention. A

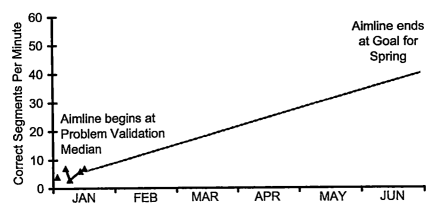

FIGURE 5.5. Establishing an aimline based on current level of performance and desired end-of-year goal.

graph with an aimline for Jeremy is depicted in Figure 5.6. In this example, Jeremy's quarterly goal on Phonemic Segmentation Fluency is 40 segments per minute for the end of kindergarten. As a result of the Problem Validation phase, a decision was made to implement an intervention to improve Jeremy's skills. A vertical line on the graph separates the baseline phase from the intervention phase. By comparing Jeremy's trendline with that of the aimline during the initial intervention, it was decided that the intervention was not effective in enabling Jeremy to meet his goal of 40

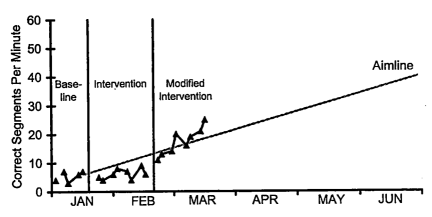

FIGURE 5.6. Modifying interventions to maintain progress consistent with aimline to attain goals.

segments per minute. A change was made in the intervention, and a second vertical line was drawn on the graph to separate the intervention and modified-intervention phases. Data were collected and graphed twice per week during the modified intervention. The modified intervention was determined to be more effective, because Jeremy's progress was judged to be adequate to meet his goal.

Problem Solution

By using DIBELS in the Problem-Solving phases described earlier, it is possible to identify kindergarten and first-grade children who are at risk for the development of reading difficulties and to evaluate the effectiveness of interventions implemented within the general education classroom on a case-by-case basis. The final decision to be made in a Problem-Solving model is whether the interventions have been sufficient to solve the problem and whether the child is no longer at risk of reading failure due to low early literacy skills.

We recommend that periodic reviews of children's performance take place in order to make Problem Solution decisions. Periodic reviews should occur on a trimester or quarterly basis, commensurate with the school grading periods. During the periodic review, the performance of children who are receiving special intervention programs, or whose progress is being monitored, should be reviewed. Essentially, a problem is judged to be solved when there no longer is a discrepancy between the performance of the target child and expectations.

Data Collection and Decision Making

In the Problem Solution phase, both normative and idiographic procedures are used to collect data and make decisions. In the first (normative) procedure, the median of the most recent three to five DIBELS probes is compared to normative expectations and the levels of skills necessary for success in learning to read. For Problem Solution decisions, the most recent three to five data points are used to provide a more reliable estimate of performance than a single data point. It is recommended that the median score be used to minimize the impact of outlying scores. In addition, idiographic data regarding the child's progress and past performance collected during the Evaluating Solutions phase are reviewed and analyzed.

In the Problem Solution phase, one of three conditions may be identified. The first condition is that there no longer is a significant discrepancy between the child's performance and current expectations for performance based on normative data. If a child's performance is commensurate with expectations, the problem would be judged to be "solved," and special intervention strategies may be discontinued. The child's progress and skills would still be monitored, although less frequently, to ensure that his or her performance and progress remains consistent with expectations. In the second condition, a discrepancy remains, but data indicate that the child's current progress is sufficient for the child to meet expectations. In the second condition, the current intervention strategies would be continued, along with the collection of ongoing progress-monitoring data. The third condition is that the child's performance is not commensurate with expectations, and his or her progress is not sufficient to meet expectations. In the third condition the Problem-Solving model would continue with the Exploring Solutions phase.

SUMMARY

In this chapter we have focused on the use of DIBELS in a Problem-Solving model to prevent serious reading problems. We have not addressed referral and eligibility decisions for special education. The decision that a kindergarten or first-grade child has educational needs that are beyond the scope of regular education and should be referred for special education is a complex and difficult one, the discussion of which is beyond the scope of this chapter. Although DIBELS can provide useful information to contribute to a decision for referral to special education, it is important to remember that the DIBELS measures are *indicators*. Just as a thermometer as an indicator of general health would not be the sole measure to diagnose illness and prescribe treatment, to make important educational decisions, additional assessment is necessary. For example, teacher ratings of early literacy and language skills, additional norm-referenced assessments, and/or observational assessment of early literacy skills, as demonstrated during routine classroom activities, may all be used in conjunction with DIBELS for making important educational decisions.

The importance of early identification and intervention with children at risk for development of reading difficulties cannot be overstated. This chapter presented strategies for using Dynamic Indicators of Basic Early Literacy Skills in assessing early literacy skills of kindergarten and first-grade children within a Problem-Solving model of service delivery. DIBELS can be used to identify children who are not making progress in the acquisition of critical early literacy skills and who may benefit from special instructional modifications within the general education classroom. Furthermore, DIBELS can be used in ongoing evaluation of the effectiveness of interventions for individual children. The use of DIBELS within a consistent decision-making framework allows for timely changes in a child's instruction and may facilitate the acquisition of early literacy skills necessary in learning to read and prevent the occurrence of later reading difficulties.

ACKNOWLEDGMENTS

This work was supported in part by U.S. Department of Education grants *Serving Young Children with ADHD: A Management and Prevention Approach* (No. H024P40062), *Training Early Intervention School Psychologists* (No. H029Q30023-95), and *Early Childhood Research Institute on Program Performance Measures: A Growth and Development Approach* (No. H024360010).

REFERENCES

Adams, M. J. (1990). *Beginning to read: Thinking and learning about print.* Cambridge, MA: MIT Press.

Anderson, R. C., Hiebert, E. H., Scott, J. A., & Wilkinson, I. A. G. (1984). *Becoming a nation of readers: The report of the Commission on Reading.* Washington, DC: National Institute of Education.

Blachman, B. A. (1994). What we have learned from longitudinal studies of phonological processing and reading, and some unanswered questions: A response to Torgesen, Wagner, and Rashotte. *Journal of Learning Disabilities, 27,* 287–291.

Bowey, J. A. (1995). Socioeconomic status differences in preschool phonological sensitivity and first-grade reading achievement. *Journal of Educational Psychology, 87,* 476–487.

Byrne, B., & Fielding-Barnsley, R. (1991). *Sound foundations: An introduction to prereading skills.* Sydney, Australia: Peter Leyden Educational.

Byrne, B., & Fielding-Barnsley, R. (1993). Evaluation of a program to teach phonemic awareness to young children: A 1-year follow-up. *Journal of Educational Psychology, 85,* 104–111.

Byrne, B., & Fielding-Barnsley, R. (1995). Evaluation of a program to teach phonemic awareness to young children: A 2- and 3-year follow-up and a new preschool trial. *Journal of Educational Psychology, 87,* 488–503.

Clay, M. M. (1979). *Reading: The patterning of complex behavior.* (2nd ed.). Auckland, New Zealand: Heinemann Educational Books.

Deno, S. L. (1985). Curriculum-based measurement: The emerging alternative. *Exceptional Children, 52,* 217–232.

Deno, S. L. (1986). Formative evaluation of individual student programs: A new role for school psychologists. *School Psychology Review, 14,* 358–374.

Deno, S. L. (1989). Curriculum-Based Measurement and special education services: A fundamental and direct relationship. In M. R. Shinn (Ed.), *Curriculum-based measurement: Assessing special children* (pp. 1–17). New York: Guilford Press.

Deno, S. L. (1990). Individual differences and individual difference: The essential difference of special education. *Journal of Special Education, 24,* 160–173.

Fuchs, L. S., & Deno, S. L. (1981). *A comparison of reading placements based on teacher judgment, standardized testing and curriculum-based assessment* (Research Rep. 56). Minneapolis: University of Minnesota, Institute for Research on Learning Disabilities.

Fuchs, L. S., & Deno, S. L. (1992). Effects of curriculum within curriculum-based measurement. *Exceptional Children, 58,* 232–243.

Fuchs, L. S., & Fuchs, D. (1986). Effects of systematic formative evaluation: A meta-analysis. *Exceptional Children, 53,* 199–208.

Fuchs, L. S., Fuchs, D., & Deno, S. L. (1985). The importance of goal ambitiousness and goal mastery to student achievement. *Exceptional Children, 52,* 63–71.

Fuchs, L. S., & Shinn, M. R. (1989). Writing CBM IEP objectives. In M. R. Shinn (Ed.), *Curriculum-based measurement: Assessing special children* (pp. 130–152). New York: Guilford Press.

Good, R. H., & Kaminski, R. A. (1996). Assessment for instructional decisions: Toward a proactive/prevention model of decision making for early literacy skills. *School Psychology Quarterly, 11*(4), 1–11.

Howell, K. W., Fox, S. L., & Morehead, M. K. (1993). *Curriculum-based evaluation: Teaching and decision making.* Pacific Grove, CA: Brooks/Cole.

Iverson, S., & Tunmer, W. E. (1993). Phonological processing skills and the reading recovery program. *Journal of Educational Psychology, 85,* 112–126.

Johnston, P., & Allington, R. (1991). Remediation. In R. Barr, M. Kamil, P. Mosenthal, & P. D. Pearson (Eds.), *Handbook of reading research* (Vol. II, pp. 984–1012). New York: Longman.

Jorm, A. F., Share, D. L., Maclean, R., & Matthews, R. (1986). Cognitive factors at school entry predictive of specific reading retardation and general reading backwardness: A research note. *Journal of Child Psychology and Psychiatry, 27,* 45–54.

Juel, C. (1988). Learning to read and write: A longitudinal study of 54 children from first through fourth grades. *Journal of Educational Psychology, 80,* 437–447.

Kaminski, R. A., & Good, R. H. (1996). Toward a technology for assessing basic early literacy skills. *School Psychology Review, 25,* 215–227.

Koehler, K. (1996). *The effect of phonological awareness and letter naming fluency interventions on reading skills of first grade students.* Unpublished Doctoral Dissertation, University of Oregon, Eugene.

Lundberg, I., Frost, J., & Petersen, O. P. (1988). Effects of an extensive program for stimulating phonological awareness in preschool children. *Reading Research Quarterly, 23,* 263–284.

Marston, D. B. (1989). A curriculum-based measurement approach to assessing academic performance: What it is and why do it. In M. R. Shinn (Ed.), *Curriculum-based measurement: Assessing special children* (pp. 18–78). New York: Guilford Press.

Masland, R. L., & Masland, M. W. (1988). *Pre-school prevention of reading failure.* Parkton, MD: York Press.

Meisels, S. J. (1985). *Developmental screening in early childhood: A guide.* Washington, DC: National Association for the Education of Young Children.

Meisels, S. J. (1989, April). High-stakes testing in kindergarten. *Educational Leadership,* pp. 16–22.

Meisels, S. J., & Provence, S. (1989). *Identifying and assessing disabled and developmentally vulnerable young children and their families: Recommended guidelines.* Washington, DC: National Center for Clinical Infant Programs.

Moats, L. C. (1995). The missing foundation in teacher education. *American Educator, 19*(2), 9, 43–51.

O'Connor, R. E., Jenkins, J. R., Leicester, N., & Slocum, T. A. (1993). Teaching phonological awareness to young children with learning disabilities. *Exceptional Children, 59,* 532–546.

Otterstedt, J. R. H. (1993). *The reliability and validity of rhyming and onset recognition tasks as measures of phonological awareness.* Unpublished master's thesis, University of Oregon, Eugene.

Shinn, M. R. (Ed.). (1989a). *Curriculum-based measurement: Assessing special children.* New York: Guilford Press.

Shinn, M. R. (Ed.). (1989b). *Identifying and defining academic problems: CBM screening and eligibility procedures.* In M. R. Shinn (Ed.), *Curriculum-based measurement: Assessing special children* (pp. 90–129). New York: Guilford Press.

Shinn, M. R., & Hubbard, D. D. (1992). Curriculum-based measurement and problem solving assessment: Basic procedures and outcomes. *Focus on Exceptional Children, 24*(5), 1–20.

Shinn, M. R., Nolet, V., & Knutson, N. (1990). Best practices in Curriculum-Based Measurement. In A. Thomas & J. Grimes (Eds.), *Best practices in school psychology—II* (pp. 287–307). Washington, DC: National Association of School Psychologists.

Shinn, M. R., Tindal, G. A., & Spira, D. A. (1987). Special education referrals as an index of teacher tolerance: Are teachers imperfect tests? *Exceptional Children, 54,* 32–40.

Simmons, D. C., Gleason, M. M., Smith, S. B., Baker, S. K., Sprick, M., Thomas, C., Chard, D., Plasencia-Peinado, J., Peinado, R., & Kameenui, E. J. (1995, April). *Applications of phonological awareness research in basal reading programs: Evidence and implications for students with reading disabilities.* Paper presented at the meeting of the American Educational Research Association, San Francisco, CA.

Torgesen, J. K., & Bryant, B. R. (1994). *Phonological awareness training for reading.* Austin, TX: PRO-ED.

Torgesen, J. K., Wagner, R. K., & Rashotte, C. A. (1994). Longitudinal studies of phonological processing and reading. *Journal of Learning Disabilities, 27,* 276–286.

Yopp, H. K. (1995). A test for assessing phonemic awareness in young children. *The Reading Teacher, 49,* 20–29.

CHAPTER 6

◆◆◆

Curriculum-Based Measurement and Its Use in a Problem-Solving Model with Students from Minority Backgrounds

◆

MARK R. SHINN
VICKI L. COLLINS
SUSAN GALLAGHER

Extensive documentation clearly shows that America's schools are failing to meet the academic needs of significant numbers of students. According to the 1992 Education Research Report, one out of every ten 9-year-olds in the United States cannot carry out simple reading tasks. Less than half (41%) of 17-year-olds can find, understand, summarize, and explain relatively complicated information in a test. Nearly one out of every five (18%) 9-year-olds cannot add and subtract two-digit numbers or recognize relationships among coins. The lack of educational skills is reflected in the country's overall rates of literacy. It has been estimated that between 21% and 23% of American adults are illiterate (Office of Educational Research and Improvement, 1992) and that the literacy scores of young adults are 11–14 points lower than in 1985.

The consequences of illiteracy are clear. It is associated highly with school dropout rate, unemployment, and crime. High school dropout rates currently are around 30% nationally (Center for the Study of Social Policy, 1991). The effects of school dropout are serious. Students without a high school education have twice the unemployment rate and have experienced a 42% decrease in earning power between 1973 and 1986 in constant 1986 dollars (Carnegie Council on Adolescent Development, 1989). According to figures cited by Adams (1990), it is estimated that 75% of unemployed persons are illiterate. Adams also reports that 60% of prison inmates and 85% of adjudicated youth are functionally illiterate.

For many students from minority backgrounds, the effects of schooling are even less positive than for the nation as a whole. According to The Condition of Education report (Alsalam, Ogle, Rogers, & Smith, 1992), at ages 9, 13, and 17, Black and Hispanic students scored an average of 1⅓ standard deviations below the mean of White students on published reading and math achievement tests. Average science test scores were two standard deviations lower for Black and Hispanic students than for White students.

The mean performance of Black children consistently is reported to be low on every major criterion of academic achievement. On average, they score the lowest on intelligence and achievement tests (Humphreys, 1988) and are more likely to be enrolled in general level or vocational classes than in more academically rigorous classes (Oakes, 1988). About two of every five Black and Hispanic students are at least one grade below their expected grade placement based on their age, more than double the rate for White students (Alsalam et al., 1992). This lack of achievement skills may explain the high illiteracy (40%) and dropout rates among minority youth (Adams, 1990). For example, students from Hispanic backgrounds are almost 2½ times more likely to drop out of school than White students (33% vs. 12.4%) as reported by the Youth Indicators report (Office of Educational Research and Improvement, 1991). School districts with a majority of Hispanic students report dropout rates as high as 50%. In major urban settings, this figure can approach 70% (Arias, 1986).

Unfortunately, it appears that general education is doing little to reduce the achievement gaps between members of the dominant culture and students from minority backgrounds. According to the Trends in Academic Progress report (National Assessment of Educational Progress, 1991), with few exceptions, the gap between White students' skills and those of Black and Hispanic students has not narrowed since 1982. Nine- and 13-year-old students from Hispanic backgrounds read at the same level in 1990 as in 1975. During the last 20 years, Hispanic students have made little progress compared to White students, despite an increase in programs designed to meet their needs.

SPECIAL EDUCATION AS THE "SOLUTION" TO ACHIEVEMENT PROBLEMS

Perhaps the major mechanism used to meet the academic needs of *all* students who are failing to perform within the expectations of general education is special education. Using special education to meet the needs of children with serious academic needs historically has been controversial (e.g., Dunn, 1968) and remains so today. For example, a special investigative report published in *US News and World Report* (Shapiro, Roeb, & Bowermaster, 1993) concluded that "the law (the Individuals with Disabilities Education Act) hurts many of the very children it is intended to help even as it costs taxpayers billions" (p. 46).

The use of special education to meet the needs of students from minority backgrounds is *especially* controversial and equally long standing. The predominant issue regarding special education and students from minority backgrounds has been disproportionality. More students from minority backgrounds are placed in special education, especially in specific categories of disabilities, than would be expected given the proportion of these students in the population at large. For example, Black students are more than twice as likely than White students to be labeled mildly mentally retarded (Reschly & Wilson, 1990).

DISCRIMINATORY ASSESSMENT AS THE "CAUSE" OF DISPROPORTIONAL PLACEMENT

Discriminatory assessment practices—testing practices that in some way are biased toward members of specific cultural groups—have been the most frequently cited reason for disproportionality of minority students in special education. With overrepresentation viewed as problematic and testing practices viewed as the cause, many educators have called for a moratorium on the use of specific types of measures (e.g., intelligence tests) with students from minority backgrounds. Some states (e.g., California, Louisiana) actually have imposed such a moratorium. Numerous others have called for the creation of "unbiased" tests that reflect "true" performance of minority students and thus do not lead to disproportionate placement. A full discussion of discriminatory assessment is beyond the scope of this chapter, but extensive resources are available on this topic. See, for example, Heller, Holtzman, and Messick (1982) and the work of C. Reynolds (1990) and Reschly (1982; Reschly & Grimes, 1990; Reschly, Kicklighter, & McKee, 1988a, 1988b, 1988c).

Despite the attention given to the topic of disproportional placement and discriminatory assessment practices, we have observed few widespread significant changes in assessment practices in the last 10 years with students from minority backgrounds. In the late 1970s and early 1980s Ysseldyke (e.g., Mercer & Ysseldyke, 1977; Ysseldyke & Regan, 1980) described four basic approaches to making tests for minority students less biased: (1) creating new devices that have lower mean score differences between members of different cultural groups, (2) using tests that minimize language to reduce culture bias, (3) test modifications such as translations or limit testing, and (4) dynamic assessment where testing takes a test–teach–test approach. These same approaches are offered today with apparently little change in assessment outcomes.

THESE NEW SOLUTIONS ARE MISGUIDED

Unfortunately, Figueroa (1990) described the first three assessment approaches as problematic. We, too, argue that *all* of these assessment approaches are misguided, because they place their emphasis solely on *identification* of processes and potential disabilities within the student. The primary reason for this type of assessment is to find the *cause* of the student's academic problem and to get that student "eligible for special education."

We find this approach philosophically unsatisfying in that it is not based on the "least dangerous assumption" about the nature of students' learning difficulties. The criterion of the least dangerous assumption maintains that "in the absence of conclusive data, educational decisions should be based on assumptions, which if incorrect, will have the least dangerous effect on the student" (Donnellan, 1984, p. 142).

Traditional assessment practices are based on what we believe to be a most dangerous assumption: that intelligence is a measurable, immutable, internal characteristic that "causes" achievement and, therefore, is critical to special education decision making. We believe this assumption is dangerous, because amelioration of problems would be difficult if intelligence is immutable. Given this assumption, provision of services beyond what is necessary to maintain relative standing would not be recommended, because the services would be unlikely to have any impact. The assumption that the problem locus is within the child (i.e., when intelligence testing drives assessment and decision making) allows schools to ignore the learning environment, including instruction, as a target for assessment and intervention. This assumption leads to the conclusion that students "ability" is the problem, rather than the educational program(s) they receive.

The assumption that intelligence is critical to special education decision making requires that "intelligence" be measured and that students be classified as mentally retarded or learning disabled to receive services to improve their educational outcomes. Measurement of intelligence also can result in classification of a student as a "slow learner," an educationally acceptable euphemism for "not eligible" or not even being "worthy" of help, because the investment of additional assistance will not be repaid in significant student learning. Finally, we believe that intelligence-testing-driven decision making is dangerous in that teachers may reduce their expectations regarding what students can learn and for all classifications emphasize "capacity to learn" as a determinant of ultimate student outcomes.

In addition to an implicit tie to dangerous assumptions about the nature of student learning difficulties, current assessment approaches collectively are inadequate because they lack diagnostic utility and treatment validity—they contribute little to improving instruction. Baker, O'Neil, and Linn (1993) maintain that in order for assessment to improve instruction, the results must be useful diagnostically. This means providing "sufficient detail regarding a student's performance . . . to form hypotheses for the design of an improved program of learning" (p. 1213). Baker et al. propose that improving instruction relies on assessment activities that can be used formatively, "in which revisions in instructional plans and processes" will be made (p. 1213). They conclude that to meet these goals, "information . . . includes performance data of the students and a reasonable description of the characteristics and sequence of the teaching program or the students' opportunity to learn the material" (p. 1213).

Current assessment practices fail to provide this information. The tasks measured are inappropriate because they are "instructionally aloof" (Jitendra & Kameenui, 1993) and contain too few items for sufficient profiling of student skills. The information yielded by the tests "are far removed from classroom tasks, and therefore the generalizability . . . is limited" (p. 14).

A SHIFT IN FOCUS: TOWARD A NEEDS-BASED AND EFFECTIVE-SERVICES SOLUTION

Changes in assessment practices for students from minority backgrounds cannot be based solely on changes in the tests administered. Instead, the changes also must be accompanied by a shift in *why* we are assessing, from assessing *"disabilities"* to assessing *instructional needs* (see Chapter 3 by Good & Jefferson, this volume). This shift requires us to do two important things. First, we must reexamine the issue of biased assessment, leading to overrepresentation of students from minority backgrounds, and identify whether the topic has distracted professionals from assessment efforts that may improve student outcomes. Second, we must identify a viable alternative approach to assessment and decision making that would provide the information we need to improve student outcomes.

Rethinking Overrepresentation

We argue that biased assessment practices leading to overrepresentation of students from minority backgrounds in special education per se are not the *real* problem. Although specific circumstances are of serious concern (e.g., the higher proportion of Black students who are labeled educable mentally retarded), overrepresentation as prima facie evidence of biased testing practices has not been upheld in the courts. Testing practices resulting in overrepresentation were deemed discriminatory *only* when (1) placement decisions were based primarily on ability measures, (2) data showing students were not benefiting from general education were not provided, and (3) data showing students were making progress in special education programs were not provided (Reschly, Kicklighter, & McKee, 1988a, 1988b, 1988c). Assessment practices that have resulted in overrepresentation have been upheld when placement decisions were based on *achievement* data showing that students were not benefiting from general education instructional efforts, and evidence that assessment led to placement in effective programs, as demonstrated by student progress on achievement measures in areas of concern (Reschly, Kicklighter, & McKee, 1988a, 1988b, 1988c).

These findings have established a court directive defining nondiscriminatory assessment as assessment practices that increase the likelihood that children are placed in *effective* programs. From this new perspective, assessment practices that lead to placement of students in ineffective programs would be deemed discriminatory. Therefore, overrepresentation of students from minority backgrounds would be problematic only if they are placed in ineffective programs.

Assessment Alternatives

We argue that a *needs-based,* validated assessment approach is needed to improve special education services for all students, especially those students from minority backgrounds. This assessment system should allow for (1) identification of students with severe academic needs in areas important for success in school and in the community, (2) identification of instructional programs that are likely to meet students' needs, and (3) evaluation of the effectiveness of these instructional programs. Identification must be tied to a needs-based approach—to base decisions about receiving any type of "extra resources" (e.g., Title 1 or special education) only on severe academic deficiencies in the general education classroom. Schools already make decisions based on severe academic deficits in general education curricula and student academic needs (Shinn, Tindal, & Spira, 1987; Shinn, Tindal, Spira, & Marston, 1987). Students who are placed in programs for learning disabilities and educable mental retardation typically perform around the third to fifth percentile in the general education curriculum compared to typical local community students when measured on tasks drawn from that curriculum.

A needs-based approach is based on a less dangerous assumption that severe academic problems are a function of limited opportunities and prior knowledge and/or ineffective previous instruction. From this perspective, student performance would be expected to improve if learning conditions were improved.

Developing and implementing effective programs requires the identification and development of measures consisting of socially important variables that are direct and can be implemented on a frequent and continuous basis. Because academic needs are based on curriculum content, "assessment should be tied to classroom tasks" (Jitendra & Kameenui, 1993, p. 15). Among the most important classroom tasks, especially for those students who historically have received special education, are basic skills or literacy skills. These types of tasks—reading, spelling, written expression, and mathematics computation—are described as cultural imperatives, tasks that are necessary for success in a democratic society and the workplace (M. C. Reynolds, 1988).

Alternative assessment also requires a shift in its purpose, from primarily determining special education eligibility to identifying and validating effective programs for individual students. Assessment results should have *treatment* validity; they should lead to development of interventions that will result in significantly improved student outcomes. Improving the assessment approach also will require a shift to formative evaluation, collecting data on an ongoing basis, so that an intervention's effectiveness can be determined. Formative evaluation is required, because we cannot know in advance what instructional program will work for any *individual* student (Deno, 1986). Therefore, all interventions should be treated as testable hypotheses; data evaluating the efficacy of the program must be collected.

CURRICULUM-BASED MEASUREMENT
AND THE PROBLEM-SOLVING MODEL

As reviewed by Shinn in Chapter 1, this volume, and detailed in a number of articles (e.g., Deno, 1992; Fuchs & Fuchs, 1992) and books (e.g., Shinn, 1989), Curriculum-Based Measurement (CBM) is a series of specific, standardized, short-duration measures of student performance in the basic skills of reading, spelling, written expression, and math computation. The measures function as DIBS, dynamic indicators of basic skills. CBM is used in a Problem-Solving model that meets the standards for a validated, needs-based approach. In brief:

1. CBM and a Problem-Solving model base decisions for additional resources on severity of student academic need in the general ed-

ucation curriculum relative to local achievement expectations (Deno, 1986, 1989; Deno, Marston, & Tindal, 1985)

2. CBM employs measurement tasks that are tied to basic skills and literacy (Deno, 1989; Shinn, 1995).

3. Using CBM formatively results in significantly improved student achievement outcomes when teachers collect student progress data and adjust their instructional programs accordingly (Fuchs, Deno, & Mirkin, 1984; Fuchs & Fuchs, 1986; Fuchs, Fuchs, & Hamlett, 1989; Fuchs, Fuchs, Hamlett, & Allinder, 1991; Fuchs, Fuchs, Hamlett, & Stecker, 1991).

CBM is used in a Problem-Solving model that dictates that specific information is collected for each of five related, but different sequential steps: Problem Identification, Problem Certification, Exploring Solutions, Evaluating Solutions, and Problem Solution. The Problem-Solving model differs from current practice in that one particular type of information, published, norm-referenced test data, is not used for purposes for which it was not developed (e.g., determining instructional plans, monitoring student progress). See Marston (1989), Shinn, Nolet, and Knutson (1990), and Shinn (1995) for more information on this topic. In a Problem-Solving model, data collected during one step of the model may be used to facilitate decision making at subsequent steps. Descriptions of the Problem-Solving model decisions and corresponding CBM procedures are presented in Table 6.1. How CBM is used specifically in the Problem-Solving model with students from minority backgrounds will be detailed later in the chapter.

The need for additional assessment information is determined on a sequential basis. Sometimes assessment activities stop after the first decision (i.e., Problem Identification) if a problem is not validated. Other times, assessment and decision making may occur on a repeated basis, spanning years throughout a student's educational career.

As described by Deno (1989), the Problem-Solving model is predicated on three assumptions. First, a problem is defined as a discrepancy between *what is expected* and *what occurs*. In an academic context, a problem exists when a student does not perform the academic behavior(s) expected of him or her in a particular curriculum. The implication of this definition is that problems are *situational* and may not be the student's "internal problem." A problem in one context may not be a problem in another context.

In addition to defining problems situationally, the Problem-Solving model assumes that within specific environments, there is a subset of students whose discrepancies are so significant that it may be unreasonable for them to achieve satisfactorily with the resources of general education

TABLE 6.1. CBM Problem-Solving Model Decisions, Measurement Activities, and Evaluation Activities

Problem-solving decision	Measurement activities	Evaluation activities	Specific tasks
Problem Identification	Observe and record student differences, if any, between actual and expected performance.	Decide that a performance discrepancy exists.	Peer-Referenced Assessment Conduct.
Problem Certification	Describe the magnitude of differences between actual and expected performance in the context of likelihood of general education alone solving the problem.	Decide if discrepancies are important enough that special services may be required for problem resolution.	Conduct Survey-Level Assessment and identify alternative intervention options.
Exploring Solutions	Determine options for annual goals.	Decide on annual goal(s) and actual content of intervention to be implemented.	Write annual goal based on Survey-Level Assessment; Identify specific skills or strategy deficits.
Evaluating Solutions	Monitor intervention implementation and changes in student performance.	Determine if intervention is effective or should be modified.	Collect progress monitoring data and compare with aimline.
Problem Solution	Observe and record student differences, if any, between actual and expected performance.	Decide if current discrepancies, if any, are not enough and special services may be reduced or eliminated.	Repeat Peer-Referenced Assessment and Survey-Level Assessment.

unless their programs are modified significantly (for more detail, see Deno, 1989). Currently, it remains a value judgment as to when the discrepancy is so severe that special services are warranted, despite repeated attempts to make it quantifiable using a battery of tests and regression formulas. A Problem-Solving model allows the determination of whether additional resources such as special education may be required to help students benefit from their education program to be based on *need*.

The final assumption of the Problem-Solving model is that educators must "generate many possible plans of action prior to attempting problem solution" (Deno, 1989, p. 11) and evaluate the effects of the program actually implemented. Presently, we lack the assessment technology to say with certainty what instructional program will work with any student. We cannot say that Maurice will benefit from special education (or peer tutoring or Title 1) in School A *before* we try it out. Therefore, we need to treat all of our interventions as testable hypotheses that must be evaluated formatively for each individual student. Interventions that show strong positive effects when they are evaluated are maintained; ineffective interventions are discarded and/or modified (Stoner & Green, 1992).

USING CBM IN A PROBLEM-SOLVING MODEL

Two case studies illustrate how CBM is used as dynamic indicators of basic skills (i.e., DIBS) within a needs-based, Problem-Solving model to resolve academic concerns in the areas of mathematics and reading with students from minority backgrounds. The students, Anthony and Dewanna, were in the fifth grade and attended a fairly low-income and ethnically diverse school in a large Rocky Mountain urban school district. The students each have different minority backgrounds and were assessed at different times in the school year from one another. Anthony came from a Hispanic background and was evaluated during fall quarter of the academic year. Dewanna was Black and was evaluated during winter quarter of the same year.

Problem Identification

The first decision of the Problem-Solving model involves collection of data to determine whether a problem warranting further investigation exists. A problem is defined as a discrepancy between expected and actual student performance in the area of concern. When CBM is used within a Problem-Solving model, *expected performance* represents the academic skill level that typical general education students display in typical general education curricula at the time a specific student is referred for a potential problem. This expected skill level is estimated by deriving same-grade local norms that represent students with similar acculturation or learning opportunities. *Actual performance* represents the academic skill level of the referred student in the same material used to generate the local norms. A potential problem exists when a referred student earns a score significantly below the typical performance of same-grade peers. If the referred student's performance is not significantly different from how typical peers perform in typical material, why would one believe a special education problem exists?

The Case of Anthony

For an illustration of the Problem Identification procedures, consider the case of Anthony, a fifth-grade Hispanic student whose low math and reading skills prompted his mother to request that he be tested for special education eligibility. In response to this referral, members of the school's multidisciplinary team (MDT) collected information that allowed them to make a Problem Identification decision. Anthony was evaluated using grade-level CBM math and reading materials. His scores on these measures then were compared to the typical performances of fifth-grade peers. For Problem Identification decisions, these same-grade local norms could have been developed at the classroom, school, or district level. In this instance, the comparison sample was comprised of fifth graders who had been sampled randomly across Anthony's school district at that time of the school year. This norming process took place during the fall, winter, and spring of the school year. For more information on developing local norms for use in the Problem-Solving model, see Habedank (1995) or Shinn (1989).

Anthony was tested over a period of 3 to 5 days using repeated samples of CBM math and reading measures. Repeated measurement of this nature generated a broad sample of Anthony's skills, provided information on the variability of his performance, and reduced the effects of "good" days, "bad" days, and examiner familiarity. For math, Anthony completed three randomly selected math probes derived from the computational objectives of the district's general education fifth-grade math curriculum. He completed one math probe per assessment day. The median number of correct digits (CD) Anthony completed on the math probes (32 CD) was determined and compared to fifth-grade math norms (26 CD). For reading, Anthony read three different randomly selected passages each day from Level 5 of the district's typical general education reading curriculum, *Houghton Mifflin*. The median number of words read correctly (WRC) and errors were determined on each day. Anthony's reading performance during the entire Problem Identification testing was summarized by computing the median of each day's median. This overall median (79 WRC) then was compared to fifth-grade reading norms (115 WRC).

Anthony's Problem Identification scores compared to his fifth-grade peers from the school district's norming sample are presented in Table 6.2. To facilitate decision making among administrators, teachers, and parents, these data are displayed graphically in Figure 6.1. Three types of information are included on the graph: (1) Anthony's daily math scores and median reading scores, represented by the black dots; (2) the median performances of his fifth-grade peers, represented by the heavy dark lines; and (3) the critical value or *cutting score* that Anthony's skills consistently had to

TABLE 6.2. Results of CBM Problem Identification Testing for Anthony, a Fifth Grader

Academic area tested	Day 1	Day 2	Day 3	Overall median	Peer median
Math grade 5 probes					
CD	32	30	35	32 CD	26 CD
Reading grade 5 passages					
WRC Passage 1	77	89	68		
WRC Passage 2	80	85	70		
WRC Passage 3	79	78	75		
WRC daily median	79	85	70	79 WRC	115 WRC

Note. WRC, words read correctly; CD, correct digits.

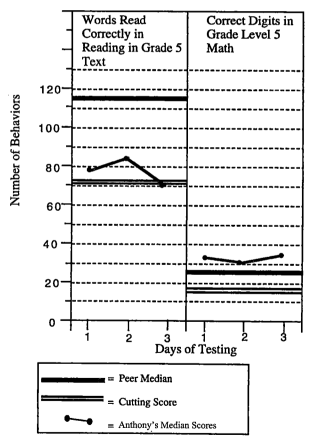

FIGURE 6.1. Results of Anthony's Problem Identification testing in grade 5 reading and math probes, compared to same-grade peers.

fall below to be considered significantly discrepant, represented by the double lines. In this example, the cutting scores were based on the 16th percentile and were the raw scores that corresponded to that rank. In Anthony's district, cutting scores corresponded to the 16th percentile. The cutting scores for math (18 CD) and reading (72 WRC) were based on fall norms, because Anthony was assessed during fall quarter. For more information on determining cutting scores for use in the Problem-Solving model, see Shinn (1989).

To answer the question of whether a significant skills discrepancy warranting further academic assessment exists, one first must compare the referred student's median performances to the cutting scores. If the student's performance is *above* the cutting score, a significant skills discrepancy warranting further academic assessment may not exist. If the student's performance is *below* the cutting score, a problem that may need to be assessed in further detail to be resolved exists. Before reaching this conclusion, however, it is necessary to rule out alternative explanations for the academic skill discrepancy such as hearing, vision, health, school attendance, and behavior.

Anthony's daily math scores consistently were *above* the math cutting score, indicating that a significant math problem was not identified. In fact, Anthony's performance exceeded the typical performance of his fifth-grade peers on these measures. Therefore, a more intensive assessment of his math performance was not warranted. In reading, Anthony's daily medians also were above the cutting score. These results indicate that a significant reading problem was not identified, and further academic assessment to resolve the problem was not warranted. This conclusion does not ignore, however, the obvious finding that all of Anthony's data fell below the *typical* performance of other fifth graders in the district. Because CBM tasks rely on production rather than selection responding, the MDT was able to observe directly Anthony's reading skills. This information facilitated identification of skills deficiencies and strategies that may be contributing to his reading difficulties. Reading characteristics of interest to the MDT included (1) reading accuracy, (2) type of reading errors, (3) self-correction of reading errors, and (4) speed of word recognition. Research has shown that successful and unsuccessful readers differ significantly on these reading characteristics (Golinkoff, 1975–1976). Based on the results of their analysis of Anthony's reading performance, the MDT offered recommendations to Anthony's general education teacher for resolving his reading problem in the general education classroom. For more information on conducting an error analysis for the purpose of intervention planning, see Howell, Fox, and Morehead (1993).

An analysis of the errors Anthony made during reading from the fifth-grade text revealed considerable information about his reading skills.

First, Anthony read with a high degree of accuracy (96%). During the 3 days of testing, he averaged only three errors. Second, Anthony's reading errors seldom changed or interfered with the original meaning of the passages. Most of his errors involved omission of word endings ("ing" and "s") or articles ("a" and "the"). Third, Anthony frequently self-corrected his occasional reading errors, a behavior that suggests he was reading for meaning. Fourth, Anthony read slowly. Slow reading potentially is problematic, because it could prevent students from completing in a timely manner school work that involves reading and can interfere with reading comprehension (Laberge & Samuels, 1974). To improve Anthony's reading rate, it was suggested that he engage in repeated reading activities to supplement his classroom reading instruction (Dahl & Samuels, 1974).

The Case of Dewanna

In Anthony's case, assessment terminated after the Problem Identification decision of the Problem-Solving model. The data collected were sufficient for determining a potential intervention for meeting his educational needs in the general education environment. However, not all problems are resolved by making general education modifications. For an example, consider the case of Dewanna, a fifth-grade Black student, whose difficulties in math and reading prompted her general education teacher to seek assistance from the MDT. The MDT responded to this teacher referral by collecting information that allowed them to make a Problem Identification decision. The procedures used to assess and summarize Dewanna's math and reading skills were identical to those described for Anthony. First, Dewanna's math and reading skills were assessed using typical fifth-grade math and reading material. Second, these results again were compared to the typical math and reading performances of fifth-grade peers comprising the school district's norming sample. Dewanna's Problem Identification scores compared to her same-grade peers are presented in Table 6.3. Again, to facilitate decision making, these data are displayed graphically in Figure 6.2. Included on the graph are (1) Dewanna's daily math scores and median reading scores, (2) the median math and reading performances of her same-grade peers, and (3) the cutting scores for math (26 CD) and reading (93 WRC). Because Dewanna was tested during the winter quarter, the cutting scores were based on winter norms from fifth graders sampled randomly from her school district.

Dewanna's math and reading scores were compared to the math and reading cutting scores to determine whether they differed significantly from fifth-grade expectations to warrant further academic assessment. As shown in Figure 6.2, Dewanna's math scores fell at or below the math cutting score. Moreover, the percentile rank of her median math score (10th

TABLE 6.3. Results of CBM Problem Identification Testing for Dewanna, a Fifth Grader

Academic area tested	Day 1	Day 2	Day 3	Overall median	Peer median
Math grade 5 probes					
CD	26	22	19	22 CD	41 CD
Reading grade 5 passages					
WRC Passage 1	52	43	50		
WRC Passage 2	46	45	49		
WRC Passage 3	43	41	42		
WRC daily median	46	43	49	46 WRC	128 WRC

Note. WRC, words read correctly; CD, correct digits.

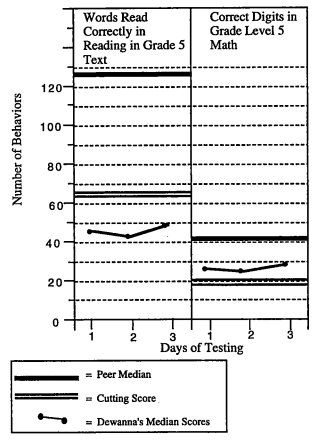

FIGURE 6.2. Results of Dewanna's Problem Identification testing in grade 5 reading and math probes, compared to same-grade peers.

percentile) was below the 16th percentile cutting score. These data indicate that a significant math problem was identified and that additional testing might be necessary to resolve the problem. Similar results were found in reading. All of Dewanna's daily median reading scores fell below the reading cutting score, indicating that a significant reading problem existed. Because no obvious alternative explanations for these skill discrepancies were found, the MDT decided that additional academic testing was necessary to determine the extent of Dewanna's educational needs and that additional resources for resolving her math and reading difficulties should be provided.

Problem Certification

The second decision in a Problem-Solving model involves collecting data to determine the *severity* of the problem. If a problem is of sufficient magnitude, additional resources (e.g., special education) may be necessary to resolve it. A problem is considered serious when a significant discrepancy between what is expected and what occurs is observed at grade level and lower levels of the general education curriculum. To measure this discrepancy and determine problem magnitude, a Survey-Level Assessment (SLA) using CBM is conducted in each academic area in which a problem has been identified. SLA involves testing the student in successive levels of the general education curriculum until a level is found where the student performs successfully. A survey-level *math* assessment involves testing the student on math probes with items selected randomly from each successive grade-level computational objectives. For example, a fifth-grade student would be tested on a fifth-grade computational probe, a fourth-grade computational probe, and so on, until the level of math curriculum in which the student was successful is identified. Dewanna was tested on fifth- and fourth-grade computational probes. A survey-level *reading* assessment involves testing the student on reading passages that were selected randomly from each successive book (or level of text) in the general education reading curriculum. The reading curriculum used in Dewanna's district (*Houghton Mifflin*) had one fifth-grade text, one fourth-grade text, two third-grade texts (3-2, 3-1), two second-grade texts (2-2, 2-1), and two first-grade texts (1-2, 1-1). Dewanna was tested in Levels 5 through 2-1.

Testing in successive levels of the general education curriculum continues until a level is found where the student performs successfully. *Success* can be defined according to (1) instructional placement standards or (2) normative performance. When instructional placement standards are used, success is defined by the "highest level of curriculum where the student meets the instructional placement standards for that level" (Fuchs & Shinn, 1989). To meet instructional placement standards in reading for grades one and two, the student must read 40 to 60 words correctly per minute with four or fewer errors on passages sampled randomly from first- and second-grade texts. To meet instructional placement standards for grades three to six, the student must read 70 to 100 words correctly per minute with six or fewer errors on passages sampled randomly from third-, fourth-, fifth-, or sixth-grade texts.

When normative performance is used, success is defined by the level of curriculum where the student performs within the average range of the local norm at that level. Definitions of "average" vary and should be decided in advance. Two definitions of "average" that have been used include (1) scores that fall between the 25th and 75th percentiles, or (2) scores that fall between the 16th and 84th percentile ranks (plus or minus one standard deviation). The latter definition of average was used in Dewanna's district. Normative Problem Certification decisions typically are based on local normative sample sizes of at least 100 students per grade level to ensure stability and representativeness of the norms.

Dewanna's math and reading SLA scores compared to fifth-, fourth-, third-, and second-grade norms are presented in Table 6.4. To facilitate communication and decision making, these data are displayed graphically in Figures 6.3 (math) and 6.4 (reading). Included on each graph are (1) Dewanna's scores in successive levels of the general education curriculum, as represented by the black dots, and (2) successive grade-level norms, as represented by the boxes.

In math, according to the normative performance definition, Dewanna performed successfully in the computational curriculum for grade 4. Her performance of 37 CD fell within the average range of the grade 4

TABLE 6.4. Results of Problem Certification Testing Using Survey-Level Assessment for Dewanna

Academic area	Curriculum level	Dewanna's median performance	Grade-level peer performance	Dewanna's percentile rank
Math	5	22	41	10th
	4	37	26	75th
Reading	5	46	128	2nd
	4	46	108	4th
	3-2	38	a	a
	3-1	37	90	7th
	2-2	59	a	a
	2-1	79	79	50th

[a]Local norms were developed only from one level of curriculum per grade level. Therefore, no norms are available for these curriculum levels.

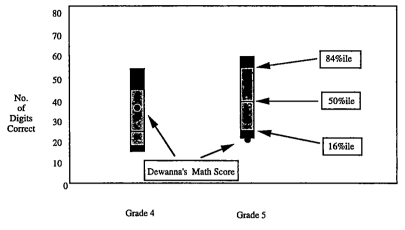

Curriculum Levels and Grade-Level Normative Ranges

FIGURE 6.3. Results of Dewanna's Survey-Level Assessment in math comparing her performance to same- and other-grade general education students.

math norm (75th percentile). In reading, Dewanna performed successfully in Levels 2-2 and 2-1 of *Houghton Mifflin.* Her performance of 59 WRC on Level 2-2 passages fell within the instructional placement standard for grade 2. Her performance of 79 WRC on Level 2-1 passages fell within the average range of the grade 2 reading norm (50th percentile).

Problem Certification decisions are based on student eligibility and need. In Dewanna's district, she could be determined eligible for special education services if her performance in the areas of concern fell below the 16th percentile in material one grade level below (fourth grade) her current grade placement of fifth grade. To determine whether Dewanna needed special education services to benefit from her education, the MDT had to consider whether resources available in general education alone could resolve her problem.

Dewanna's performance on the fourth-grade math probe was *above* the eligibility cutting score and exceeded the typical performance of the grade 4 norm sample. These data indicate that Dewanna would not be considered eligible for special education because of mathematics needs. Again, because CBM math tasks rely on production rather than selection responses, the MDT was able to use the data collected during Problem Identification and Certification to identify math skill and strategy deficits, and develop a general education intervention for resolving her math problem. Dewanna completed many of the math problems from the Problem Identification and Certification assessments inaccurately. She frequently

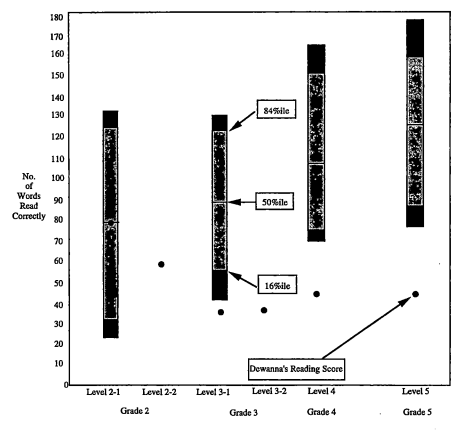

FIGURE 6.4. Results of Dewanna's Survey-Level Assessment in reading comparing her performance to same- and other-grade general education students.

miscounted by 1 on addition problems, and added when she was supposed to subtract and multiply. However, she accurately solved addition, subtraction, and single-digit multiplication problems when only problems of each type were given to her. This outcome indicates that on probes containing mixed problems, Dewanna did not attend to the sign and worked carelessly. Dewanna did not accurately solve multiple-digit multiplication problems, however. To improve Dewanna's math skills, it was suggested that she be taught and given adequate opportunity to practice systematic strategies for (1) self-monitoring the accuracy of her work and (2) solving multiple-digit multiplication problems.

Dewanna's median performance on the fourth-grade reading passages fell below the eligibility cutting score. Thus, she could be found eligible for special education if the MDT decided that general education resources only were insufficient to resolve the reading problem. The MDT considered several sources of information when making this decision. First, they considered the magnitude of Dewanna's reading problem by noting her curriculum discrepancy (i.e., the difference between her expected grade-level material and the curriculum level where she performed successfully). The 2-2 book was the highest level of *Houghton Mifflin* in which Dewanna read successfully. This book was four levels below her expected grade-level material. Second, the MDT examined the type of errors Dewanna made during the reading assessment. Overall, Dewanna read inaccurately (74% correct on fifth-grade passages), made a number of meaning distortion errors (i.e., changed the passage meaning), seldom corrected her reading errors, and read very slowly. Collectively, these reading skills were considered very problematic because they interfered with reading comprehension. Dewanna read more fluently, and made fewer errors as the material became easier. However, she continued to make meaning distortion errors when encountering unfamiliar words. The MDT hypothesized that Dewanna lacked a problem-solving strategy for determining correct pronunciations of unfamiliar words she encountered while reading. To improve Dewanna's reading skills, it was suggested that she be instructed in a level of the curriculum where she could be successful, a recommendation that would not likely be implemented in general education. The MDT also recommended that Dewanna be taught a systematic strategy for decoding unfamiliar words, and that she be given opportunities to practice reading from connected text daily. After considering the magnitude of Dewanna's reading problem and the resources necessary for implementing the recommendations, the MDT decided that Dewanna's reading problem likely would not be resolved using general education resources only, and thus found her eligible for special education with an Individualized Education Plan (IEP) objective needed in reading.

Exploring Solutions

During this third decision in a Problem-Solving model, intervention goals, content, and implementation methods are specified. CBM is most useful for establishing intervention goals. Although not useless for intervention planning, as shown previously, other CBA models (e.g., Curriculum-Based Evaluation; Howell, Fox, & Morehead, 1993) are more suitable for that purpose.

CBM goals are established using data collected during Problem Identification and Certification. These goals provide a basis for evaluating intervention success and are documented in the student's IEP. When CBM is used within a Problem-Solving model, successful interventions are defined as those that result in students becoming more proficient in the general education curriculum over time. Students have become more proficient in the general education curriculum when the curriculum level where they perform successfully at the time of their next review is higher in the curriculum sequence than it was at the time of their previous review, and their curriculum discrepancy is reduced. To facilitate implementation of successful interventions, it is necessary to establish goals that specify clearly the (1) behavior to be measured, (2) conditions for evaluating goal attainment, and (3) criterion for determining intervention success. As shown in Table 6.5, CBM goals are written in a format that contains each of these components.

The goal process begins by identifying the academic area in which the goal is to be written. The dynamic indicator for that content area (i.e., oral reading for reading) becomes the behavior to measure. Because Dewanna required an annual goal in reading, the MDT specified oral reading fluency as the behavioral component of her IEP goal.

TABLE 6.5. Basic Format for CBM Annual IEP Goals in Reading, Math, Written Expression, and Spelling

Academic area	Conditions	Behavior	Criterion
Reading	In *(number of weeks until annual review)*, when given a randomly selected passage from *(level and name of reading series)*,	Student will read aloud	At *(number of words per minute correct/# of errors)*.
Math	In *(number of weeks until annual review)*, when given a randomly selected problem from *(level and name of math series)*, for 2 minutes,	Student will write	*(Number of correct digits)*.
Written expression	In *(number of weeks until annual review)*, when given a story starter or topic sentence and 3 minutes in which to write,	Student will write	A total of *(number of words or letter sequences)*.
Spelling	In *(number of weeks until annual review)*, when dictated randomly selected words from (level and name of spelling series), for 2 minutes,	Student will write	*(Number of correct letter sequences)*.

Note. From Fuchs and Shinn (1989, p. 136). Copyright 1989 by The Guilford Press. Reprinted by permission.

The conditional components of the goal, time frame and evaluation material, are established next. *Time frame* specifies when the goal is expected to be accomplished and is written in units of weeks. In Dewanna's district, IEP goals expire on their anniversary date, 1 year after the goal was written. Thus, Dewanna's annual goal began, *"In 36 weeks (1 academic year). . . ." Evaluation material* refers to the general education curriculum level that the student's performance will be evaluated in at the time of the annual review and is where the student is expected to perform proficiently within a year's time. For a discussion of why long-term goal material is appropriate for evaluating goal attainment, see Fuchs and Deno (1991). For a discussion of general goal-setting procedures, see Fuchs and Shinn (1989). When determining evaluation material, the MDT considers both where in the general education curriculum the student currently performs successfully and where the student will perform within 1 year if the intervention is successful. Dewanna read successfully in Level 2-2 of *Houghton Mifflin*. After checking *Houghton Mifflin*'s scope-and-sequence chart, the MDT identified Level 3-2 as the general education curriculum level where she would be expected to perform proficiently within 1 year if the program is successful. This initial evaluation material was adjusted upward to Level 4, so that Dewanna's curriculum discrepancy would be reduced by two curriculum levels rather than one. With specification of the time frame, evaluation material, and behavior, Dewanna's IEP goal read, *"In 36 weeks, when given a randomly selected passage from Level 4 of* Houghton Mifflin, *Dewanna will read aloud. . . ."*

The final component of the IEP goal, criterion of success, indicates how well the student must perform in the evaluation material in 1 year for the intervention to be considered successful. In Dewanna's case, the MDT had to determine how proficiently they wanted her to read Level 4 material of *Houghton Mifflin*. This criterion of success can be determined using local norm or professional judgment approaches. When local norms are available, the criterion of success can correspond to the performance level of typical peers in the evaluation material. In the winter, typical fourth graders in Dewanna's district read 108 words correctly per minute. In the spring, they improved to 118 words correct per minute. When local norms are not available, criteria of success can be determined using data-based professional judgment. The MDT decides that the student will perform at a higher level of proficiency in the evaluation material in 1 year than he or she did at the time of the initial evaluation. Thus, Dewanna would have to read more than 46 words correctly per minute in Level 4, her performance at the initial review. Because Dewanna's goal is in reading, her criterion of success also could be determined using instructional placement standards. The criterion of success for fourth-grade evaluation material would fall between 70 and 100 words correct per minute.

Local norms were available in Dewanna's district and thus were used to determine her criterion of success. The MDT chose the performance of typical fourth graders during spring. With specification of the time frame, evaluation material, behavior, and criterion of success, Dewanna's IEP goal read, *"In 36 weeks, when given a randomly selected passage from Level 4 of* Houghton Mifflin, *Dewanna will read aloud 118 words correctly per minute with 5 or fewer errors."* The accuracy criterion indicates that Dewanna will read fourth-grade passages with 95% accuracy. This IEP goal will have Dewanna reading as proficiently as end-of-the-year fourth graders during winter quarter of sixth grade. In a years time, her reading performance discrepancy will be decreased from four to two levels below her expected grade-level material.

The IEP components can be graphed to facilitate communication. As shown in Figure 6.5, behavior is recorded on the vertical axis and time frame is recorded on the horizontal axis. The student's initial performance in the evaluation material is plotted at the beginning of the time frame, and the criterion of success is recorded at the end of the time frame. The line connecting these two data points is the expected rate of progress. This aimline represents the amount of improvement per week that the student will need to make in order to meet the criterion of success.

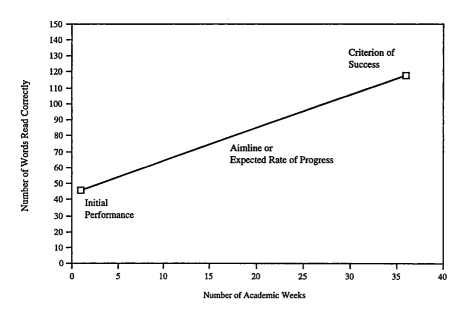

FIGURE 6.5. Graphic display of Dewanna's IEP goal translated into expected rate of student progress.

Evaluating Solutions

The fourth decision in the Problem-Solving model involves collection of data to determine intervention effectiveness. Effective interventions are those that result in students making progress toward meeting or exceeding the criterion of success specified on their IEP graph. When CBM is used within a Problem-Solving model, students are tested once or twice weekly throughout the time frame of their goal on CBM probes selected randomly from their evaluation material (Fuchs, 1989; Fuchs, Hamlett, & Fuchs, 1990). These data are graphed and compared routinely to the student's expected rate of progress. When actual rate of progress exceeds the expected rate of progress, the goal is raised. When actual and expected progress rates are equal, interventions are considered effective and, therefore, maintained. When actual rate of progress falls below the expected progress rate, interventions are considered ineffective and, consequently, modified.

To determine whether Dewanna was making sufficient progress towards her IEP goal in reading, she was tested twice weekly on passages selected randomly from Level 4 of *Houghton Mifflin* over a period of 36 weeks. Dewanna read a different passage each assessment day. To meet the criterion of success in her IEP goal (118 WRC), Dewanna needed to improve her reading rate by 2 words each week. Her actual and expected progress rates were compared after 10 reading samples had been collected, which is the minimum number of data points necessary to calculate a reliable slope (Good & Shinn, 1990). As shown in Phase 1 on Figure 6.6, Dewanna's slope was below the expected rate of progress. This outcome suggests that an instructional change was needed in order for Dewanna to meet her IEP goal.

Evaluating whether intervention suggestions have been implemented as intended is a good place to begin the instructional modification process. Three recommendations for improving Dewanna's reading skills were offered as a result of the Problem Identification and Certification assessments:

1. Provide reading instruction in material where Dewanna is successful.
2. Teach Dewanna a systematic strategy for decoding unfamiliar words.
3. Provide Dewanna with opportunities to practice reading connected text of appropriate difficulty independently.

Suggestions 1 and 2 were addressed adequately. The last suggestion, however, perhaps was not implemented in a beneficial way. Dewanna was giv-

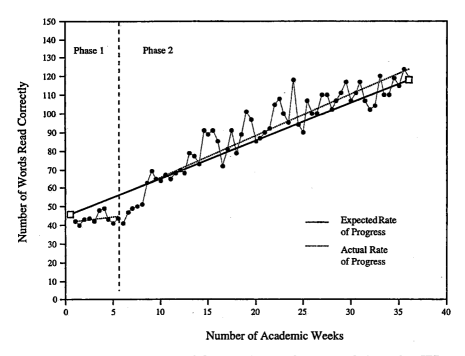

FIGURE 6.6. Graphic display of Dewanna's rate of progess relative to her IEP goal.

en an opportunity to practice reading connected text independently at the end of each week from material of her choosing. The difficulty level of the material was not controlled, nor were the types of words reviewed in the stories. The team hypothesized that the practice opportunities would be more beneficial if (1) they were offered more frequently, and (2) the stories were of appropriate difficulty and contained words that allowed Dewanna to practice the phonetic rules from her instructional lessons. After implementing these instructional modifications for 5 weeks, Dewanna's slope of progress was compared to her expected rate of progress. As shown in Phase 2 of Figure 6.6, Dewanna's rate of progress equaled her expected rate of progress. This outcome continued throughout the remainder of the 36 weeks.

Because the effects of the intervention on Dewanna's performance were evaluated systematically and continuously throughout the IEP time frame, her teacher was able to make data-based decisions about continuing or modifying the intervention. Consequently, an ineffective program was not prolonged, and an effective program was not discarded. Research has shown that increased student achievement occurs when CBM progress-monitoring procedures are used to maintain or modify instructional programs (Fuchs, Deno, & Mirkin, 1984; Fuchs & Fuchs, 1986).

Problem Solution

The fifth decision in the Problem-Solving model involves determining whether a significant academic problem still exists. Several sources of information are used to make this decision, including (1) the student's rate of progress toward the IEP goal, (2) initial peer-referenced data from Problem Identification and Certification, and (3) new peer-referenced data. The most logical times to make Problem Solution decisions are during periodic and annual reviews, which are required by law (Rothstein, 1990).

Periodic Reviews

Determining whether skill discrepancies still exist at the time of periodic reviews involves evaluation of whether students are making *meaningful progress* towards their IEP goal. Students have made meaningful progress toward their IEP goal when their rate of progress is at or above their expected rate of progress *and* their skill discrepancy in typical grade-level material is reduced. The former criterion is determined by evaluating a student's actual rate of progress relative to the aimline, using the procedures described in Evaluating Solutions. The latter criterion is determined by collecting peer-referenced data, using the procedures described in Problem Identification. Skills discrepancies can be evaluated using percentile ranks or discrepancy ratios. When percentiles are used, the skills discrepancy has decreased if the percentile at the periodic review is higher than it was at the initial review. When discrepancy ratios are used, the skills discrepancy has decreased when the discrepancy ratio at the periodic review is lower than it was at the initial review.

A periodic review of Dewanna's performance was conducted approximately 10 weeks after she was certified to receive special education reading support (spring quarter). During the last 5 weeks of this time period, Dewanna's rate of progress approximated her aimline (see Figure 6.6). The importance of this progress was determined by testing Dewanna on three randomly selected passages from typical grade-level material, Level 5 of *Houghton Mifflin*. The summarized scores and percentile ranks from the initial and periodic reviews are summarized in Table 6.6. Although the number of words Dewanna read correctly increased from 46 to 58, her skills discrepancy increased (went from the 2nd percentile at the initial review to the 1st percentile at the periodic review). This periodic review process was repeated during fall quarter of Dewanna's sixth-grade year.

Annual Review

Determining whether skills discrepancies still exist at the time of the annual review is similar to the periodic review, except more comprehensive. The question of whether the student has made meaningful progress toward the IEP goal remains the critical question, yet more data are included in the evaluation. The student's actual rate of progress over the entire IEP time frame is compared to the aimline. Additionally, peer-referenced data are collected at grade level and in subsequently lower levels of the general education curriculum to evaluate whether the skills discrepancy has decreased in magnitude. The SLA procedures described in Problem Certification are used to make the latter decision.

An annual review for Dewanna was conducted during winter quarter of sixth grade. Her rate of reading progress over the entire IEP time frame approximated her aimline, although it was less steep initially. To determine whether the magnitude of Dewanna's reading discrepancy decreased over the time frame of the IEP, a reading SLA was conducted on passages selected randomly from Levels 6 through 2-1 of *Houghton Mifflin*. The results of the SLA are presented in Table 6.6.

Dewanna's skills discrepancy relative to same-grade peers decreased. A year earlier, her reading performance was at the 2nd percentile. At the

TABLE 6.6. Periodic Review Reading Assessment as Part of Problem Solution Decisions for Dewanna in Reading

Level of curriculum	Dewanna's winter median WRC[a]	Dewanna's spring median WRC[b]	Dewanna's fall median WRC[b]	Dewanna's winter median WRC[a]
6	NA	NA	50 (6%ile)	60 (8%ile)
5	46 (2%ile)	58 (1%ile)		80 (10%ile)
4	46 (4%ile)			110 (52%ile)
3-2[c]	38			89
3-1	37 (7%ile)			90 (50%ile)
2-2[c]	59			95
2-1	79 (50%ile)			100 (66%ile)

[a]Based on Survey-Level Assessment.
[b]Peer-Referenced Testing compared to same-grade students only.
[c]Local norms were developed only from one level of curriculum per grade level. Therefore, no norms are available for these curriculum levels.

time of the annual review, it was at the 8th percentile. Dewanna's reading skills relative to peers in subsequently lower levels of *Houghton Mifflin* also improved. Her reading skills were below the normative range for grades 4 and 3 at the initial review but were within the normative range at the annual review. Overall, the magnitude of Dewanna's reading problem decreased considerably. At the time of the annual review, she read successfully in Level 4 of *Houghton Mifflin*, which is two, rather than four, curriculum levels below her expected grade-level material. Because a significant reading problem still existed, the team used the new SLA data to establish new intervention goals for the subsequent year. With the new intervention goal established, the MDT followed the procedures described in Evaluating Solutions and Problem Solution until Dewanna's reading problem was resolved. If the results of Dewanna's periodic and annual reviews had revealed that a significant problem no longer existed, the MDT would have concluded that she no longer needed additional resources to benefit from the reading instruction provided in her general education environment.

SUMMARY

Significant numbers of students from minority backgrounds are failing to acquire the basic academic skills necessary for success in school and life. On the whole, general education efforts to resolve this problem often are not successful, and special education placement is the only alternative. However, special education placement is controversial for reasons of potentially discriminatory assessment practices and limited effectiveness of the services themselves. Assessment practices that place sole emphasis on identification of potential disabilities within the student have contributed to the problem, because they are linked to dangerous assumptions about the nature of student learning difficulties, especially with students from minority backgrounds. Furthermore, current assessment practices do not increase the likelihood that students will be placed and maintained in *effective* programs.

CBM, when used within a needs-based Problem-Solving model, is a viable approach to assessment and decision making that is not tied to dangerous assumptions about the nature of student learning. A Problem-Solving model defines problems situationally. Local norms reflecting community expectations are employed in normative decisions. This local standard allows for issues of acculturation to be incorporated into decision making as any particular student is compared to other students who likely have similar, though not necessarily identical, learning experiences and opportunities.

    CBM with a Problem-Solving model provides consistent and contin-
uous dynamic indicators of basic skills outcomes. Its use in writing goals
and objectives and continuously monitoring student outcomes has been
shown to increase the likelihood that children benefit academically from
their instructional programs. These improved outcomes should be the focus of all educators' activities, especially for those students most at risk for
poorer educational outcomes—students from minority backgrounds.

ACKNOWLEDGMENTS

Sections of this chapter are reprinted from Shinn (1995). Copyright 1995 by the National Association of School Psychologists. Reprinted by permission.

    The development of this chapter also was supported in part by Grant No.
8029D80051-92 from the U.S. Department of Education, Special Education Programs, to provide leadership training in Curriculum-Based Assessment and by Grant
No. H023C10151 from the U.S. Department of Education, Office of Special Education Research, to conduct research in using Curriculum-Based Measurement to facilitate reintegration of students with mild disabilities into general education classrooms.
The views expressed within this chapter are not necessarily those of the U.S. Department of Education.

REFERENCES

Adams, M. J. (1990). *Beginning to read: Thinking and learning about print*. Cambridge,
    MA: MIT Press.
Alsalam, N., Ogle, L. T., Rogers, G. T., & Smith, T. M. (1992). *The condition of edu-
    cation* (NCES 92-096). Washington, DC: U.S. Department of Education, Of-
    fice of Educational Research and Improvement.
Arias, M. B. (1986, November). The context of education for Hispanic students:
    An overview. *American Journal of Education*, pp. 26–57.
Baker, E. L., O'Neil, H. F. Jr., & Linn, R. L. (1993). Policy and validity prospects
    for performance-based assessment. *American Psychologist, 48*(12), 1210–1218.
Carnegie Council on Adolescent Development. (1989). *Turning points: Preparing
    American youth for the 21st century: The report of the task force on education of young
    adolescents*. New York: Carnegie Corporation.
Center for the Study of Social Policy. (1991). *Kids count data book*. Washington, DC:
    Author.
Dahl, P. R., & Samuels, S. J. (1974). *A mastery based experimental program for teaching
    poor readers high speed word recognition skill*. Unpublished manuscript.
Deno, S. L. (1986). Formative evaluation of individual student programs: A new
    role for school psychologists. *School Psychology Review, 15*, 358–374.
Deno, S. L. (1989). Curriculum-based measurement and alternative special edu-

cation services: A fundamental and direct relationship. In M. R. Shinn (Ed.), *Curriculum-based measurement: Assessing special children* (pp. 1–17). New York: Guilford Press.

Deno, S. L. (1992). The nature and development of curriculum-based measurement. *Preventing School Failure, 36*(2), 5–10.

Deno, S. L., Marston, D., & Tindal, G. (1985). Direct and frequent curriculum-based measurement: An alternative for educational decision making. *Special Services in the Schools, 2,* 5–28.

Donnellan, A. M. (1984). The criterion of the least dangerous assumption. *Behavioral Disorders, 9,* 141–150.

Dunn, L. (1968). Special education for the mentally retarded—Is much of it justifiable? *Exceptional Children, 35,* 5–22.

Figueroa, R. A. (1990). Best practices in assessment of bilingual children. In A. Thomas & J. P. Grimes (Eds.), *Best practices in school psychology II* (pp. 93–106). Washington, DC: National Association of School Psychologists.

Fuchs, L. S. (1989). Evaluating solutions: Monitoring progress and revising intervention plans. In M. R. Shinn (Ed.), *Curriculum-based measurement: Assessing special children* (pp. 155–183). New York: Guilford Press.

Fuchs, L. S., & Deno, S. L. (1991). Paradigmatic distinctions between instructionally relevant measurement models. *Exceptional Children, 57,* 488–500.

Fuchs, L. S., Deno, S. L., & Mirkin, P. (1984). The effects of frequent curriculum based measurement and evaluation on pedagogy, student achievement and student awareness of learning. *American Educational Research Journal, 21,* 449–460.

Fuchs, L. S., & Fuchs, D. (1986). Effects of systematic formative evaluation on student achievement: A meta-analysis. *Exceptional Children, 53,* 199–208.

Fuchs, L. S., & Fuchs, D. (1992). Identifying a measure for monitoring student reading progress. *School Psychology Review, 21*(1), 45–58.

Fuchs, L. S., Fuchs, D., & Hamlett, C. L. (1989). Effects of instrumental use of curriculum-based measurement to enhance instructional programs. *Remedial and Special Education, 10*(2), 43–52.

Fuchs, L. S., Fuchs, D., Hamlett, C. L., & Allinder, R. M. (1991). Effects of expert system advice within curriculum-based measurement on teacher planning and student achievement in spelling. *School Psychology Review, 20*(1), 49–66.

Fuchs, L. S., Fuchs, D., Hamlett, C. L., & Stecker, P. M. (1991). Effects of curriculum-based measurement and consultation on teaching planning and student achievement in mathematics operations. *American Educational Research Journal, 28,* 617–641.

Fuchs, L. S., Hamlett, C. L., & Fuchs, D. (1990). *Monitoring basic skills progress.* Austin, TX: PRO-ED.

Fuchs, L. S., & Shinn, M. R. (1989). Writing CBM IEP objectives. In M. R. Shinn (Ed.), *Curriculum-based measurement: Assessing special children* (pp. 130–152). New York: Guilford.

Golinkoff, R. M. (1975–1976). A comparison of reading comprehension processes in good and poor comprehenders. *Reading Research Quarterly, 11,* 623–659.

Good, R. H. III, & Shinn, M. R. (1990). Forecasting accuracy of slope estimates for reading curriculum-based measurement: Empirical evidence. *Behavioral Assessment, 12,* 1–15.

Habedank, L. K. (1995). Best practices in developing local norms for problem solving in schools. In A. Thomas & J. Grimes (Eds.), *Best practices in school psychology III* (pp. 701–716). Washington, DC: National Association of School Psychologists.

Heller, K. A., Holtzman, W., & Messick, S. (1982). *Placing children in special education: A strategy for equity.* Washington, DC: National Academy Press.

Howell, K. W., Fox, S. L., & Morehead, M. K. (1993). *Curriculum-based evaluation: Teaching and decision making* (2nd ed.). Belmont, CA: Brooks/Cole.

Humphreys, L. G. (1988). Trends in levels of academic achievement of Blacks and other minorities. *Intelligence, 12*(3), 231–260.

Jitendra, A. K., & Kameenui, E. J. (1993). Dynamic assessment as a compensatory assessment approach: A description and analysis. *Remedial and Special Education, 14*(5), 6–18.

Laberge, D., & Samuels, S. J. (1974). Toward a theory of automatic information processing in reading. *Cognitive Psychology, 6,* 293–323.

Marston, D. (1989). Curriculum-based measurement: What is it and why do it? In M. R. Shinn (Ed.), *Curriculum-based measurement: Assessing special children* (pp. 18–78). New York: Guilford Press.

Mercer, J. R., & Ysseldyke, J. E. (1977). Designing diagnostic-intervention programs. In T. Oakland (Ed.), *Psychological and educational assessment of minority children* (pp. 70–90). New York: Brunner/Mazel.

National Assessment of Educational Progress. (1991). *Trends in academic progress: Achievement of American students in science, 1969–1970 to 1990, mathematics, 1973–1990, reading, 1971–1990, writing, 1984–1990, 1991.* Washington, DC: U.S. Department of Education.

Oakes, J. (1988). Tracking: Can schools take a different route? *NEA Today (Issues '88), 6*(6), 41–47.

Office of Educational Research and Improvement of the U.S. Department of Education. (1991). *Youth Indicators.* Washington, DC: U.S. Government Printing Office.

Office of Educational Research and Improvement of the U.S. Department of Education. (1992). *Meeting goal 3: How well are we doing?* (OR 92-3071). Washington, DC: U.S. Government Printing Office.

Reschly, D. J. (1982). Assessing mild retardation: The influence of adaptive behavior, sociocultural status and prospects for nonbiased assessment. In C. Reynolds & T. Gutkin (Eds.), *The handbook of school psychology* (pp. 232–257). New York: Wiley.

Reschly, D. J., & Grimes, J. P. (1990). Best practices in intellectual assessment. In A. Thomas & J. P. Grimes (Eds.), *Best practices in school psychology II* (pp. 425–440). Washington, DC: National Association of School Psychologists.

Reschly, D. J., Kicklighter, R., & McKee, P. (1988a). Recent placement litigation, Part I: Regular education grouping: Comparison of Marshall (1984, 1985) and Hobson (1967, 1969). *School Psychology Review, 17,* 9–21.

Reschly, D. J., Kicklighter, R., & McKee, P. (1988b). Recent placement litigation,

Part II: Minority EMR overrepresentation: Comparison of Larry P. (1979, 1984, 1986) with Marshall (1984, 1985) and S-1 (1986). *School Psychology Review, 17,* 22–49.

Reschly, D. J., Kicklighter, R., & McKee, P. (1988c). Recent placement litigation, Part III: Analysis of differences in Larry P., Marshall, and S-1 and implications for future practices. *School Psychology Review, 17,* 39–50.

Reschly, D. J., & Wilson, M. S. (1990). Cognitive processing versus traditional intelligence: Diagnostic utility, intervention implications, and treatment validity. *School Psychology Review, 19*(4), 443–458.

Reynolds, C. (1990). Test bias in psychological assessment. In T. Gutkin & C.R. Reynolds (Eds.), *The handbook of school psychology* (pp. 487–525). New York: Wiley.

Reynolds, M. C. (1988). Alternative educational delivery systems: Implications for school psychology. In J. Graden, J. Zins, & M. Curtis (Eds.), *Alternative educational delivery systems: Enhancing instructional options for all students* (pp. 555–662). Washington, DC: National Association of School Psychologists.

Rothstein, L. G. (1990). *Special Education Law.* New York: Longman. Library of Congress.

Shapiro, J. P., Loeb, P., & Bowermaster, D. (1993, December 13). Separate and unequal. *US News and World Report, 115,* 46–50.

Shinn, M. R. (1989). Identifying and defining academic problems: CBM screening and eligibility procedures. In M. R. Shinn (Ed.), *Curriculum-based measurement: Assessing special children* (pp. 90–129). New York: Guilford Press.

Shinn, M. R. (1995). Curriculum-Based Measurement and its use in a Problem-Solving model. In A. Thomas & J. Grimes (Ed.), *Best practices in school psychology III* (pp. 547–568). Washington, DC: National Association of School Psychologists.

Shinn, M. R., Nolet, V., & Knutson, N. (1990). Best practices in curriculum-based measurement. In A. Thomas & J. Grimes (Eds.), *Best practices in school psychology II* (pp. 287–308). Washington, DC: National Association of School Psychologists.

Shinn, M. R., Tindal, G., & Spira, D. (1987). Special education referrals as an index of teacher tolerance: Are teachers imperfect tests? *Exceptional Children, 54,* 32–40.

Shinn, M. R., Tindal, G., Spira, D., & Marston, D. (1987). Practice of learning disabilities as social policy. *Learning Disability Quarterly, 10*(1), 17–28.

Stoner, G., & Green, S. K. (1992). Reconsidering the scientist practitioner model for school psychology practice. *School Psychology Review, 21*(1), 155–166.

Ysseldyke, J. E., & Regan, R. (1980). Non-discriminatory assessment: A formative model. *Exceptional Children, 46,* 465–468.

CHAPTER 7

◆◆◆

The Use of Curriculum-Based Measurement with Language-Minority Students

◆

SCOTT K. BAKER
JUDITH PLASENCIA-PEINADO
VIVIAN LEZCANO-LYTLE

This chapter provides a rationale for using Curriculum-Based Measurement (CBM) and a Problem-Solving model with students for whom English is not their native language. Evidence for using CBM to make educational decisions about language-minority students' acquisition of fundamental academic skills is based on (1) studies with bilingual students in the United States who speak Spanish and English, (2) monolingual Spanish-speaking students in Mexico, and (3) three brief case studies illustrating how CBM has been used with language-minority students in school settings. Our focus is primarily on aspects of CBM related to the development of literacy skills, in particular, reading acquisition. We begin by describing important contextual factors that establish a rationale for a chapter on the needs of language-minority students. Then we discuss important issues that characterize the current instructional and assessment climate of language-minority students in the country. We conclude the chapter by presenting three brief case studies demonstrating the use of CBM with language-minority students.

BACKGROUND ON DEMOGRAPHIC AND ACHIEVEMENT FACTORS

Public schools are constantly struggling to adequately meet the needs of language-minority students, who by far are the most rapidly growing segment of the student population. Much of the population increase is accounted for by immigration, which currently is the highest in U.S. history (U.S. Department of Education, National Center for Education Statistics, 1993). During the past decade, for example, immigrants accounted for 39% of the country's population growth (Portales, 1994). Not surprisingly, the majority of immigrants to this country arrive with limited English skills.

Individuals from Spanish-speaking countries (i.e., Hispanics) represent the largest immigrant group in the country (U. S. General Accounting Office, 1993). In addition, after African Americans, the combination of immigrant and U.S.-born Hispanics accounts for the second largest minority group overall. Presently, Hispanics represent about 9% of the total U.S. population. By the year 2020, they are projected to surpass African Americans to become the largest minority group in the country (U.S. Bureau of Census, 1992; Reddy, 1993).

Increases in immigration and higher than average birthrates in many families for whom English is a second language have resulted in more limited-English-proficient (LEP) students in the United States than ever before. LEP students are language-minority students whose learning in the mainstream is adversely affected by their lack of English-language exposure. These students require instructional programs that are sensitive to their language needs. During the past decade, it is estimated that the number of LEP students has increased 26% (U. S. General Accounting Office, 1994).

Spanish-speaking students comprise approximately 78% of the overall language-minority population. The remaining 22% speak many different non-English native languages (U.S. Department of Education, 1993). For example, over 100 native languages are spoken by students in the Los Angeles Unified School District alone (Barber, 1993).

The rapidly growing number of language-minority students is not itself a concern. What is a concern is that many language-minority children fare poorly in U.S. schools and consequently struggle as adults to share in the economic, social, and political opportunities that typically reward those who are successful in school. Many language-minority individuals are unable to reverse the effects of unsuccessful school experiences and consequently live in poverty and on the fringes of society throughout their lives.

The manifestations of unrewarding school experiences for language-minority students are evident in many ways. For example, compared to African American students and White students, Hispanic students leave school earlier, are less likely to complete high school, and are less likely to enter college (Alva & Padilla, 1995; De La Rosa & Carlyle, 1990; Rumberger, 1983, 1995). The school dropout rate for Hispanic students (49%)

is much higher than the dropout rate for White students (23%) or African Americans (37%) (Gersten & Woodward, 1994; U.S. Department of Education, National Center for Education Statistics, 1992, 1993; Rumberger, 1995).

The most publicized and important effect of public school's failure to effectively meet the needs of language-minority students, however, is low academic achievement. For example, Hispanic students achieve substantially below their White counterparts in math, science, reading, and writing (U.S. Department of Education, National Center for Education Statistics, 1992, 1993). The average reading scores for Hispanic 17-year-old students are at about the same level as White 13-year-old students (U.S. Department of Education, National Center for Education Statistics, 1995a; Ornstein & Levine, 1989). In grades 1 through 4, 24.5% of Hispanic students are enrolled below grade level; by grades 11 and 12, the percentage increases to 47.8% (De La Rosa & Carlyle, 1990). The achievement discrepancy between Hispanic and White students has improved little over many decades (Arias, 1986; Fradd & Correa, 1989; Millis, Campbell, & Farstrup, 1993; National Council of La Raza, 1990). In fact, across the nation, there was a decline in average proficiency reading scores from 1992 to 1994 for fourth-grade Hispanic students (U.S. Department of Education, National Center for Education Statistics, 1995b).

COMMON INSTRUCTIONAL APPROACHES WITH LANGUAGE-MINORITY STUDENTS

Since 1968, the Bilingual Education Act has been responsible for ensuring that many language-minority students are provided with instruction that addresses their language needs (Stewner-Manzanares, 1988). However, debate about the effectiveness of bilingual education programs has been waged consistently since 1968 (Baker & de Kanter, 1983; Lam, 1992; Rossell, 1988; Willig, 1985).

The primary goal of programs funded through bilingual education has been to help students acquire the English and academic skills necessary for them to perform successfully in mainstream general education classrooms. For most of the nearly 30 years of bilingual education funding, this goal has been interpreted to mean that students need to become proficient in their native language before receiving instruction in the mainstream.

Whether instruction should be primarily in the student's native language or in English has dominated research with language-minority students (Crawford, 1989; Gersten & Woodward, 1994). However, there is beginning to be a focus on conducting research with language-minority students that looks at effective instructional strategies that cut across language of instruction (Fitzgerald, 1995; Gersten, 1996a).

Instruction in the Native Language

The most common model of bilingual education, Transitional Bilingual Education (TBE), stipulates that students should receive primarily native-language instruction during their first few years of school. Concurrently, they should also receive 30–60 minutes of instruction in English as a Second Language (ESL). The amount of ESL instruction increases gradually until students develop sufficient English-language skills to be transitioned into general education mainstream settings (Gersten & Woodward, 1994).

Wong-Fillmore and Valdez (1985) suggested the rationale for early native-language instruction is strongest in the area of reading. Essentially, Wong-Fillmore and Valdez argued that because students find it easier to read in a language they already know than in one they are learning, native instruction is best. Part of the argument these authors and other have made (e.g., Cummins, 1979, 1984) is that reading skills can be transferred relatively easily from one language to another (Gersten, 1996b). Research is beginning to show, however, that this type of transfer is much more difficult for children than was previously believed (Jiménez, García, & Pearson, 1995; Gersten, 1996). For example, in reading it seems that even proficient readers work hard and deliberately to transfer knowledge from one language to another (Jiménez, García, & Pearson, 1995, 1996). Proficient bilingual readers seem to use a number of specific, deliberate strategies to help them transfer what they know from Spanish into English. For less proficient readers, these problems of transferring knowledge from one language to another may be immense (Gersten, 1996; Jiménez et al. 1995, 1996).

Instruction in English

The strongest contrast to native-language instruction is immersion, in which students receive all, or nearly all, of their instruction in English from the outset. Advocates of an immersion approach to bilingual education invariably point to the success of immersion programs in Canada for support. This approach was well publicized in the 1970s and 1980s (Genesee, 1984; Lambert & Tucker, 1972). The essence of these reports suggests that native English-speaking students acquired a good command of French rapidly during their early school years through an instructional method that used French to teach all academic subject areas.

By necessity, districts have begun to experiment with structured immersion programs, or "sheltered English," as it is sometimes referred to in the United States (Northcutt & Watson, 1986). For example, the large in-flux of Southeast Asian students from many different countries in the 1980s and 1990s have made it extremely difficult for some schools to pro-vide native-language support for all of their eligible students, because so many different language groups are represented. Not only are qualified teachers who speak these languages unavailable, but also in many cases there may be insufficient numbers of students who speak a specific lan-guage to warrant full-time instruction in that language.

Empirical studies of sheltered-English approaches have produced positive results in both elementary schools (Gersten, 1985; Gersten, Tay-lor, Woodward, & White, 1984) and secondary schools (Chamot & O'Mal-ley, 1989). However, because of the lack of native-language instruction, sheltered-English approaches have not been viewed positively in the tradi-tional bilingual education community (Crawford, 1989; Mackey, 1978).

Effective Instructional Strategies across Languages

It may be that the actual type of program used with language-minority students is not as critical to academic success as the quality of the instruc-tional practices within a given program. A combination of instructional practices that have been documented to be effective with native English-speaking students and specialized instructional practices that are sensitive to the unique circumstances of language-minority students may produce the most positive results. Educators have begun to identify high-quality in-structional practices with language-minority students that cut across issues related to the language of instruction (Gersten, 1996a).

For example, Fitzgerald (1995) recently completed an integrative re-view of research on the cognitive reading strategies of students who are learning ESL. Fitzgerald investigated studies addressing a range of issues, including the relation between vocabulary knowledge and reading perfor-mance, the word recognition and metacognitive strategies of ESL stu-dents, and the influence of prior knowledge and text structure in facilitat-ing reading comprehension.

Two findings from Fitzgerald's investigation have significant implica-tions for reading instruction with language-minority students and future research with these students. First, there was substantial individual vari-ability among ESL students in their use of vocabulary knowledge and word-recognition strategies to facilitate reading comprehension. Recent research by Jiménez and his colleagues (1995, 1996) has described in vivid detail how more and less successful ESL Hispanic readers used their knowledge of vocabulary in two languages to comprehend text. Second, Fitzgerald found that ESL students used substantively the same cognitive reading strategies as those of native English speakers, but that selected facets of those strategies may be used less or may operate more slowly for ESL students than for native English learners. Fitzgerald's (1995) review suggests that in reading instruction, many practices associated with positive outcomes for native English-speaking students are relevant to language-minority students, but that the unique language circumstances of language-minority students requires an intense and distinct focus on identifying specific instructional practices that are effective with them.

One of the clear advantages of a direct measure of academic skills, such as CBM, is its potential to provide important information regarding the effectiveness of programs to help language-minority students develop the skills they need to be successful in school. In addition to being a direct measure of student academic performance, CBM also has the potential to function as an *intervention* to improve student acquisition of academic skills, and as a *research tool* to help empirically evaluate the effectiveness of different instructional approaches to improve the academic performance of language-minority students.

CBM as a Student Performance Outcome Measure

Improving Assessment Practices

The unique language and cultural circumstances of language-minority students require the use of assessment practices that consider the influence of developing proficiency in a second language on overall academic achievement. For students referred for possible special education placement, for example, this means collecting data that will help a multidisciplinary team (MDT) determine whether academic problems are caused primarily by disabilities or issues involved in learning a second language. Federal law stipulates that the data used to help make decisions about the existence of disabilities must be based on more than one source. Research indicates, however, that even for native English-speaking students, MDTs do not find the data provided in many special education eligibility decisions very helpful. This problem with data credibility is more pronounced for minority students (Marston 1989; Ysseldyke & Thurlow, 1984), especially language-minority students (Gottlieb, Alter, Gottlieb, & Wishner, 1994).

Making decisions about the existence of disabilities is complex. With language-minority students, several factors are important. To reiterate, learning a second language requires determining the degree to which students' academic problems in English are influenced by relatively normal issues of learning a second language versus more chronic learning difficulties. One way educators should address this is by assessing students' academic skills in both languages.

It is also important to understand what influence language factors in the student's home play in facilitating student success in school (Goldenberg, Reese, & Gallimore, 1992). For example, parents of language-minority students may have strong personal beliefs about the school's use of native- or English-language instruction for their children. Also, the extent that English and the student's native language is used in the home has an obvious bearing on the kinds of opportunities students have to practice learning a new language, or improve skills in their native language. The process of collecting meaningful information to address these questions takes time and a very different decision-making model than one that operates from a "child-centered" problem focus.

More and more educators are becoming aware that a "child's problem" is caused and influenced to a high degree by environmental circumstances completely beyond the control or responsibility of the child. School psychologists, in particular, are probably more aware of how extensive these influences are. However, because the tools at their disposal to assess problems (e.g., the Woodcock–Johnson test batteries, Wechsler Intelligence Scale for Children—III) are so limited in scope and time-consuming to administer, they have few opportunities to collect information beyond that which tends to reinforce the perspective that problems operate primarily in the context of a child-centered focus.

Extensive background data collection is especially relevant for the many language-minority immigrant students, for example, who enter U.S. schools with varying degrees of formal educational experiences. An understanding of these experiences, though a time-consuming process, is critical in developing educational programs that address student needs. A student who has attended school sporadically because of the need to support his or her family financially may have very different educational, social, and emotional needs than a student who has attended school sporadically because of growing up in a country divided by civil war. Being able to investigate these factors is critical for some students, and if educators are serious about collecting and understanding this information, more time than is currently available needs to be allocated to expanded data-collection effort.

If the only tools school psychologists use to evaluate the current and potential achievement of language-minority students are a battery of published, norm-referenced reading tests (PNRTs), such as the Woodcock–Johnson (Woodcock, 1981) and the Wechsler Intelligence Scale for Children—Revised (WISC-R; Wechsler, 1974), not only will the data be essentially irrelevant in making many important decisions about students, but also the time and resources available to collect other data relevant to the individual circumstances of the child will likely be minuscule. CBM procedures allow for the collection of meaningful achievement information in a time-efficient manner, and thus fit very well in a data-collection framework designed to construct a comprehensive understanding of the educational needs of language-minority students.

Program Evaluation

CBM data can be used as an important source in evaluating educational programs for language-minority students. For example, CBM reading measures in the early grades can be used to document the range of reading skills for students from different backgrounds and to monitor individual student reading progress. In Figure 7.1, normative English reading fluency scores are presented for all first- and second-grade bilingual students in a rural school district. The figure demonstrates that the reading program in English is resulting in higher reading scores for second-grade students. In grade 1, 61% of bilingual students read between 0 and 10 words correctly on a CBM reading probe. By grade 2, the percentage of students in this range dropped to 18%. This kind of information can be used to keep track of the general success of programs as students move through the grades, and it also allows for a meaningful comparison among students who have similar cultural and language backgrounds. Developing local norms is an important feature of CBM and Problem-Solving Assessment (Shinn, 1988; Habedank, 1995) and may be especially applicable for language-minority students (Shinn & Baker, 1996).

CBM as an Intervention

The use of systematic procedures to monitor student academic progress results in significant achievement gains. Fuchs and Fuchs (1986) conducted a meta-analysis of 21 studies to determine the effects of systematic formative evaluation of educational programs on academic achievement. The use of such procedures resulted in a mean effect size of 0.70. An effect size of 0.70 raises typical achievement outcomes from the 50th to the 76th percentile. As shown in Figure 7.2, the reading progress over time of Miguel and Carmen, two bilingual second-grade students, presents a compelling picture of how CBM can provide clear, formative evaluation data.

CBM as a Research Tool

Finally, CBM data can play an important role in future research with language-minority students. Whether traditional questions are posed concerning language of instruction (i.e., English or the student's native language) and the opportune time for transitioning students into English-

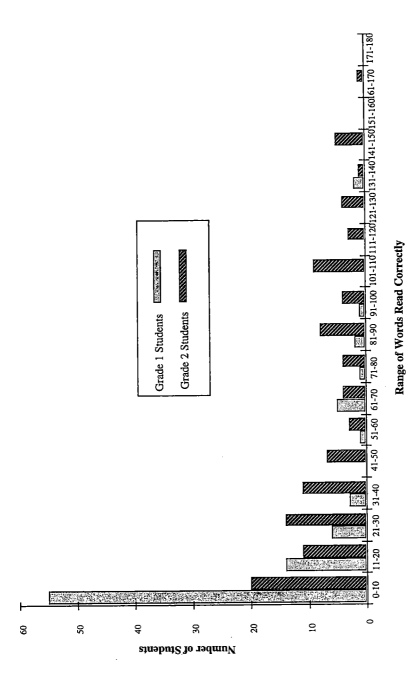

FIGURE 7.1. English reading fluency scores for all first- and second-grade bilingual students in a rural school district.

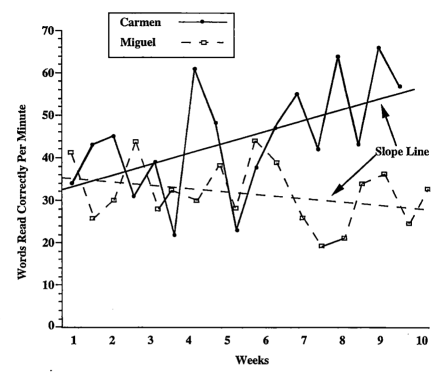

FIGURE 7.2. English reading fluency progress of two bilingual students.

language classrooms, or more contemporary topics are pursued concerning the balance of instructional approaches that will help language-minority students become successful learners, CBM can be used as a dependent measure to help answer these important questions. For example, there is evidence that CBM can be used to evaluate language-minority students' attainment of native and English reading skills (Baker & Good, 1995; Good, Baker, Baker, & Berber, 1990). Goldenberg and Gallimore (1991) have suggested that a well-balanced literacy program for students who are not native English speakers should include early and intense native-language reading instruction. There is some support for using CBM reading data to investigate the effects of native-language reading programs.

More subtle aspects of native- and English-language instruction could be clarified by using CBM as a dependent measure. For example, notions of how easy it is for students to transfer reading skills from one language to another could be investigated by closely examining the relation between the strength of students' native-language skills and the progress made on CBM reading measures (Cummins, 1979; Fuchs, Fuchs, Hamlett, Walz, & Germann, 1993; Jiménez et al., 1995, 1996)

Research on language-minority students is focusing on specific instructional strategies that lead to academic success. Some evidence suggests that differences in reading skills between language-minority and native-English students result from less efficient use of strategic reading strategies by language-minority students. For example, in reviewing research on the cognitive reading strategies, Fitzgerald (1995) found that ESL students used reading strategies less well than native-English students. Studies indicated that ESL students used fewer metacognitive strategies and verbalized metacognitive strategies less, recalled subordinate ideas less well, and monitored comprehension more slowly. The degree to which the effective use of these higher order reading comprehension strategies is influenced by how "automatic" (Laberge & Samuels, 1974) and fluent the reading process has become for students is not clear. In future research, CBM reading-fluency measures may be able to help untangle whether reading strategy differences between language-minority students and native English speakers are due to factors associated with learning two languages simultaneously (Gersten, 1996b), or due to the overall attainment of fundamental reading skills.

Another important research direction is to determine the parameters of literacy growth that can be expected of language-minority students. Educators frequently criticize studies with language-minority students that invariably highlight achievement discrepancies between language-minority students and middle-class White students, without providing insights into solutions or better measures. Research is desperately needed on factors that facilitate the *progress* language-minority students are making on acquiring important academic skills.

Individual and normative indices of academic progress are a strength of CBM data (Fuchs et al., 1993; Hasbrouck & Tindal, 1992; Shinn, 1989). For example, Fuchs et al. (1993) examined aggregated data from many school districts that were using CBM data to monitor the progress of their students and reported average yearly growth indicators in reading fluency, reading maze tasks, spelling, and mathematics computation. In other words, in addition to being able to determine at any fixed point in time how well a student has acquired basic skills compared to other students, by collecting data frequently, individually referenced student growth over time can be monitored.

Future research should investigate typical growth rates for language-minority students. In terms of decision making, the individual progress of a specific language-minority student could be compared to other students of a similar cultural and language background to determine if the student's academic growth appears to be adequate, or if more intensive intervention procedures are necessary to help increase the student's growth.

The issue is not so much that students from diverse language and cultural backgrounds who are referred for services are having academic difficulties—almost invariably they are. The more important question is what can be done to increase the trajectory of their academic progress. Students whose rates of progress can be increased sufficiently will eventually move out of the "at-risk" category, however implicitly or explicitly this category is defined, regardless of where their skills happen to be at any given point in time. One crucial job of educators is to determine what those important skills are and to help students achieve healthy rates of progress as soon as possible.

USING TRADITIONAL ASSESSMENT PROCEDURES TO VALIDATE INSTRUCTIONAL APPROACHES

In contrast to the divergent views about what constitute effective instructional practices for language-minority students, there is a strong consensus that assessment practices have not served these students well. Many problems exist in trying to address the assessment needs of language-minority students. Most solutions merely threaten to reconfirm the usual approach of using published tests to make educational decisions. The tendency has been to search for the "right" test or procedure and to think only cursorily about the purposes behind data collection (Shinn & Baker, 1996).

One of the primary criticisms of assessment practices with language-minority students is that eligibility decisions are premised on distinguishing learning difficulties that are due to insufficient exposure to English from those that are due to difficulty learning (Cummins, 1984; Duran, 1989; Erickson & Walker, 1983; Langdon, 1989; Rueda, 1989). However, by their very nature, published tests, the hallmark of educational assessment practices, are unable to make that difficult distinction. Thus, many language-minority students are identified incorrectly as having mild disabilities and placed in special education programs designed for students with pervasive learning or language problems (Barnes; 1983; Langdon, 1989). Indeed, conditions of overidentification and misidentification of language-minority students have resulted in new assessment problems with language-minority students, namely, a reluctance on the part of schools to refer language-minority students for special services in an effort to *avoid* potential problems associated with inappropriate assessment practices (Gersten & Woodward, 1994). It is clear that a number of popular assessment practices are problematic specifically for language-minority students.

Translating Tests to Assess Students in Their Native Language

A common assessment solution with language-minority students has been to translate English tests such as the WISC-R (Wechsler, 1974) and the Woodcock–Johnson Psychoeducational Assessment Battery (Woodcock, 1981) into other languages (Caterino, 1990; Figueroa, 1990). Educators have long pointed out the numerous problems associated with this practice. Figueroa (1990) summarized these problems by concluding that a "translated test is a mystery test whose scores defy interpretation." Olmedo (1981) demonstrated that one of the most serious difficulties was that "translated items may exhibit psychometric properties substantially different from those of the original English items" (p. 1083). To address these and other problems, the *Standards for Educational and Psychological Testing* (1985) advise that "when a test is translated from one language or dialect to another, its reliability and validity for the uses intended in the linguistic groups to be tested should be established" (p. 75). Establishing the reliability and validity of translated tests is done rarely, if ever (Figueroa, 1990).

Technically, translating tests is extremely difficult, because it is impossible to directly translate many English words and concepts into other languages (Esquival, 1988; Zirkel, 1972). Consequently, not only might the item domains sampled by the two language versions have little overlap, but the psychometric properties that led to the development of the original version might be significantly different in the translated version (Olmedo, 1981; Standards for Educational and Psychological Testing, 1985).

Adjusting Scores to More Accurately Assess Performance

Adjusting student scores on the basis of race, ethnicity, or socioeconomic status (SES) has also been proposed as a means to obtain more accurate and useful assessment information on language-minority students. For example, Mercer (1979) proposed the System of Multicultural Pluralistic Assessment (SOMPA) to determine in a culturally fair way the performance potential of low-income students. The SOMPA modified students' WISC-R scores on the basis of age and sociocultural background to predict student potential. In general, the modified WISC-R scores predict achievement *less* well than traditional WISC-R scores (Figueroa & Sassenrath, 1989). Critics of this procedure also contend that separate norms based on student profiles are very costly to develop, do not provide for important comparisons with the general population, and do not in truth take into account the complexity of cultural identity, despite giving the appearance of doing so (Mercer, 1979; Samuda, 1975).

Comparing Language-Minority Students to Other Students

Obtaining appropriate norms is a critical issue in efforts to compare language-minority students to a representative group. Although many norm-referenced tests in non-English languages exist, they have been standardized on students living in foreign countries, who may or may not know any English at all. Their use with language-minority students in the United States, where the degree of student knowledge of English and the native language may be heavily influenced by their residency in the United States, is highly questionable. To date, no tests have been adequately normed on language-minority students in the United States (Figueroa, 1989).

At least two significant problems limit the possibilities of developing norms that can be used to make valid comparisons with language-minority students. First, language-minority groups in the country differ significantly in factors that would question the validity of comparisons. For example, Hispanic communities in the United States differ dramatically in language dominance, rates of English adoption, public and private language use, SES, attitudes toward education, and history of educational opportunities and achievement (Figueroa, 1990; Kanellos, 1993; Laosa, 1975; Luz Reyes, 1992; Reddy, 1993). These factors affect the validity of developing appropriate norms for single-language minority groups.

In other words, for Hispanics, as for any other linguistic or culturally different group, assessment procedures are needed that are sensitive to the local context of the communities in which they live (Baker & Good, 1995; Habedank, 1995; Shinn, 1988). The second problem in developing useful normative profiles is the difficulty of developing *local norms*, given the current availability of assessment tools. Standard assessment practices that utilize published tests do not represent a realistic option for the development of local norms. A big hurdle is that published tests are too time consuming to administer to a sufficient number of students to generate reliable normative information.

The Importance of a Decision-Making Model

Finally, data provided by published tests are not useful for making many educational decisions (Reschly, 1988; Salvia & Ysseldyke, 1988; Ysseldyke & Thurlow, 1984); that is, different types of tests are needed for making decisions regarding student referral and program eligibility, instructional planning, student progress, and program termination (Reschly, 1988; Shinn, 1995). Consequently, test data frequently play a limited role in the way many decisions are made (García & Pearson, 1994). For example, studies indicate that multidisciplinary teams often disregard assessment data and place students in special education, even when they do not meet formal eligibility criteria (Glaser & Silver, 1994; Marston, 1989).

Educators need information they can collect to make a *range* of educational decisions (Shinn & Baker, 1996). García and Pearson (1994) echoed this perspective when they said that "multiple assessment systems, in which different types of assessments are useful for different purposes, might be the best resolution for some of the daunting problems we face . . . as long as we do not try to adapt [information] to a purpose for which it was never intended" (p. 380). Educators need to carefully consider what data are needed to help make a specific decision, and how to efficiently collect them.

In traditional assessment practices, the tendency is for children referred for evaluation to be administered the same battery of tests, regardless of need, and regardless of the decision to be made. Rather than collecting specific information to make a specific decision, the data are collected first and then used to make numerous decisions (Reschly & Grimes, 1995; Shinn, 1995). The danger of this practice is that data are used for inappropriate purposes, or for purposes for which they are not intended (García & Pearson, 1994; Shinn & Baker, 1996).

CBM WITH LANGUAGE-MINORITY STUDENTS

The long-standing and continuing achievement difficulties of language-minority students have been documented thoroughly. Clearly, educational decision making could be enhanced by direct measures of academic skills indicating the degree to which language-minority students are meeting important learning objectives. These measures could play a powerful role in documenting the degree to which different instructional programs are effective for language-minority students (Deno, 1990).

Evaluating the effectiveness of instructional programs is precisely the role CBM has played best for many years with English-speaking special education students. CBM has the ability to monitor the acquisition of fundamental academic skills in reading, writing, math, and spelling. One of the strongest advantages of CBM is that it can provide critical evidence concerning the effectiveness of instructional programs focusing on the acquisition of essential skills and knowledge. For example, CBM data could be used to offer evidence in the debate between whole-language or phonics by clearly showing how well each type of program leads to the acquisition of important reading-fluency skills during the early years of reading instruction. Published validation studies with CBM have been restricted exclusively to English, however, and the students in these studies have not included language-minority students as a matter of specific focus.

CBM and the Development of Spanish Reading Skills

In bilingual education not only is the acquisition of knowledge and skill an issue, but also the language to which these skills apply. One obvious question concerns the importance of reading fluency as a critical component of reading programs in non-English languages, such as Spanish.

Spanish Oral-Reading Fluency

It may be that the relation between Spanish reading fluency and overall Spanish reading proficiency has a different psychometric relationship than the relation between English reading fluency and overall English reading proficiency. This proposition is tenable, given that the degree of orthographic structure is very different in Spanish and English. Spanish is almost completely phonetic, and English words, especially a high percentage of words used most frequently, have irregular spellings.

To examine the meaning of reading fluency in Spanish, Good et al. (1990) investigated the relation between Spanish reading fluency and overall Spanish reading proficiency with 61 native Spanish-speaking students living in Mexico City. These students read three passages from their fourth-grade classroom reading books, administered according to standard CBM reading procedures (Shinn, 1989). Three criterion measures were used to evaluate student reading comprehension: (1) the Woodcock–Johnson Reading Comprehension (WJRC) subtest (Woodcock, 1981); (2) a short reading comprehension test from the Secretary of Education in Mexico City (SEP); and (3) the classroom teacher ratings of each student's reading skills compared to other students in the same grade.

The intercorrelations among all the measures are reported in Table 7.1. Spanish reading fluency was significantly correlated with all other reading comprehension measures and was consistently the highest in magnitude compared to the other measures. A factor analysis identified one

TABLE 7.1. Correlations among Spanish Reading Measures

	Spanish CBM reading fluency	WJRC subtest	SEP
WJRC subtest	.47**		
SEP	.46**	.32*	
Teacher ratings	.55**	.38**	.30*

Note. Correlations based on $n = 61$ subjects. WJRC, Woodcock–Johnson Reading Comprehension; SEP, reading comprehension test from the Secretaría de Educación Pública.
*$p < 0.05$; **$p < 0.01$.

TABLE 7.2. Factor Loading on Reading Comprehension

Spanish reading comprehension variable	Reading comprehension factor
Spanish CBM reading fluency	.96
WJRC subtest	.50
SEP	.48
Teacher rating	.58

Note. WJRC, Woodcock–Johnson Reading Comprehension; SEP, reading comprehension test from the Secretaría de Educación Pública.

primary factor that best fit the data. This factor was conceptualized as a *global* measure of reading proficiency, because it appeared to be the primary construct each of the measures was attempting to assess. The loadings for each of the measures on this factor are reported in Table 7.2. Spanish reading fluency clearly had the largest loading on the global index of reading proficiency.

The alternate-form reliability of the reading fluency measures was .89, representing a very stable estimate and comparable in magnitude to reported reliability estimates in English. Perhaps most importantly, Spanish reading fluency provided adequate discrimination between levels of student performance allowing a precise statement of relative standing.

Spanish Reading Programs in the United States

Goldenberg and Gallimore (1991) argued that native Spanish reading programs should be an important component of Spanish bilingual programs and that this critical literacy skill had been largely ignored. A school district in the Pacific Northwest was considering the implementation of a Spanish reading program as part of its expanding bilingual education program. The student population was approximately 60% Hispanic, of which a high percentage were native Spanish speakers.

During a 10-week period, 16 second-grade students in the district who could read in both Spanish and English had their reading fluency skills monitored in both languages using CBM administration procedures (Baker & Good, 1995). This information was gathered to explore issues of reading fluency for bilingual students, to collect data on the effectiveness of the English reading program, and to provide some baseline data on Spanish reading fluency. These 16 students were receiving at least 30 minutes of direct English reading instruction per day and no direct Spanish reading instruction. Thus, it was expected that their progress in English reading would surpass their progress in Spanish, providing some evidence for the extent of the effectiveness of the English reading instructional program. In addition, the Spanish reading progress of the 16 students was to serve as a baseline for the implementation of the Spanish reading program that was being considered.

As expected, the reading performance of the 16 students in English was superior to Spanish in both level of performance and rate of progress. The *mean* number of words read correctly (WRC) over the 10 weeks for the 16 students was 90.8 WRC in English and 43.1 WRC in Spanish. The *increase* in the number of WRC per week during the 10 weeks was 1.5 words per week in English and 0.4 in Spanish. The low rate of progress in Spanish was understandable, given that these students were not receiving Spanish reading instruction. The implementation of a Spanish reading program could be used to make a meaningful comparison to conditions prior to implementation. Again, Spanish reading fluency proved to be a very stable measure, with alternate-form reliability estimates averaging 0.96 across the 10 weeks.

These two examples suggest it may be valid to use CBM procedures to assess the reading fluency skills of students in Spanish. Not only might CBM reading data provide important information on the effectiveness of reading instruction, but also the information could help determine when students have developed sufficient native literacy skills to transition into full-time English language classrooms (Shinn, Baker, Habedank, & Good, 1993).

CBM and the Development of English Reading Skills

Perhaps the primary benefit of a direct assessment approach such as CBM with language-minority students is to determine the degree to which students are acquiring English skills, especially important literacy skills such as reading. The majority of these studies documenting the reliability and validity of CBM were conducting with native English-speaking students. Although language-minority students may have been included, the studies did not investigate directly how reliable and valid the measures were with them. If assessment data are going to be used to make decisions about language-minority students, however, then these types of investigations are necessary to establish that the measures are appropriate for use with them (Figueroa, 1989).

Data at the Group Level

Baker and Good (1995) explored whether the reliability and validity of measures of CBM reading fluency in English were as high for second-grade bilingual students (native Spanish speakers) as monolingual English speakers. To ensure that reading growth could be measured accurately during the study, all students had reading fluency scores of at least 20 words per minute in grade-level material. All students in the bilingual group were Hispanic, had at least some proficiency in English and Spanish, and were evaluated by the district for ESL services. Thirty-three of the 50 bilingual students were provided with ESL services.

For 10 weeks, the 50 second-grade bilingual students and 26 students who spoke English only were administered grade-level reading passages twice a week. Students were also administered a battery of criterion measures, including the Stanford Diagnostic Reading Test (SDRT; Karlsen & Gardner, 1985), teacher ratings of reading proficiency, and, for a sample of the bilingual students, the Language Assessment Scales (LAS) in English and Spanish.

Descriptive data on student performance are presented in Table 7.3. The CBM reading fluency measure represents the mean score during the 10-week study. Although performance of the English-only students was higher than the performance of the bilingual students, it is interesting that the difference was not statistically significant. This finding is noteworthy, because most comparisons in reading between Hispanic and White students invariably demonstrate that Hispanic students lag significantly behind their White counterparts (De La Rosa & Carlyle, 1990). On the two criterion measures of reading proficiency, the SDRT and teacher ratings of reading proficiency, the differences between the groups were significant. It may be that when language minority and White students are tested on material sampled directly from the classroom, as was the case with

TABLE 7.3. Mean English Reading Scores by Group

Variables	English-only students			Bilingual students			
	n	Mean	SD	n	Mean	SD	$t(df)$
Reading							
Curriculum-Based Measurement—mean score	26	76.7	34.6	50	69.5	38.9	0.8(56.3)
Stanford Diagnostic Reading Test total score	24	129.2	22.9	19	108.0	16.7	4.4(35.7)**
Teacher rating of reading	26	4.4	1.3	25	3.4	1.8	2.2(43.0)*

Note. Test statistic is the Behrens–Fisher *t*-test for independent groups with unequal sample sizes using Welch's solution for *df*.
*$p < .05$; **$p < .01$.

the students in the Baker and Good (1995) study, student performance differences are less extensive than when the test material includes unfamiliar content.

The reliability of the CBM reading fluency measures is presented in Table 7.4. Point reliability represents an average of 20, 1-week alternate-form reliabilities of adjacent CBM data points. Thus, they represent an estimate of the reliability of a 1-minute CBM reading fluency probe. Split-half reliability was calculated by correlating the mean CBM scores for even and odd data points for all students. The split-half reliability estimates were extremely high for both groups (.99). In addition, a 1-minute measure provides a very stable estimate of reading fluency for both groups: .92 for students in the bilingual group and .87 for students in the English-only group.

Evidence for the validity of the CBM reading fluency measures for the bilingual students is also presented in Table 7.4. Correlations between the CBM reading fluency and (1) the total score on the SDRT, (2) the reading comprehension subtest of the SDRT, and (3) teacher ratings of reading proficiency indicate that correlations were significant for the bilingual group and not significantly different from the students in the English-only group. The most important finding was that the validity coefficients

TABLE 7.4. Reliability and Validity of CBM English Reading Measures by Group

Criterion	English-only students	Bilingual students	Test difference[a]
	Reliability		
Point[a]	.87** (26)	.92** (50)	4.17*
Level[b]	.99** (26)	.99** (50)	0.00
Slope[b,c]	.39 (26)	.49** (50)	1.14
	Convergent construct validity		
Stanford Diagnostic Reading Test—total score[b]	.51* (24)	.53* (19)	0.08
Stanford reading comprehension subtest—pretest[b]	.56** (25)	.73** (21)	0.93
Teacher rating of reading[b]	.82** (26)	.80** (25)	0.20

Note. The number of subjects is reported in parentheses.
[a]Test statistic for reliability coefficient differences is the t-test for independent sample means. The means were derived using Fisher Z transformation.
[b]Test statistic for differences between correlations for CBM reading and criterion reading and language measures is the z-test for independent correlations.
[c]Reliability is based on Spearman–Brown prophecy formula.
*$p < 0.05$; **$p < 0.01$.

ranged from .51 to .82. For the bilingual students, three of the four corre-lations were above .70, indicating a strong relationship between CBM reading fluency and the criterion reading measures. None of the differ-ences in the correlations between students in the bilingual and English-only groups was significant, indicating that the magnitude of the relations between CBM reading fluency and the criterion reading measures was comparable for both groups of students.

The convergent validity evidence for CBM reading fluency was com-parable for bilingual and English-only students and was similar to other technical adequacy studies of CBM reading (Marston, 1989; Shinn, Good, Knutson, Tilly, & Collins, 1992). For example, Shinn et al. (1992) reported correlations between CBM reading and the reading comprehen-sion subtest of the SDRT of .57 to .60 for 114 third-grade students. The convergent validity evidence for CBM English reading for bilingual stu-dents also was within the range of commonly reported correlations be-tween published measures of reading achievement. For example, correla-tions between the SDRT and the reading subtests on the Stanford Achievement Test were reported in the SDRT test manual to range from approximately .60 to .85 (Karlsen & Gardner, 1985).

The Baker and Good (1995) study suggests that the CBM measure of reading fluency may work as well as an overall measure of reading profi-ciency for language-minority students as it does for native English-speak-ing students. If future research continues to support this conclusion, there are important implications for decision making at the group level and at the individual-student level. A valid measure of reading can help educa-tors determine the overall effectiveness of reading programs for groups of students.

Data at the Individual-Student Level

A second way of appreciating what CBM reading data can offer in the context of improving educational programs for language-minority stu-dents can be illustrated in analyzing the data of individual students. Two students in the Baker and Good (1995) study will be used to illustrate this point. Carmen and Miguel were two of the 50 bilingual students whose progress was monitored for 10 weeks. In terms of Spanish-language profi-ciency, both students were rated by the teacher that delivered Spanish na-tive language instruction as 6 on a 7-point scale, with 1 representing *Way below Average*, and 7 representing *Way above Average*. On the Spanish version of the LAS, Carmen scored at Level 3 and Miguel at Level 2, both of which are classified in the LAS manual as limited proficiency. Both Car-men and Miguel could read in Spanish. Thus, in addition to monitoring their reading fluency in English for 10 weeks, their Spanish reading fluency was also monitored. On measures of Spanish reading fluency collected over 10 weeks, Carmen demonstrated a mean score that was nearly two times higher than Miguel's mean score, 86.5 to 47.9.

On overall reading proficiency in English, both students were rated by their teacher as 1 on a scale of 1 to 6, meaning *way below average.* They both received a level rating of 1 on the English version of the LAS, which is interpreted to mean *non-English speaking.* On the SDRT, both Carmen's and Miguel's performance (raw scores = 94 and 97, respectively) performed more than 0.5 standard deviations below other students in the bilingual group (mean = 108; SD = 20.5) and more than 1.5 standard deviations below students in the English-only group (mean = 129.2).

It is also useful to look at the performance of Carmen and Miguel in relation to winter normative information. Reading-fluency data were collected with all second-grade students in the district (n = 236), some of whom had very little English and/or reading skills. The overall reading fluency mean for the second-grade students was 67.5 WRC per minute (SD = 42.2). Carmen's score (38) and Miguel's (33) scores were 0.70 and 0.82 standard deviations below the second-grade winter mean. The mean score for language-minority students in the second grade (n = 109) was 54.5 (SD = 44.2). Thus, Carmen and Miguel's reading fluency scores were 0.37 and 0.49 standard deviations below the mean for other language-minority students.

The multiple sources of information present a converging picture that both Carmen and Miguel had fairly low English academic skills compared to other students in their district. This kind of level information provides a snapshot of Carmen and Miguel's performance at various single points in time. Another very important source of information is the rate of progress students are making over time. With Carmen and Miguel, an examination of their individual progress over time presents a very different picture than does their performance at single points in time compared to other students.

Figure 7.2 shows the rate of growth Carmen and Miguel made during a 10-week period in which their reading fluency progress was monitored two times per week. The graph indicates that Carmen's progress, 2.3 words per week improvement during the 10-week period, was adequate (cf. Fuchs et al., 1993). In contrast, Miguel made no growth and actually *decreased,* at about 0.65 words per week during the 10-week study.

The example in Figure 7.2 is especially relevant, because Carmen and Miguel began the study reading at about the same level on the CBM reading measure, were in the same classroom, and received their reading instruction from the same teacher under highly similar instructional circumstances. In addition, other information collected indicated that these students were similar in other assessment areas, with the exception of

Spanish reading fluency. However, when CBM English reading fluency measures were used to determine reading progress, different conclusion about the effectiveness of the reading program would be drawn for *each* student (Deno, 1990). This picture of *individually referenced* growth over time complicates our understanding of learning by demonstrating that normative information on student performance provides a limited perspective of learning.

The efficiency of CBM data-collection procedures provides realistic opportunities for meaningful data collection from multiple sources. This data-collection possibility is an important point for all students, but it may be especially critical for language-minority students; educators at the minimum should (1) assess native language proficiency, (2) carefully document previous educational experiences, and (3) determine the language and cultural variables in the home that may enhance school–home collaboration to strengthen students opportunities to learn. In addition, data from multiple sources may paint a different picture of student performance than data from only one or two sources.

ILLUSTRATIVE EXAMPLES OF CBM
AND PROBLEM-SOLVING ASSESSMENT
WITH LANGUAGE-MINORITY STUDENTS

Excerpts from three case studies of language-minority students will be presented to illustrate the use of CBM and Problem-Solving Assessment across grades and languages. Although the array of educational decisions in each case was based on many sources of information, only data pertaining to CBM and specific types of educational decisions will be presented.

Problem Identification

During Problem Identification decisions, data are collected to help determine whether a problem is of sufficient magnitude to warrant a comprehensive investigation. Using the Problem-Solving model, a problem is defined as a discrepancy between a student's expected performance and his or her actual performance in the area of concern. *Expected performance* is defined as the level attained by typical general education students in the general education curriculum. *Actual performance* is defined as the level attained by the referred student on the same general education curriculum materials. A problem is considered to be of sufficient magnitude to warrant further assessment when the referred student's skills are significantly below the typical performance of same-grade peers (Shinn & Baker, 1996).

The Case of Su-Rai

Su-Rai's case illustrates the Problem Identification process. Su-Rai, a Cambodian student who spoke Kmai and was learning English as a second language, was referred for special education eligibility by her second-grade teacher. Su-Rai had been in her present school since kindergarten. Su-Rai's teacher had concerns about her listening comprehension, reading, written expression, and math. Su-Rai's parents were concerned that she might not be doing well in school because of her limited English proficiency. At the time of referral, Su-Rai was receiving daily remedial services as well as ESL support services every other day.

Using CBM Problem Identification assessment procedures (Shinn, 1989), Su-Rai was evaluated in reading, writing, and mathematics. Su-Rai's performance on materials selected from the general education curriculum was compared to students who were similar to Su-Rai in many ways. Su-Rai's performance was compared to the performance of 52 Southeast Asian LEP second-grade students in her district whose acculturation (i.e., past experiences, language, length of residence in the United States) was similar to Su-Rai's. The performance of the peer sample on the same tasks served as an index of average performance for LEP students. A discrepancy ratio of 2.0 between Su-Rai's performance and her peer's performance was used as a cutoff, with a cutoff score above 2.0 indicating the need for a comprehensive evaluation to determine eligibility for special education services.

Both Su-Rai and her peers were administered four different types of measures: oral reading fluency, maze, written expression, and mathematics computation probes. Su-Rai was tested on each of the measures for

TABLE 7.5. Results of CBM Problem Identification Testing for Su-Rai and Her Peers

Measure	Su-Rai's median	Peers' median	Su-Rai's discrepancy	Range of peer scores
Oral reading fluency				
Words read correctly	38	42	1.1	17–123
Maze reading				
Correct answers	2	2	1.0	0–7
Written language				
Total words written	18	26	1.4	10–50
Correct writing sequences	14	19.5	1.4	6–45
Second-grade math				
Correct digits	22	25.5	1.2	0–29

three consecutive days to ensure that a representative sample of her behavior in each skill area was collected. Table 7.5 and Figure 7.3 summarize Su-Rai's scores compared to her peers.

The data indicated that Su-Rai's performance in reading, written language, and math was not more than two times discrepant than the performance of other LEP second-grade students in her district. Thus, further assessment for special education services was not conducted.

However, specific recommendations for the general education classroom were made on the basis of the data collected in the Problem Identification process. For example, an analysis of Su-Rai's errors across the dif-

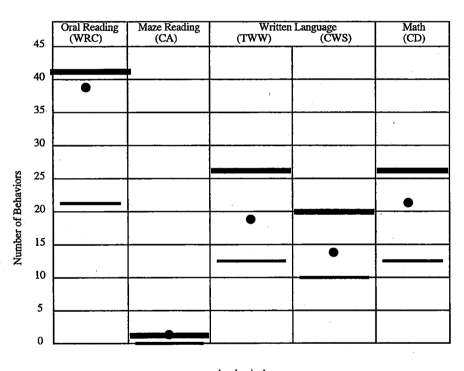

FIGURE 7.3. Su-Rai's Problem Identification data in reading, written expression, and math.

ferent probes administered in reading, written expression, and math was conducted to identify strengths, strategies, and deficiencies that may have been contributing to her academic difficulties. Modifications were made in the instruction she received in the general education classroom. Short-term, weekly objectives related to these modifications were established in reading, writing, and math. A progress-monitoring program was implemented to evaluate the effectiveness of these modifications over time.

Problem Certification

The second decision in the Problem-Solving model is Problem Certification, the focus of which is a comprehensive assessment to determine the severity of the problem. Problems are considered sever if they require additional resources beyond general education (e.g., special education) to adequately address them. Additional resources are typically provided when there is a significant discrepancy between expected and actual behavior at grades below the student's actual grade level. To measure the magnitude of the discrepancy, a procedure called a Survey-Level Assessment (SLA) is conducted. An SLA involves testing the student in successively lower levels of the curriculum until a level is found in which the student performs comparable to peers at that grade (Shinn & Baker, 1996).

Grade-level proficiency can be determined by actually comparing the performance of the referred student to the performance of peers at lower grades or by using instructional placement standards that help determine what typical performance should be in certain academic areas at each grade (Shinn, 1989). Currently, there are commonly identified instructional placement standards in reading at the elementary grades. SLA data can also help to (1) determine appropriate instructional materials, (2) write IEP goals if needed, and (3) analyze the kinds of errors the target student makes in each academic area, for the purpose of developing interventions (Shinn, 1989, 1995).

The Case of José

José's case will exemplify the Problem Certification process. José is a third-grade student who was referred by his general education teacher due to concerns regarding his difficulty with oral expression, reading, spelling, and writing. At the time of referral, José was in a Transitional Bilingual Education Program. According to José's bilingual teacher and his school records, José did not speak English when he entered school in kindergarten. However, by the beginning of second grade, José was found to have near native language proficiency in English. Although José received a higher score in English than Spanish, he continued to be classified as LEP. According to his bilingual education teacher, José was able to express himself better in Spanish than in English, and his general classroom teacher believed he needed much more work developing his English vocabulary.

The first step in José's case, Problem Identification, indicated that his skills in reading and written expression were significantly below (i.e., more than 2.0 times discrepant) the skills of other Hispanic LEP third graders. Thus, Jose moved to the second step, Problem Certification, to determine if the problem was of sufficient severity to warrant additional resources to adequately address them. We will discuss José's SLA data in reading.

Jose's reading was assessed in third-, second-, and first-grade material. One purpose of the data was to determine where in the curriculum José would be appropriately placed for instruction (Gickling & Armstrong, 1978; Taylor, Harris, & Pearson, 1988). One method commonly used to determine the appropriate reading-instruction level is to identify the highest level in first- or second-grade curricula in which the student reads 40–60 words correctly per minute or the highest level in third grade curricula and above in which the student reads 70–100 words correctly (Fuchs & Deno, 1982).

José read three randomly selected passages from each level of his reading curriculum, *Silver Burdett Ginn*, Levels 1 through 3. Table 7.6 and Figure 7.4 present José's SLA scores.

The SLA data indicated that José's current instructional material (Level 3) was too difficult for him. Level 1 was determined to be the best material for instructional purposes because José read between 40–60 words correctly.

The SLA error analysis revealed that José had difficulty reading both regular (e.g., lamp, hot) and irregular (e.g., was, none) words. Furthermore, as the difficulty of the material increased, José appeared to have more severe errors. For example, at Level 1, José used contractions when the word was not a contraction (e.g., *didn't* for *did*, *can't* for *can*). In Level 2, José omitted some words (e.g., who, I, see, lot) and substituted others (e.g., *to* for *look*, *with* for *what*). In Level 3, most of José's errors were more serious omissions

TABLE 7.6. Results of Survey-Level Assessment for José, a Third Grader

Curriculum	Grade level	Words read correctly	Errors
Silver Burdett Ginn	3	27	6
Silver Burdett Ginn	2	31	3
Silver Burdett Ginn	1	49	2

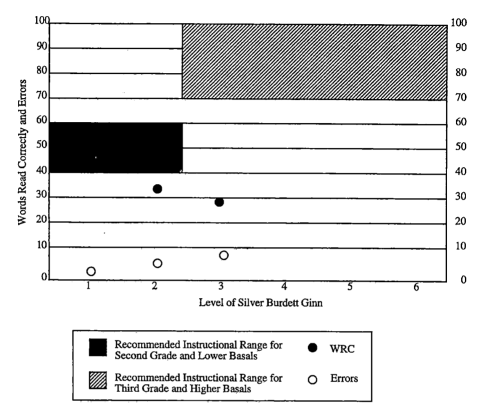

FIGURE 7.4. José's Survey-Level Assessment data in reading.

(e.g., wind, went, said, came). However, when he did attempt to read difficult words, he usually correctly identified the initial and ending sounds.
From the error-analysis data, the examiner concluded that José was still
learning some of the basic sound/letter associations, and that more controlled vocabulary and easier material would allow him to make more
rapid progress in mastering those associations.

Based on the Problem Certification data, the multidisciplinary team
determined that second-language issues could not be ruled out as an explanation for José's academic difficulties. However, the data collected during the assessment provided important information about how to better
plan José's program in the general education classroom to meet his academic needs. The CBM data played an integral part in this planning
process.

Exploring and Evaluating Solutions

The third step of the Problem-Solving model, Exploring Solutions, involves three steps: (1) designing intervention goals; (2) planning "what to teach," that is, the content of the interventions; and (3) specifying "how to teach," that is, determining the methods to be used in the implementation. In the Exploring Solutions step, CBM is very useful and efficient in helping to set clear, measurable goals, because the assessment information collected during Problem Identification and Problem Certification are directly related to this task (Shinn, 1989). The goals established using CBM provide a basis for evaluating whether the interventions are successful.

In the fourth step of the Problem-Solving model, Evaluating Solutions, the effectiveness of the intervention is evaluated. Success is based on whether the student's progress toward the goal has met or exceeded the criterion for success.

Even though the Problem-Solving model includes five "steps" that can be used in sequence to help make a range of related decisions about students, it is possible to use some of these steps in a nonsequential way. Especially in Exploring and Evaluating Solutions, it is possible to implement interventions to increase academic achievement and evaluate the effects of these interventions without having to conduct Problem Identification and Certification decisions. We will use Victor's case to illustrate some of the essential features of Exploring and Evaluating Solutions.

The Case of Victor

Victor is a second-grade student who was referred by his general education teacher because of concerns regarding his academic progress, "work habits," lack of retention, and distractibility. His teachers reported that Victor also had difficulty listening and following directions. Victor's teachers were concerned about his hearing, because his mother reported that he had a history of chronic ear infections. Information from Victor's records indicated that he and his family had lived in the United States for 3 years. Victor entered kindergarten speaking only Spanish. During the time of the assessment, Victor was receiving ESL, Chapter 1, and Migrant Tutorial services.

To determine if Victor was making adequate progress in the general education curriculum, CBM measures in reading and writing were administered. Victor's performance was compared to the performance of Hispanic, LEP, second-grade students in his school on three different occasions.

Victor's and his peers' progress in reading and written expression is summarized in Table 7.7 and Figure 7.5.

In October, there was a significant discrepancy between Victor and his peers in reading (2.6) and written expression (2.4). An Exploring Solutions decision was made using Problem Identification data, and interventions were implemented in Victor's general education classroom. Simultaneously, Victor's progress was monitored to evaluate the effectiveness of the interventions. Although Victor had made some gains by January, he continued to be discrepant from his same-grade peers in both reading and written expression. The interventions in Victor's general education classroom were modified, and by March, when compared to his grade-level peers, Victor had made considerable gains and was no longer significantly discrepant in either reading or written expression. Victor's teachers reported that he was doing much better during classroom instruction. They also reported that Victor had made excellent progress in reading and spelling and that he appeared more sure of himself. Thus, monitoring Victor's academic progress assisted in evaluating the effectiveness of the interventions and making changes in Victor's general education instruction without the need for special education services. In the general education classroom, Victor's progress in reading and writing continued to be monitored.

TABLE 7.7. Results of Exploring and Evaluating Solutions Testing for Victor and His Peers

	October			January			March		
Measure	Victor	Peers	Discrep.	Victor	Peers	Discrep.	Victor	Peers	Discrep.
Reading *SB Ginn*									
WRC	8	21	2.6×	20	43	2.2×	41	63	1.5×
Errors	13	9	1.4×	9	7	1.3×	5	6	1.2×
Reading common passage									
WRC	4	23	5.8×	14	42	3.0×	30	53	1.8×
Errors	16	9	1.8×	13	7	1.9×	8	5	1.6×
Written e×pression									
TWW	5	12	2.4×	10	21	2.1×	16	28	1.8×
CWS	0	6	6.0×	3	9	3.0×	7	14	2.0×

Note. WRC, words read correctly; TWW, total words written; CWS, correct writing sequences.

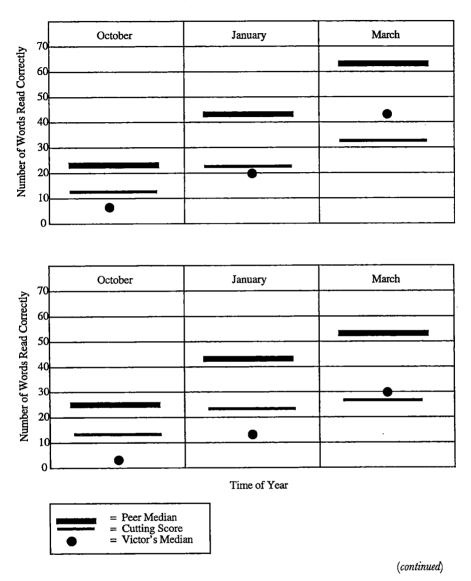

FIGURE 7.5. Victor's progress-monitoring data in reading and written expression.

(*continued*)

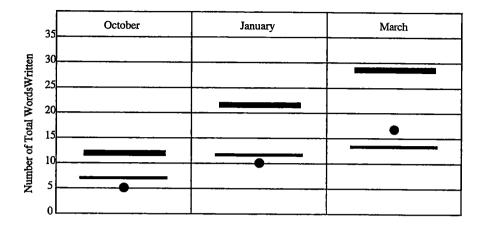

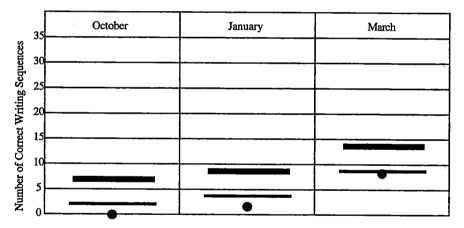

Time of Year

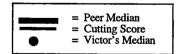
= Peer Median
= Cutting Score
= Victor's Median

FIGURE 7.5. *cont.*

SUMMARY

CBM and its use in a Problem-Solving model has been examined empirically and used in applied settings for 20 years. CBM has been used extensively with students from language minority backgrounds since 1990 (Minnesota Department of Education, 1987). Empirical support for the use of CBM with language-minority students has lagged behind the extensive research with English-speaking students in large part because of the lack of research funds to conduct investigations. However, research support is accumulating (Baker & Good, 1995; Good et al., 1990; Shinn & Baker, 1996), and initial evidence supports the use of CBM and Problem-Solving Assessment with these students.

The limitations of using PNRTs for educational decision making (Marston, 1989) provides a clear rationale for the exploration of alternative assessment practices such as CBM with language-minority students. Given its record of improving achievement outcomes with native English-speaking students, CBM should be at the forefront of this exploration. It is useful to conceptualize the advantages of a direct measure of student performance, such as CBM, with language-minority students in three general ways: (1) first, as a direct measure of student performance for evaluating the effectiveness of individual programs for students, (2) as an intervention to increase learning outcomes because of the benefits associated with greater understanding of teachers and students of student academic growth, and (3) as a dependent measure for evaluating research outcomes that target improving educational practices with language-minority students.

Extensive evidence suggests that language-minority students in the United States are at greater risk for long-term academic problems that many other groups of students. Academic comparisons between language-minority students and native English-speaking students have consistently documented achievement discrepancies that become more severe over time. Also, many language-minority students are recent immigrants to the United States and have attended school sporadically in their native countries. Even in their native language, many of these students have not had the opportunity to develop high levels of literacy, especially in reading and writing. The academic prognosis for many of these students is bleak in the absence of strategic interventions. Finally, the burden of learning two languages simultaneously should not be minimized (Gersten, 1996b), even for language-minority students with strong native-language skills, let alone for students who have low levels of literacy in both languages.

Research evidence supports the importance of early literacy development as a foundation for lifelong learning and shows clearly what the linkages are between early literacy development and successful school experiences. Kameenui (1993) talks about the "tyranny of time" for those students who begin school behind their peers in critical areas and fall further and further behind as time goes by. Juel's (1988) longitudinal study showed very clearly how likely it was that low readers in first grade will still be low readers in fourth grade. Our clearest understanding of why many students fall further and further behind in reading was explained by Stanovich (1986), who also described how early reading difficulties lead to other long-term problems, including areas of limited vocabulary and cognitive development.

It is obvious that strategic interventions are needed for those students who begin school already behind their peers, or who are otherwise at risk for academic problems. Many language-minority student fall into this camp. Educators can have a positive effect by developing and implementing intense instructional programs designed to meet the literacy needs of language-minority students. One of the most critical of these literacy areas is reading, certainly reading in English, and also, in many school districts around the country, reading in the native language (Goldenberg & Gallimore, 1991). The initial evidence suggests that CBM reading measures can be used to monitor the effectiveness of these English reading programs and some native-language reading programs such as Spanish to help shape the development and validation of instructional programs that meet the literacy needs of language-minority students.

REFERENCES

Alva, S. A., & Padilla, A. M. (1995). Academic invulnerability among Mexican Americans: A conceptual framework. *Journal of Educational Issues of Language-Minority Students, 15,* 27–47.

Arias, M. B. (1986). The context of education for Hispanic students: An overview. *American Journal of Education, 95*(1), 26–57.

Baker, K., & de Kanter, A. (1983). Federal policy and the effectiveness of bilingual education. In K. Baker & A. de Kanter (Eds.), *Bilingual education* (pp. 33–86). Lexington, MA: Lexington Books.

Baker, S. K., & Good, R. (1995). Curriculum-Based measurement of English reading with bilingual Hispanic students: A validation study with second-grade students. *School Psychology Review, 24*(4), 561–578.

Barber, M. B. (1993). With schools becoming towers of Babel, California stumbles along without a state bilingual education program. *California Journal, 24,* 17–18.

Barnes, R. (1983). The size of the eligible language minority population. In K. Baker & A. de Kanter (Eds.), *Bilingual education: A reappraisal of federal policy* (pp. 3–22). Lexington, MA: Lexington Books.

Caterino, L. C. (1990). Step-by-step procedure for the assessment of language-minority children. In A. Barona & E. E. Garcia (Eds.), *Children at risk: Poverty, minority status, and other issues of educational equality* (pp. 269–282). Washington, DC: National Association of School Psychologists.

Chamot, A. U., & O'Malley, J. M. (1989). The cognitive academic language learning approach. In P. Rigg & V. Allen (Eds.), *When they don't all speak English* (pp. 108–125). Urbana, IL: National Council of Teachers of English.

Crawford, J. (1989). *Bilingual education: History, politics, theory, and practice.* Trenton, NJ: Crane.

Cummins, J. (1979). Linguistic interdependence and the educational development of bilingual children. *American Education Research Journal, 49,* 222–251.

Cummins, J. (1984). *Bilingualism and special education: Issues in assessment and pedagogy.* Clevedon, UK: Multilingual Matters.

De La Rosa, D., & Carlyle, M. E. (1990). *Hispanic education: A statistical portrait.* Washington, DC: National Council of La Raza.

Deno, S. L. (1990). Individual differences and individual difference: The essential difference of special education. *Journal of Special Education, 24*(2), 160–173.

Duran, R. P. (1989). Assessment and instruction of at-risk Hispanic students. *Exceptional Children, 56,* 154–158.

Erickson, J. G., & Walker, C. L. (1983). Bilingual exceptional children: What are the issues? In D. R. Omark & J. G. Erickson (Eds.), *The bilingual exceptional child* (pp. 3–24). San Diego, CA: College Hill Press.

Esquival, G. (1988). Best practices in the assessment of limited English and bilingual children. In A. Thomas & J. Grimes (Eds.), *Best practices in school psychology* (pp. 113–125). Washington, DC: National Association of School Psychologists.

Figueroa, R. A. (1989). Psychological testing of linguistic-minority students: Knowledge gaps and regulations. *Exceptional Children, 56,* 145–152.

Figueroa, R. A. (1990). Best practices in the assessment of bilingual children. In A. T. Thomas & J. Grimes (Eds.), *Best practices in school psychology—II* (pp. 93–106). Washington, DC: National Association of School Psychologists.

Figueroa, R. A., & Sassenrath, J. M. (1989). A longitudinal study of the predictive validity of the System of Multicultural Pluralistic Assessment (SOMPA). *Psychology in the Schools, 26,* 5–19.

Fitzgerald, J. (1995). English-as-a-second-language learners' cognitive reading processes: A review of research in the United States. *Review of Educational Research, 65*(2), 145–190.

Fradd, S. H., & Correa, V. I. (1989). Hispanic students at risk: Do we abdicate or advocate? *Exceptional Children, 56,* 105–110.

Fuchs, L. S., & Deno, S. (1982). *Developing goal and objectives for educational programs.* Washington DC: American Association of Colleges for Teacher Education.

Fuchs, L. S., & Fuchs, D. (1986). Effects of systematic formative evaluation on student achievement: A meta-analysis. *Exceptional Children, 53,* 199–208.

Fuchs, L. S., Fuchs, D., Hamlett, C. L., Walz, L., & Germann, G. (1993). Formative evaluation of academic progress: How much growth can we expect? *School Psychology Review, 22*(1), 27–48.

García, G. E., & Pearson, P. D. (1994). Assessment and diversity. In L. Darling-

Hammond (Ed.), *Review of research in education* (20th ed., pp. 337–391). Washington, DC: American Educational Research Association.

Gersten, R. G. (1985). Structured immersion for language-minority students: Results of a longitudinal evaluation. *Educational Evaluation and Policy Analysis, 7*(3), 187–196.

Gersten, R. G. (1996a). Literacy instruction for language-minority students: The transition years. *Elementary School Journal, 96*(3), 227–244.

Gersten, R. G. (1996b). The double demands of teaching English language learners. *Educational Leadership, 53*(5), 18–22.

Gersten, R. G., Taylor, R., Woodward, J., & White, W. A. T. (1984). *Structured English immersion for Hispanic students in the U.S.: Findings from the fourteen-year evaluation of the Uvalde, Texas Program: Technical Report 84-1.* Eugene: Follow Through Project, University of Oregon.

Gersten, R., & Woodward, J. (1994). The language-minority student and special education: Issues, trends, and paradoxes. *Exceptional Children, 60,* 310–322.

Gickling, E. E., & Armstrong, D. L. (1978). Levels of instructional difficulty as related to on-task behavior, task completion, and comprehension. *Journal of Learning Disabilities, 11,* 559–566.

Glaser, R., & Silver, E. (Eds.). (1994). *Assessment, testing, and instruction: Retrospect and prospect.* Washington, DC: American Educational Research Association.

Goldenberg, C., & Gallimore, R. (1991). Local knowledge, research knowledge, and educational change: A case study of early Spanish reading improvement. *Educational Researcher, 20*(8), 2–14.

Goldenberg, C., Reese, L., & Gallimore, R. (1992). Effects of literacy materials from school on Hispanic children's home experiences and early reading achievement. *American Journal of Education, 100,* 497–536.

Good, R. H., Baker, S. K., Baker, D. L., & Berber, A. (1990). [The reliability and validity of Spanish reading fluency]. Unpublished raw data.

Gottlieb, J., Alter, M., Gottlieb, B. W., & Wishner, J. (1994). Special education in urban America: It's not justifiable for many. *Journal of Special Education, 27*(4), 453–465.

Habedank, L. (1995). Developing local norms for problem solving in the schools. In A. Thomas & J. Grimes (Eds.), *Best practices in school psychology III* (pp. 701–716). Washington, DC: National Association of School Psychologists.

Hasbrouck, J. E., & Tindal, G. (1992). Curriculum-based oral reading fluency norms for students in grades 2 through 5. *Teaching Exceptional Children, 24*(3), 41–44.

Jiménez, R. T., Garcia, G. E., & Pearson, P. D. (1995). Three children, two languages, and strategic reading: Case studies of bilingual and monolingual readers. *American Educational Research Journal, 32,* 67–97.

Jiménez, R. T., Garcia, G. E., & Pearson, P. D. (1996). The reading strategies of bilingual Latina/o students who are successful English readers: Opportunities and obstacles. *Reading Research Quarterly, 31*(1), 90–112.

Juel, C. (1988). Learning to read and write: A longitudinal study of 54 children from first through fourth grades. *Journal of Educational Psychology, 80,* 837–847.

Kameenui, E. J. (1993). Diverse learners and tyranny of time: Don't fix blame; fix the leaky roof. *The Reading Teacher, 46*(5), 376–383.

Kanellos, N. (1993). *The Hispanic-American almanac.* Detroit, MI: Gale Research.

Karlsen, B., & Gardner, E. (1985). *Stanford Diagnostic Reading Test* (3rd ed.). San Antonio, TX: Psychological Corporation.

Laberge, D., & Samuels, S. J. (1974). Toward a theory of automatic information processing in reading. *Cognitive Psychology, 6,* 293–323.

Lam, T. C. (1992). Review of practices and problems in the evaluation of bilingual education. *Review of Educational Research, 62,* 181–203.

Lambert, W. E., & Tucker, G. R. (1972). *Bilingual education of children: The St. Lambert experiment.* Rowley, MA: Newbury House.

Langdon, W. H. (1989). Language disorder or difference? Assessing the language skills of Hispanic students. *Exceptional Children, 56*(2), 160–167.

Laosa, L. M. (1975). Bilingualism in three United States Hispanic groups: Contextual use of language by children and adults in their families. *Journal of Educational Psychology, 67,* 617–627.

Luz Reyes, M. (1992). Challenging venerable assumptions: Literacy instruction for linguistically different children. *Harvard Educational Review, 62,* 427–446.

Mackey, W. F. (1978). The importation of bilingual education models. In J. E. Alatis (Ed.), *International dimensions of bilingual education* (pp. 1–18). Washington, DC: Georgetown University Press.

Marston, D. (1989). Curriculum-based measurement: What is it and why do it? In M. R. Shinn (Ed.), *Curriculum-based measurement: Assessing special children* (pp. 18–78). New York: Guilford Press.

Mercer, J. (1979). *SOMPA: Technical and conceptual manual.* New York: Psychological Corporation.

Millis, I. V. S., Campbell, J., & Farstrup, A. (1993). *National Assessment of Educational Progress 1992 Reading Report Card for the nation and the states: Data from the national and trial states assessment.* Washington, DC: U.S. Department of Education, National Center for Education Statistics.

Minnesota Department of Education. (1987). *A resource handbook for the assessment and identification of limited English proficient students with special education needs.* Minneapolis: Minnesota Department of Education, Curriculum Services Center.

National Council of La Raza. (1990). *Hispanic education: A statistical portrait.* Washington, DC: National Council of La Raza.

Northcutt, L., & Watson, D. (1986). *Sheltered English teaching handbook.* Carlsbad, CA: Northcutt, Watson, Gonzalez.

Olmedo, E. L. (1981). Testing linguistic minorities. *American Psychologist, 36,* 1078–1085.

Ornstein, A. C., & Levine, D. U. (1989). Social class, race, and school achievement: Problems and prospects. *Journal of Teacher Education, 40,* 17–23.

Portales, A. (1994). Introduction: Immigration and aftermath. *International Migration Review, 28,* 632–639.

Reddy, M. (Ed.). (1993). *Statistical record of Hispanic Americans.* Detroit, MI: Gale Research.

Reschly, D. (1988). Special education reform: School psychology revolution. *School Psychology Review, 17,* 459–475.

Reschly, D. J., & Grimes, J. P. (1995). Intellectual assessment. In A. Thomas & J. Grimes (Eds.), *Best practices in school psychology III* (pp. 775–788). Washington, DC: National Association of School Psychologists.

Rossell, C. H. (1988). The problem with bilingual research: A critique of the Walsh and Carballo study of bilingual education projects. *Equity and Excellence, 23*(4), 25–29.

Rueda, R. (1989). Defining mild disabilities with language-minority students. *Exceptional Children, 56*(2), 121–128.

Rumberger, R. W. (1983). Dropping out of high school: The influence of race, sex, and family background. *American Educational Research Journal, 202,* 199–220.

Rumberger, R. W. (1995). Dropping out of middle school: A multilevel analysis of students and schools. *American Educational Research Journal, 32*(3), 583–626.

Salvia, J., & Ysseldyke, J. E. (1988). *Assessment in special and remedial education* (4th ed.). Boston: Houghton Mifflin.

Samuda, R. J. (1975). *Psychological testing of American minorities: Issues and consequences.* New York: Harper & Row.

Shinn, M. R. (1988). Development of curriculum-based local norms for use in special education decision making. *School Psychology Review, 17,* 61–80.

Shinn, M. R. (Ed.). (1989). *Curriculum-based measurement: Assessing special children.* New York: Guilford Press.

Shinn, M. R. (1995). Curriculum-Based measurement and its use in a problem-solving model. In A. Thomas & J. Grimes (Eds.), *Best practices in school psychology III* (pp. 547–568). Washington, DC: National Association of School Psychologists.

Shinn, M. R., & Baker, S. K. (1996). The use of Curriculum-based measurement with diverse learners. In L. A. Suzuki, P. J. Meller, & J. G. Ponterro (Eds.), *Handbook of multicultural assessment: Clinical, psychological, and educational applications* (pp. 179–222). San Francisco: Jossey-Bass.

Shinn, M. R., Good, R. H., Knutson, N., Tilly, W. D., & Collins, V. (1992). Curriculum-Based reading fluency: A confirmatory analysis of its relation to reading. *School Psychology Review, 21,* 458–478.

Standards for educational and psychological testing. (1985). Washington, DC: American Psychological Association.

Stanovich, K. E. (1986). Matthew effects in reading: Some consequences of individual differences in the acquisition of literacy. *Reading Research Quarterly, 21,* 360–406.

Stewner-Manzanares, G. (1988). The Bilingual Education Act: Twenty years later. *Focus: The National Clearing House for Bilingual Education, 6,* 1–8.

Taylor, B., Harris, L. A., & Pearson, P. D. (1988). *Reading difficulties: Instruction and assessment.* New York: Random House.

U.S. Bureau of the Census. (1992). *Population projections of the United States, by age, sex, race, and Hispanic origin: 1992 to 2050* (No. P25-1092). Washington, DC: U.S. Government Printing Office.

U.S. Department of Education. (1993). *Fifteenth annual report to congress: 1993*. Washington, DC: Office of Special Education and Rehabilitative Services.

U.S. Department of Education, National Center for Education Statistics. (1992). *The Condition of Education 1992*. Washington, DC: Office of Educational Research and Improvement.

U.S. Department of Education, National Center for Education Statistics. (1993). *The Condition of Education 1993*. Washington, DC: Office of Educational Research and Improvement.

U.S. Department of Education, National Center for Education Statistics. (1995a). *The Condition of Education 1995*. Washington, DC: Office of Educational Research and Improvement.

U.S. Department of Education, National Center for Education Statistics. (1995b). *NAEP 1994 reading: A first look*. Washington, DC: Office of Educational Research and Improvement.

U.S. General Accounting Office. (1993). *School age demographics: Recent trends pose new educational challenges*. (GAO/HRD-93-105BR). Washington, DC: U.S. Government Printing Office.

U.S. General Accounting Office. (1994). *Limited English proficiency: A growing and costly educational challenge facing many school districts*. (GAO/HEHS-94-38). Washington, DC: U.S. Government Printing Office.

Wechsler, D. (1974). *Manual for the Wechsler Intelligence Scale for Children—Revised*. New York: Psychological Corporation.

Willig, A. C. (1985). A meta-analysis of selected studies on the effectiveness of bilingual education. *Review of Educational Research, 55*(3), 269–317.

Wong-Fillmore, L., & Valdez, C. (1985). Teaching bilingual learners. In M. C. Wittrock (Ed.), *Handbook of research on teaching* (pp. 648–685). New York: Macmillan.

Woodcock, R. W. (1981). *Bateria Woodcock do proficiencia en el idioma: Version en Espanol*. Hingham, MA: Teaching Resources.

Ysseldyke, J. E., & Thurlow, M. L. (1984). Assessment practices in special education: Adequacy and appropriateness. *Educational Psychologist, 9*, 123–136.

Zirkel, P. A. (1972). Spanish-speaking students and standardized tests. *Urban Review, 5/6*, 32–40.

CHAPTER 8

◆◆◆

Curriculum-Based Measurement for Secondary Students

◆

CHRISTINE A. ESPIN
GERALD TINDAL

One of the most important questions to be addressed in the development of a Curriculum Based Measurement (CBM) system is the question of "what to measure" (Deno & Fuchs, 1987). At the elementary-school level, efforts to answer this question have focused on the identification of measures that can serve as "critical indicators" of performance in reading, spelling, written expression, and arithmetic (Deno, 1985). The "curriculum" is defined as student performance in these four basic skill areas, with little disagreement that growth in these skill areas is essential for elementary-school-aged children. At the secondary level, however, the question of "what to measure" becomes more complex. Few agree on an appropriate curriculum for secondary students, particularly for those with disabilities; thus, it is difficult to determine in what areas student progress should be measured.

We begin this chapter by reviewing issues related to curriculum choices for secondary students with mild disabilities. We conclude the first section with a proposal for a two-pronged approach to the development of Curriculum Based Measures (CBMs) at the secondary level, with a dual focus on progress measurement in basic skill and content areas (e.g., social studies, science, etc.). In the second section of the chapter, we review the research conducted on CBM at the secondary level. In the final section, we propose a framework for decision making at the secondary level that is informed by the use of CBM. We illustrate this framework through use of a case study.

THE "CURRICULUM" FOR SECONDARY STUDENTS WITH MILD DISABILITIES

At the secondary level, the focus of instruction turns away from an emphasis on basic skills toward the *use* of those skills to acquire content-area information (Alley & Deshler, 1979). Unfortunately, the level of proficiency in basic skills for secondary students with mild disabilities is often so low as to inhibit their ability to perform more advanced learning tasks successfully (deBettencourt, Zigmond, & Thornton, 1989; Deshler, Schumaker, Alley, Warner, & Clark, 1982; Levin, Zigmond, & Birch, 1985; Warner, Schumaker, Alley, & Deshler, 1980; Zigmond, 1990). A not unexpected but rather alarming concomitant finding is that the rate of school failure, absenteeism, and dropping out of school for students with mild disabilities is two to three times higher than that of their nondisabled peers (deBettencourt et al., 1989; Levin et al., 1985; Sitlington & Frank, 1990; Wagner, 1990; Wagner, Blackorby, & Hebbeler, 1993).

What type of curriculum is best suited for students who are not yet proficient in basic skills but are in a setting that emphasizes content-area learning? Several options exist (e.g., basic skills, functional skills, learning strategies, vocational skills, content-area learning; see Deshler, Lowrey, & Alley, 1979; Halpern & Benz, 1987; Mercer, 1997), but there is little consensus on the most effective approach. Not surprisingly, then, our curriculum choices for secondary students with mild disabilities are influenced by factors other than effectiveness. Two of these factors are especially relevant to our discussion of CBM.

The first factor to influence our choice of curriculum is the extent to which students with mild disabilities participate in the general education curriculum and are held to general education graduation requirements. Wagner (1990) found that secondary students with learning disabilities spent up to 70% of their day in general education classrooms. Because at the secondary level, the "place" of instruction is to a large extent synonymous with the content of instruction (Schumaker, & Deshler, 1988), we can assume that the curriculum for secondary students with mild disabilities will place a heavy emphasis on content-area instruction.

Even when students with mild disabilities are not placed in general education classrooms for instruction, their graduation requirements are often the same as those for students without disabilities. In general, students are required to complete a certain number of credits in core academic areas, including English, mathematics, social studies, and science. Thus, in many programs for secondary students, special education teachers teach "content-area" classes so that students with disabilities can earn their credits and graduate from high school (see McKenzie, 1991a, 1991b).

Given the fact that students with mild disabilities participate to a large extent in general education curriculum, and the fact that the students are held to the same graduation standards as nondisabled students, one can conclude that an important area of instruction is content-area learning. It follows, then, that the development of measures for monitoring progress in the content areas should prove useful at the secondary level.

The second factor that influences our choice of curriculum for secondary students with disabilities is our belief regarding students' ability to progress in basic skill areas. Students with mild disabilities appear to make little to no progress in basic skills during their four years of high school (Deshler, Warner, Schumaker, & Alley, 1983; Zigmond, 1990). Some argue that this lack of progress is due to the fact that students plateau in basic skills when they reach high school (e.g., see Deshler et al., 1983). Others argue that the lack of progress is due to a lack of direct and intensive instruction in basic skill areas at the secondary level (e.g., see Zigmond, 1990).

Given (1) the importance of basic reading and written expression skills across the curriculum (Scruggs & Mastropieri, 1993; Espin & Deno, 1993b), (2) the increasing number of states requiring students to meet specific basic skill competency standards, and (3) the importance of these skills for job success following graduation (Mikulecky & Diehl, 1980), we think it is worthwhile to assume the latter explanation; that is, to assume that students can progress in basic skills if given direct and intensive instruction. This assumption can then be tested using a system of progress measurement such as CBM.

In summary, we propose a two-pronged approach to curriculum development for secondary students with mild disabilities, with a dual focus on content-area learning and basic skill improvement. The measures we develop for progress monitoring at the secondary level will also have this dual focus. In this chapter, we review the research on the development of measures in both basic skill and content areas. A summary of the studies reviewed in the chapter is presented in Table 8.1. We begin with a review of the research conducted in the basic skill areas.

CBM IN BASIC SKILLS AREAS

One of the ways that CBM procedures can be used at the secondary level is in Problem Identification (Deno & Fuchs, 1987); that is, the measures can be used to identify students with basic skill deficits in reading, written expression, or mathematics. Once these students are identified, the measures can be used to monitor students' progress in these basic skill domains.

TABLE 8.1. Summary of Studies on the Use of CBM at the Secondary-School Level

Academic area	Study	Participants	Type of measure	Outcomes
Written expression	Tindal & Parker (1989)	Compensatory and special education students in grades 6 to 8	Number of words written, written legibly, spelled correctly, written in correct sequence; percent of words written legibly, spelled correctly, written in correct sequences; mean length of correct word sequence	High correlations between holistic ratings and percent of words spelled correctly and percent of correct word sequences. Production-independent factor was a better prediction of holistic ratings than production-dependent factor.
	Parker, Tindal, & Hasbrouck (1991)	Regular and compensatory students in grades 6, 8, and 11	Number of words written, spelled correctly, and correct word sequences; percent of correct word sequences	Low-moderate to moderate correlations between writing measures and holistic ratings of writing, with strongest relations found for correct word sequences. Correct word sequences discriminated between grade levels.
	Espin, Scierka, Skare, & Halverson (1996)	147 students in grade 10. Students were in four groups: LD, Basic, Regular, and Enriched English.	Number of words written, words spelled correctly, correct word sequences, characters written, characters per word, sentences, and mean length of correct word sequence	Low to moderate correlations between written expression measures and measures of writing proficiency. A combination of three measures—characters per word, sentences written, and mean length of correct word sequences—predicted better than any single measure.
	Espin (1997)	112 students in grades 7 and 8	Number of words written, words spelled correctly, correct word sequences, correct minus incorrect word sequences. Characters written, characters per word, sentences written. Students completed story and descriptive writing samples, and wrote for 3 or 5 minutes	No differences in validity and reliability between story writing and descriptive writing. Two measures found to have low alternate form reliability in characters per word and mean length of correct word sequences. Correct minus incorrect word sequences and sentences written were the best indicators of proficiency.

217

TABLE 8.1. *Continued*

Academic area	Study	Participants	Type of measure	Outcomes
Mathematics	Foegen (1995)	100 students in grades 6 to 8	Basic math operations task, basic estimation task, modified estimation task	Basic math operations task was the best predictor of general math proficiency. A modified estimation task in which students selected answers from rounded responses also predicted well.
Reading/content-area learning	Espin & Deno (1993b)	121 general and special education students in grade 10. Low-achieving students were students in the lowest 20th percentile of the GPA distribution. High-achieving students were in the upper 20th percentile.	Reading aloud from English and science texts	Low/moderate correlations between reading aloud and answering questions from the text. Reading measure predicted performance better for low-achieving students than for high-achieving students.
	Espin & Deno (1994–1995)	121 general and special education students in grade 10	Matching vocabulary terms with definitions. Vocabulary selected from English and science texts.	Low/moderate to moderate correlations between vocabulary task and answering questions from text. In a regression analysis, vocabulary accounted for a greater proportion of the variance than reading aloud.
	Espin & Foegen (1996)	184 general and special education students in grades 6 to 8	Reading-aloud, vocabulary-matching, and maze tasks. Tasks developed from two expository texts on volcanoes and ancient manuscripts.	Moderate to moderately high correlations between each of the three measures and comprehension, acquisition, and retention of content material. In a regression analysis, vocabulary accounted for a greater proportion of the variance than reading-aloud or maze tasks.
	Espin & Deno (1993a)	121 general and special education students in grade 10	Reading aloud from English and science texts	Discrepancy in reading performance on English and science texts could be used to identify students with general and specific reading deficits. Students

Content-area learning: science	Nolet & Tindal (1993)	64 general, Chapter 1, and special education students in grade 6	Perception probes	in content-specific group benefited more from re-reading and study of the text than students in the general deficit reading group. Perception probes reflected differences in performance between general and special education/Chapter 1 students. Strong relation between the number of times a concept was listed on the perception probe and the end-of-the-unit achievement test.
	Tindal & Nolet (1996)	74 general, Chapter 1, and special education students in grade 7	Perception probes	Perception probes differentiated the performance of general and special education/Chapter 1 students.
	Nolet & Tindal (1994)	40 general, Chapter 1, and special education students in grade 6	Perception probes and evaluation essay	General education students listed more ideas identified by the teacher as important on their perception probes and essays than did special education/Chapter 1 students. General education students produced essays with greater logical soundness and used more concept labels in their essays.
	Nolet & Tindal (in press)	27 general and special education students in grade 7	Evaluation and compare-and-contrast essays	Moderate correlations between ratings of critical thinking and the number of teacher-targeted concepts included in the essay.
Content-area learning: social studies	Tindal, Rebar, Nolet, & McCollum (1995)	150 general, Chapter 1, and special education students in grade 8	Short and extended essays that tapped application, prediction, and evaluation operations	Reliable group differences between general and special education/Chapter 1 students found on extended evaluation essay.

The question that arises in this process is whether the measures used at the elementary level can also be used at the secondary level to identify students with difficulties and, subsequently, to monitor their progress. To answer this question, research has focused on the construct validity of *critical indicators* of performance: the pattern of relations between indicators and other measures of performance in written expression, mathematics, and reading (Deno, 1985; Fuchs & Deno, 1994). One general theme emerges from the validity studies done at the secondary level: The direct and simple measures that are used at the elementary-school level are not necessarily appropriate for use at the secondary-school level. We begin this section by reviewing the research on the development of critical indicators in written expression, and then discuss the development of indicators in mathematics and reading.

Written Expression

The CBMs used most often at the elementary level in written expression are the number of words written, the number of words spelled correctly, and the number of correct word sequences. Tindal and Parker (1989) found that these measures were not the most appropriate measures for monitoring progress for students at the secondary-school level. They collected 6-minute writing samples from students in grades six through eight. The samples were scored in eight different ways, including the *number* of words written, written legibly, spelled correctly, and written in correct sequence (Videen, Deno, & Marston, 1982); the *percentage* of words written legibly, spelled correctly, and written in correct sequence; and, finally, the mean length of each continuous correct sequence. The dependent variable in the study was teachers' holistic ratings of student performance.

Moderate to strong correlations between the objective measures and teachers' holistic evaluations were obtained, with the largest coefficients found between the holistic ratings and the percent of words spelled correctly ($r = .73$) and percent of correct words sequences written ($r = .75$). In a regression analysis in which the holistic ratings were regressed on each of the independent variables, only the percent of correct word sequences entered into the equation.

Results of a factor analysis and a cluster analysis revealed two factors: (1) a production-dependent factor that consisted of the number of words written, words written legibly, words spelled correctly, and correct word sequences; and (2) a production-independent factor that consisted of the percent of legible words, words spelled correctly, and correct word sequences, as well as the mean length of correct word sequences. A regression analysis revealed that the production-independent factor scores were stronger predictors of holistic ratings than the production-dependent factors. Finally, significant differences between special education and compensatory students were found on three of the production-independent measures: percentage of correct word sequences, percentage of words spelled correctly, and the mean length of correct word sequences.

The results of Tindal and Parker (1989) support the use of production-independent measures as general indicators of student performance in the area of written expression for middle school students. The percentage measures seemed to be especially good predictors of holistic ratings of student performance and could be used to identify students who experience difficulty in written expression and are in need of additional instruction in the area. However, percentage measures present special difficulties when used as indicators of growth or for distinguishing between students (Tindal & Parker, 1989). Change across percentage values is a function of the number of opportunities to respond; thus, when converting a score to percentage for a student who writes 25 words correctly, the scale will have an interval of 4%. For a student who writes 100 words correctly, the scale will have an interval of 1%. Although both students might increase the same number of words spelled correctly (e.g., from 5 to 15) over a given period of time, the change in percentages will be radically different, with a change from 20% to 60% for the first student, and a change from 5% to 15% for the second.

Parker, Tindal, and Hasbrouck (1991) explored the use of five indices of writing for making screening and eligibility decisions. In this study, writing samples were collected from regular, compensatory, and special education students in grades 2 through 5, and from regular and compensatory students in grades 6, 8, and 11. Writing samples were scored in five ways: words written, words spelled correctly, correct word sequences, percentage of correctly spelled words, and percentage of correct word sequences. As with Tindal and Parker (1989), the dependent variable was a holistic rating of student writing.

Results of the study revealed a general pattern of increase in scores on all five indices from one grade to the next (with a slight regression on three of the measures from grades four to five). Percentile graphs with standard errors of measurement bands were created to examine the use of two measures (correct words sequences and percentage of correct word sequences) for discriminating students at different percentile levels and between grade levels. For grades six to eight, the number of correct word sequences created a nearly linear slope from the 10th to the 99th percentile, indicating that there was a clear difference in students' scores at different percentile levels. Correct word sequences was the better measure for discriminating between grade levels, although at the lower percentile levels (e.g., below the 10th percentile) *percentage* of correct word sequences discriminated better than the *number* of correct word sequences.

Correlations between objective scores and holistic ratings were calculated within each grade level. Low-moderate to moderate correlations
were found between the five indices and holistic ratings for students in
grades 6, 8, and 11. The best predictor was the number of correct word
sequences, with correlations of .52, .56, and .48 at each respective grade
level. Correlations for the other four measures ranged from .36 to .52,
with the majority of coefficients in the .40s.

Results of Parker et al. (1991) in conjunction with Tindal and Parker
(1989) indicate that two measures have promise as general outcome indicators in written expression at the secondary level: the number of correct
word sequences, and the percentage of correct word sequences. Data
from these two studies support the use of a percentage measure for students at the lowest ends of the performance continuum, but, as mentioned
previously, percentage measures present unique difficulties for differentiating students and for measuring student progress.

Espin, Scierka, Skare, and Halverson (in press) extended the work
conducted by Tindal, Parker, and colleagues to investigate the criterion-
related validity of a variety of measures that could be used for progress
monitoring. The measures included words written, words spelled correctly,
correct word sequences, mean length of correct word sequences, characters written, characters per word, and sentences written. With the exception of words spelled correctly, correct word sequences and mean length
of correct word sequences, all scoring was done via the grammar-check
component of a common word-processing program. In addition to exploring the validity of individual measures, Espin et al. examined the possibility of combining measures to represent students' writing performance.

Participants were 10th-grade students randomly selected from three
English classes: Basic English, Regular English, and Enriched English. In
addition, students receiving services for learning disabilities (LD) were included in the study. The analyses focused on the relation between the writing measures and four outcome measures: scores on the language arts section of the California Achievement Test (CAT), semester grades in English class, independent ratings of writing quality, and group placement.

Results of correlational analyses revealed that no *individual* indicator
was a very strong predictor of writing performance as measured by the
CAT, semester grades in English, or rating of writing quality. The best
predictors were correct words sequences, mean length of correct word sequences, characters per word, and sentences written. Average correlations
between these four variables and the criterion variables were low to moderate, ranging from $r = .30$ to $r = .45$.

A multivariate analysis of variance was conducted to determine
whether any measure differentiated students in the four groups: LD, Basic
English, Regular English, and Enriched English. Results indicated that

four measures differentiated at least one group from the others. These were the same measures that showed the strongest pattern of correlations with the dependent variables: correct words sequences, mean length of correct word sequences, characters per word, and sentences written.

Finally, a regression analysis was conducted to examine whether a combination of measures better predicted CAT scores than any single measure. Results revealed that three measures added to the prediction of CAT Language Arts scores: characters per word, sentences written, and mean length of correct word sequences. The multiple R for the combination of the three variables was .62, meaning that the combination of variables accounted for 38% of the variance in the dependent variable.

Results of Espin et al. (in press) indicate that a combination of measures may be better than any single measure for predicting student performance in written expression. However, the data set for the original study, which had been collected as a part of school-wide norming effort, consisted of only one sample per student; thus, reliability of the measure was not examined.

Espin (1997) examined both the validity and reliability of CBM writing measures with middle-school students. Participants completed two different types of writing probes—story writing and descriptive writing—and wrote both 3- and 5-minute samples. In addition, students wrote two samples for each type of text so that alternate-form reliability of the measures could be examined. Finally, students in this study composed directly on the computer.

The independent variables in the study were the same measures used in the 10th-grade study: words written, words spelled correctly, correct word sequences, mean length of correct word sequences, characters written, characters per word, and sentences written. One additional measure was included: correct minus incorrect word sequences.[1] Dependent variables were teachers' ratings of students' writing performance and students' scores on a district-wide writing test.

Results revealed no differences in reliability and validity of the measures for story-writing versus descriptive writing, or for 3- versus 5-minute samples; thus, only the results for the 3-minute story writing sample are summarized here. Analyses conducted on the alternate form reliability of the measures revealed that two of the measures had reliabilities too low to be considered viable measures: characters per word and mean length of correct word sequence. Reliabilities for the remaining measures ranged from .61 to .77.

[1]The idea for the correct minus incorrect measure came from Barbara Scierka, a doctoral student in special education at the University of Minnesota, who noticed in a study that she was conducting that the number of incorrect sequences in a written expression probe seemed to be almost as important as the number of correct sequences for secondary students.

Validity of the measures was examined by conducting correlational analyses between the measures with acceptable reliabilities and the dependent variables. Results revealed that three measures were valid indicators of students' general writing performance: correct word sequences, correct minus incorrect word sequences, and sentences written. Of these three, correct minus incorrect word sequences and sentences written were the best predictors of writing proficiency, with respective correlations .65 and .62 with teachers' rating of writing proficiency, and .68 and .74 with the district writing test. In a regression analysis, a combination of measures did not substantially improve the prediction of student performance over the use of a single measure.

Results of this partial replication study indicate that two measures that originally appeared to be useful predictors of students' general writing proficiency—characters per word and mean length of correct word sequences—had low alternate-form reliability. Three measures proved to be valid indicators of general writing proficiency. Of these three, correct minus incorrect word sequences was the best measure. It had slightly larger correlation coefficients than correct word sequences alone, and it is probably more sensitive to growth over time than sentences written. Additional research is needed to further examine the reliability of the measures and to examine the utility of the correct minus incorrect word sequence measure for progress monitoring.

The results of the research on developing CBM measures in written expression for secondary students indicate that monitoring students' writing progress at this level is likely to be more complex than at the elementary level. It seems likely that measurement procedures are going to have to account for multiple variables in student writing. For example, correct word sequences, which in some form was a useful indicator in all four of the writing studies reviewed here, is based on the number of words written, the number spelled correctly, and the words written in a correct grammatical sequence. Unfortunately, as the measures become more complex, so do the measurement procedures.

Mathematics

Very little work has been done in the area of progress measurement in mathematics for secondary students. Foegen (1995) conducted a study in which she compared the technical adequacy of three measures in mathematics for low-achieving students in middle school. The three measures were a basic math operations task (BMOT), a basic estimation task (BET), and a modified estimation task (MET). The BMOT consisted of 20 randomly selected basic fact problems from the areas of addition, subtraction, multiplication, and division. Problems were single-digit fact problems. Student answered each problem, and probes were scored according to the number of correct answers produced by the student. The BET consisted of 40 problems, 10 from each operation. Problems were both computation and word problems, which varied in difficulty from one-digit to three-digit problems. Students estimated the answer to the problem and selected the correct answer from a choice of three. Students had to select an exact answer.

The MET was a variation of the BET, consisting of more word problems and more division problems, and included problems involving rational numbers. In addition, basic computation problems were eliminated. The MET was given using two different response formats. The first format (MET-A) was similar to the BET. Students selected an exact answer. In the second format (MET-B), students selected a rounded response to the problem. The choices differed in magnitude by a factor of 10. Table 8.2 presents a sample problem from each type of probe.

The dependent variables in the study included math grade point average (GPA), overall GPA, teacher ratings of mathematics performance, and standardized test scores in mathematics. Results of the study indicated that the BMOT was the single best predictor of students' general math performance. Moderately strong correlations were found between the BMOT and the dependent variables, ranging from .44 to .63. The

TABLE 8.2. Sample Problems from the Basic Operations and Estimation Probes

Probe type	Computation problem	Word problem
Basic math operations task	$7 \times 8 =$ $16 - 9 =$	—
Basic estimation	$921 - 480 =$ A. 2 B. 48 C. 441	Jenny wrote 74 pages in her book. She decided to take 24 pages out. How many pages are in the book now? A. 4 B. 27 C. 50
Modified estimation, Form A	$22 \times 59 =$ A. 37 B. 711 C. 1,298	Edward makes $4 per hour doing odd jobs. If he works 11 hours, how much will he earn? A. $2 B. $15 C. $44
Modified estimation, Form B	22×59 is about A. 12 B. 120 C. 1,200	Edward makes $4 per hour doing odd jobs. If he works 11 hours, about how much will he earn? A. $4 B. $40 C. $400

MET-B also predicted fairly well, with moderately strong correlations ranging from .44 to .55. Neither the BET nor the MET-A proved to be a good predictor of general math performance.

The results of this study indicate that a simple measure of single basic-math facts, similar to measures used often at the elementary level, may prove to be an adequate measure of performance for low-achieving middle-school students. In addition, an estimation task in which students select a rounded response (e.g., the MET-B) may be useful as an indicator of student performance, and may prove to be a better predictor of math-concepts knowledge than the basic-math fact test. The estimation task does not, however, predict in-class performance as well as the basic fact test.

Reading

At the secondary level, much of the reading that students do is in the content areas; thus, the research on reading measures at the secondary level is closely tied to the research on content-area learning. That is to say, reading measures might be used both to determine a student's level of general reading proficiency and to determine how much a student is learning in a content area such as social studies or science. In this section, we review research on the development of critical indicators in reading. The use of the measures for determining general reading proficiency, as well as for measuring content learning, is examined. Later in the chapter, we discuss the development of measures focused solely on content-area learning.

The measures that have been investigated in the area of reading include reading aloud from text, maze, and vocabulary matching. A detailed description of each measure is presented in Table 8.3. We begin with a review of the reliability of the three CBMs and then discuss the validity of the measures for predicting student performance both in reading and content-area learning.

Reliability

Espin and Deno (1993a) reported on the reliability of the reading-aloud measure. Parallel-form reliability for the reading-aloud measure was, on average, .91, and ranged from .90 to .92. Test–retest reliability was on average .91, ranging from .88 to .93. Espin (1994) reported on the reliability of the reading-aloud, maze, and vocabulary measures. Alternate-form reliability was .94 for the reading-aloud measure and .75 for the maze measure. Test–retest reliability was .90 for the maze measure and .81 for the vocabulary measure.

TABLE 8.3. Description of Reading-Aloud, Maze, and Vocabulary General Outcome Measures

Measure	Construction of measure	Student behavior	Administration time	Scoring	Example
Reading aloud	Reading passages selected from students' textbooks. Passages can also be selected from newspaper articles.	Student reads aloud.	1 min.	Number of words read correctly	Volcanoes are cone-shaped hills made of lava, ash, and dust.
Maze	Passages selected from textbooks or newspapers. Every seventh word is deleted and replaced with three multiple-choice items. (The first sentence is left intact.)	Student selects the correct word.	2 min.	Number of correct selections.	Volcanoes are cone-shaped hills made of (lava/call/date), ash, and dust.
Vocabulary	Vocabulary words selected from glossary of textbook, or selected on basis of teacher judgment. Definitions selected from glossary or dictionary. Probes usually have 20 words and 22 definitions.	Student matches word with definition.	5 min.	Number of correct matches	_____ volcano _____ lava _____ magma A. melted rock below the earth's surface. B. cone-shaped hills made of lava, ash, and dust. C. melted rock released from a volcano. D. a violent outburst.

Validity

Research on the validity of the CBMs in reading has examined the pattern of relations between the CBMs and other indicators of student performance, including reading comprehension and content learning.[2] Espin and Deno (1993b) examined the validity of a reading-aloud measure for predicting students' performance on a study task in English and science. Participants were students in general and special education in 10th grade. Students read aloud for 1 minute from three English and three science passages, and the number of words read correctly in 1 minute was recorded. The English passages were selected from the American literature textbook used in the school in which the study took place. Science passages were selected from the biology textbook used in the school.

After reading aloud from the three passages, students completed a study task in which they read a longer passage from the content area and answered multiple-choice questions on the passage as they read it. Following the completion of the study task, students again read the three probe passages. All students completed these tasks in both English and science.

The analysis focused on the validity of the reading-aloud measures for predicting student performance on the study task. Correlations between the reading-aloud measure in English and performance on the study task were in the low/moderate range ($r = .37$). The same was true in the science area ($r = .37$). Additional analyses looked at the relations between reading aloud from text and other indicators of students' general school performance, including performance on a standardized achievement test and GPA (Espin, 1990). Once again, correlations were in the low/moderate to moderate range ($r = .35–.047$).

Although the use of reading-aloud measures for predicting student performance in the content areas shows some promise, one cannot ignore the small magnitude of the correlations, ranging from .30 to .40. These coefficients are much smaller than those found at the elementary level, where correlations between reading aloud from text and other measures of reading performance, range from .70 to .90 (see Deno, 1985; Deno & Fuchs, 1987; Fuchs, Fuchs, & Maxwell, 1988). The small magnitude of the correlations led to an examination of other measures that might be used as predictors of content-area performance, specifically vocabulary matching and maze measures. Espin and Deno (1994–1995) and Espin and Foegen (1996) examined the use of these other measures for predicting student performance in the content areas.

---

[2]Espin, Deno, and colleagues have referred to their measures as General Outcome Measures, a term first described by Fuchs and Deno (1994). This term reflects the fact that the measures are generic in nature and do not necessarily need to be selected from the curriculum. For simplicity's sake, we use the term Curriculum-Based Measurement (CBM) throughout the chapter.

In a reanalysis of the 10th-grade data set, Espin and Deno (1994–1995) examined the utility of a simple vocabulary-matching measure for predicting performance in the content areas. The vocabulary-matching measure consisted of 10 vocabulary items selected from the study passage and 12 definitions (two distracter definitions were included). The vocabulary items were selected from words that were highlighted or italicized in the text, or from words the researchers believed were specific to the content of the passage. Definitions were based on definitions in the text and in the *American Heritage Dictionary of the English Language.* Students were given 10 minutes to match the vocabulary terms with the correct definition.

Results of the study indicated that the vocabulary-matching measure was a slightly better measure for predicting student performance on the study task than was the reading-aloud measure. Correlations between the study task and the two CBMs were nearly equivalent in both English (r = .41 vs. r = .44 for reading aloud and vocabulary matching, respectively) and science (r = .32 vs. r = .40 for reading aloud and vocabulary matching, respectively). However, results of a regression analysis supported the use of the vocabulary task. Scores on the study tasks in English and science were regressed on the two predictor variables (vocabulary matching and reading aloud). In both the English and science areas, when vocabulary matching was entered first into the equation, it accounted for a statistically significant proportion of the variance in the study task (R^2 = .20 and .17 in English and science, respectively), and reading aloud did not add to the strength of the prediction. In contrast, when reading aloud was entered first into the equation, it accounted for a small proportion of the variance in the study task (R^2 = .13 and .07 in English and science, respectively), and vocabulary matching added to the strength of the prediction (R^2 = .09 and .11, respectively).

Espin and Foegen (1996) conducted a follow-up study with middle-school students in which they examined the strength of the relations between three CBMs and performance on content-area tasks. In this study, the authors tried to differentiate reading comprehension from learning of content-area material; thus, they included three criterion tasks: comprehension, acquisition, and retention of content material.

The CBMs in this study were reading aloud, maze, and vocabulary matching. Students first completed the CBMs. For the reading task, students read aloud from two 400-word expository passages describing volcanoes and ancient manuscripts, and the number of words read correctly in 1 minute for each passage was recorded. A maze task was developed from the same two passages used for the reading task. Every seventh word was deleted and replaced with a multiple-choice item consisting of the correct choice and two distracters. The number of correct choices made by the students in 2 minutes was recorded. The vocabulary-matching task consisted of 20 vocabulary items and 22 definitions. Students were given 5 minutes to match each word with its definition, and the number of correct matches was scored.

Following completion of the CBMs, students completed the three content-area tasks. For the comprehension task, students read a passage and then answered comprehension questions in writing. No instruction was given to the students between their reading of the passage and answering of comprehension questions. For the acquisition task, students read a passage and received instruction related to the content of the material. Following each instructional session, students were given a 10-item multiple-choice test on the material covered during that session. Instructional sessions were once a week for 5 weeks and focused on interventions to help students read and understand the material in the passages. The retention test was given 1 week following the last week of instruction. The retention test was a 25-item multiple-choice test and consisted of items selected from each of the five weekly tests.

All three of the CBMs proved to be adequate predictors of student performance on the three content-area tasks, with correlations between the CBMs and the content-area tasks ranging from .52 to .65. Interestingly, the CBMs predicted student performance on the content-area tasks as well as or better than other more commonly used measures of performance, such as GPA, performance on a pretest, and performance on the vocabulary and comprehension subtest of the CAT (CTB/McGraw-Hill, 1985).

To compare the relative strength of each of the CBMs for predicting student performance on the content-area tasks, a series of regression analyses were conducted. Results were similar to those found in Espin and Deno (1994–1995). When vocabulary was entered first into the equation, it accounted for a substantial proportion of the variance in the comprehension ($R^2 = .43$), acquisition ($R^2 = .41$), and retention tasks ($R^2 = .38$). Neither the maze task nor the oral reading task added substantially to the prediction of student performance.

The results of the Espin and Deno (1994–1995) and Espin and Foegen (1996) studies indicate that a vocabulary matching task is a better predictor of performance on reading and content-area learning tasks than reading-aloud or maze measures; however, there are other factors to consider when selecting a progress measure.

First, although the vocabulary measure clearly came through as the best predictor in the regression analysis, the correlations associated with the vocabulary, maze, and reading-aloud measures were not very different from each other. Second, it is possible that performance on the vocabulary-matching measure will not be sensitive to changes in students' reading

performance over time. Although vocabulary knowledge is highly correlated with reading comprehension, it appears to be somewhat resistant to
change (Baumann & Kameenui, 1991; Beck & McKeown, 1991). The vocabulary measure might better be used as a measure of progress in the
content areas. As students increase their knowledge in a content area such
as social studies or science, we could imagine that they would also increase
their knowledge of words specific to that area. The utility of the vocabulary-matching measure for progress monitoring in either reading proficiency or content learning has yet to be investigated.

A final consideration when selecting among the three reading measures is the skill level of the students who are being monitored. Different
measures may be appropriate for students at different skill levels. For example, in their study, Espin and Deno (1993b) compared the use of reading aloud from text for predicting performance of low- and high-achieving students. Correlations between reading aloud from text and performance on a study task, a standardized achievement test, and GPA were,
on the whole, stronger for the low-achieving students (with an average correlation of $r = .48$) than for high-achieving students (with an average correlation of $r = .30$). These results make sense if one considers the fact that
reading is an important factor related to students' ability to do well in their
content-area classes. At the lowest levels of school success, even small differences in reading may result in large differences in task performance.
Once students have become proficient readers, other factors such as background knowledge and learning strategies may begin to exert an influence
on student performance.

Thus far, we have focused our discussion on the use of CBMs to predict student performance in the content areas. CBMs also may help teachers to diagnose a student's source of difficulty and appropriately plan an
intervention.

Use of CBMs to Make Diagnostic Decisions

Espin and Deno (1993a) examined the use of CBMs for making diagnostic decisions. The authors hypothesized that students who experienced difficulty reading content-area material could be placed into two groups:
those whose difficulties were due to general reading deficits and those
whose difficulties were due to reading deficits specific to the content area.
The former group they referred to as the "general deficit" group and the
latter as the "content-specific deficit" group.

Participants in study were the 10th-grade students who participated
in the earlier study in which students read from English and science text
(Espin & Deno, 1993b). Student read three passages, completed a study

task, and read three passages again. One of the passages was selected from the study passage (referred to as the embedded passage), while the other two were selected from elsewhere in the text (referred to as nonembedded passages).

The first analyses focused on the existence of the two groups. Students were placed into the general deficit group if their reading aloud scores in both English and science were below the 40th percentile, but within 20 percentage points of each other. Students were placed into the content-specific deficit group if their reading scores in science were at or below the 40th percentile, but their scores in English were above the 40th percentile. In addition, their English and science scores could not be within 20 percentage points of each other. Results of the analysis verified the existence of the two groups. Of the 121 participants in the study, 32 students had scores that placed them in the general deficit group, and six had scores that placed them in the content-specific group.

Examination of students' scores on a background knowledge test confirmed the hypothesis that students in the content-specific group experienced difficulties related specifically to the content area. For the content-specific group, performance on a background-knowledge task in science was reliably lower than in English, whereas for the general deficit group, background knowledge in the two areas was virtually identical.

Once the groups were formed, an analysis was conducted to determine the educational value of the content-specific and general deficit subgroups. Students in the content-specific group were matched with students from the general deficit group on the basis of their prestudy reading-aloud scores on the embedded science passage. Reading-aloud scores on the poststudy embedded and nonembedded passages were examined. It was hypothesized that students in the content-specific group would improve their reading performance given the chance to study the passage, whereas the students in the general deficit group would not. It was also hypothesized that gains would be greater on the embedded passage than on the nonembedded passage.

Results revealed that, although both groups of students improved their reading performance on the embedded and nonembedded passages, the poststudy scores for the content-specific group were reliably higher than for the general deficit group. In addition, the gains for both groups on the embedded passages were one-half to one-third greater than on the nonembedded passage (see Figure 8.1).

Taken together, these results support the existence of two different educational groups, and support the educational relevance of the groups for decision making. Students in the content-specific group lacked background knowledge in science, and perhaps as a result of this background knowledge deficit, struggled with their reading in the content area. Given time to reread and study the passage, they improved their reading perfor-

Text-Embedded Passage

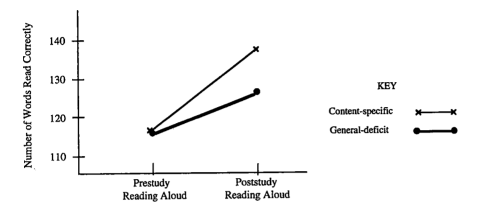

Nonembedded Passage

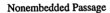

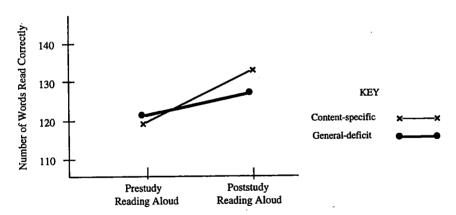

FIGURE 8.1. Performance on text-embedded and nonembedded passages for students in content-specific and general deficit groups. Adapted from Espin and Deno (1993a).

mance. Students with general deficits, on the other hand, read poorly in both content areas. Extra time to reread and study the passage did not help these students as much as it did students in the content-specific group.

Noting such discrepancies in students' reading scores on English and science reading passages should help teachers plan instruction for students. Espin and Deno (1993a) hypothesized that appropriate interventions for students in the general deficit group would be aimed at developing increased literacy skills. Interventions for students in the content-specific group, on the other hand, would be aimed at acquiring content material in an efficient and effective manner. The relative effects of these interventions for the two groups have yet to be tested.

Summary

Three types of measures were investigated in the research on reading: reading aloud, maze, and vocabulary matching. The strongest support was found for the vocabulary measure in terms of predicting student performance in reading and content learning; however, the maze and reading-aloud measures also were adequate predictors. Maze and reading aloud may have some advantages over the vocabulary measure, especially for use with low-achieving and special education students. The use of the measures for making diagnostic decisions was addressed, with results supporting the use of the reading-aloud measure for differentiating students with general and content-specific deficits.

We have thus far reviewed work conducted in the areas of written expression, mathematics, and reading. In the area of reading, we discussed the development of CBMs both for monitoring progress in general reading proficiency and content learning. In the next section, we review work conducted on critical thinking measures. These measures were developed solely for the purpose of monitoring progress in content learning.

CBM IN CONTENT-AREA LEARNING

Tindal, Nolet, and colleagues have conducted a program of research focused on the development of measures for assessing student learning in the content areas. The measures used in this approach are referred to as Critical Thinking Measures (CTMs; Tindal & Nolet, 1995) because the focus is on identifying the *critical thinking skills* that students need in order to use and understand content-area information. Whereas the reading measures we discussed earlier might help the teacher to identify students who are likely to experience difficulties in the content areas and subsequently monitor the progress of those students, CTMs provide teachers with information regarding how and what to teach students who are not progressing. We begin with a description of the essential features of critical thinking.

Three Essential Features of Critical Thinking

The assumption underlying the development of CTMs is that critical thinking skills span different content areas and different topics within a content area; thus, critical thinking skills are the "generic" skills that should be measured in relation to content-area learning. There are three essential features of critical thinking in the content areas: (1) the *forms of knowledge* present in the content areas, (2) the *type of intellectual operations* required of students in the content areas, and (3) the *classroom contexts* within which these knowledge forms are presented, and within which the intellectual operations take place (Tindal & Nolet, 1995).

Knowledge Forms

The first feature of critical thinking is the knowledge forms present in the content area. Adopting a taxonomy developed by Roid and Haladyna (1982), Tindal and Nolet (1995) classify knowledge into three forms: (1) facts, (2) concepts, and (3) principles. *Facts* are simple, one-to-one relations between names, objects, places, or events. An example of a fact is: The capitol of the United States is Washington, D.C.

At the next level of knowledge are *concepts*. Tindal and Nolet (1995) describe concepts as clusters of names, dates, objects, places, and events, each with three components: a label, a set of defining attributes or characteristics, and a set of examples and nonexamples. For example, "the Crusades" is a concept included in a unit on the Middle Ages. The label for the concept is "Crusades." The defining characteristics of "Crusades" are that they were war-like campaigns, they were fought during a specific time period, they were fought by certain groups who had something in common, and their purpose was to take over resources or defeat a common enemy. Examples of the Crusades include the Christian Crusades (in the Middle Ages), the President's Crusade against poverty, and the Children's Crusade. A nonexample is World War I.

At the next level of knowledge are *principles*. Principles are described by Tindal and Nolet (1995) as rule relations among different concepts. An "if–then" relation is often stated or implied in a principle. An example of a principle related to a unit on the Middle Ages is: If people want to gain power and enhance their ability to control land, resources, or other people, then they must mount a Crusade.

Intellectual Operations

The second feature of critical thinking identified by Tindal and Nolet (1995) is the type of intellectual operation required of the student (again adopted from the taxonomy of Roid and Haladyna, 1982). This feature is defined as the type of response expected from students on an assessment task. These responses, arranged hierarchically from simple to complex, include reiteration/summarization, illustration, prediction, explanation, and evaluation.

A *reiteration/summarization* task requires the student to produce either a verbatim response or to paraphrase the information. An *illustration* task requires the student to generate or identify new (i.e., previously not presented) examples of a concept or principle. A *prediction* task requires the student to describe or select a likely outcome given a set of conditions or circumstances that the student has not previously encountered. An *explanation* task requires that the student describe the conditions or circumstances that would result in a particular outcome. Finally, an *evaluation* task requires the student to carefully analyze a problem and then identify and use appropriate criteria to make a decision or judgment.

Classroom Contexts

The final feature of critical thinking described by Tindal and Nolet (1995) is the classroom context in which instruction occurs. The three components of classroom context included in the Tindal and Nolet model are the *curriculum material* used by the teacher, the *interactive instruction* used by the teacher, and the types of *assessment formats* used to measure student learning. The classroom context serves as a basis for defining the domain from which CTMs are selected. Assessment tasks are selected on the basis of the material presented in the textbook (i.e., the curriculum material), the activities and discourse used by the teacher to present information (i.e., the interactive instruction), and the various ways in which the students are expected to use the information they have learned (i.e., the assessment formats).

Summary

To summarize, the first essential feature of critical thinking is the knowledge forms: facts, concepts, and principles. Facts are the simplest, and principles the most complex, knowledge form. The second essential feature is the intellectual operation required of the student in order to complete an assessment task. There are five different intellectual operations. The student can reiterate or summarize what has been learned, illustrate concepts or principles, predict what will happen given a certain set of circumstances, explain what type of conditions or circumstances would lead to a certain set of outcomes, or evaluate a problem in order to make a decision. The third essential feature is the classroom context in which instruction occurs. Three features of classroom context are taken into consideration when developing assessment tasks: the curriculum material used by the teacher, the interactive instruction delivered by the teachers and the assessment format used to measure learning. This framework serves as the basis for the development of measures of critical thinking across content areas.

Development of CTMs

Tindal and Nolet have focused their efforts on the development of measures that allow teachers to examine whether students can use content information in complex intellectual operations (Tindal, Nolet, & Blake, 1992). The focus of the assessment has been primarily on concepts and principles rather than on facts, because facts lack in-depth information that can be manipulated in a complex intellectual operation (Nolet, Tindal, & Blake, 1993).

The first step in the development of CTMs is to identify key concepts and principles in the curriculum and instruction. To help teachers identify these concepts and principles, Tindal and Nolet developed a Content Planning Worksheet (Tindal, Nolet, & Blake, 1992; see Figure 8.2). The worksheet spans a 2–3 week segment of instruction, usually corresponding to one chapter of text, and it consists of three parts: concepts, important ideas, and a graphic organizer. The worksheet helps the teacher to define the content that should be included in the assessment measures.

Once the concepts and principals have been identified, the teacher formulates measures that sample students' knowledge of these concepts and principles, as well as students' ability to use the information via various intellectual operations. (For more detailed information on development of the assessment measures, one can refer to Nolet, Tindal, & Blake, 1993; Tindal & Nolet, 1995; Tindal, Nolet, & Blake, 1992.)

Description of the Assessment Tools

The assessment tools developed by Tindal and Nolet have been of two types: (1) perception probes, and (2) essay measures. Perception probes are short, simple measures designed to get a "take" on students' awareness of the material presented in class and students' ability to identify the important information. Essays are longer production measures and directly address students' ability to manipulate the information presented in the class.

Date:_____

Teacher:_____

Class: _____

Textbook: _____

Other curriculum materials: _____

APPROXIMATE SCHEDULE OF CONTENT TO BE DELIVERED

Week	Dates		Textbook Unit	Chapters	Quiz Dates	Test Dates
1	From:	To:				
2	From:	To:				
3	From:	To:				
4	From:	To:				

KEY CONCEPTS TO BE COVERED

1. _____   6. _____

2. _____   7. _____

3. _____   8. _____

4. _____   9. _____

5. _____   10. _____

IMPORTANT IDEAS FOR STUDENTS TO LEARN

1. _____

_____

2. _____

_____

3. _____

_____

FIGURE 8.2. Content Planning Worksheet.

Perception Probes

Perception probes are given on a frequent basis (every few days or once per week), and can be scored easily and quickly. The perception probes consist of three parts: listing important words, telling important ideas, and relating the words and ideas (Tindal, Nolet, & Blake, 1992). Students are first asked to pretend they are telling a friend what they have been learning in class. They are then asked to list the most important *words* related to the topic they have been studying. They have 3 minutes to complete this task. Following this, students are given 3 minutes to write three important *ideas* that are related to the topic they have been discussing. Students use their listed words to formulate their ideas. Finally, students are given 2 minutes to tell how the words and ideas they have listed are *related* to one another. Students are invited either to write a short paragraph or illustrate the relations using a sketch. A sample perception probe form is presented in Figure 8.3.

Perception probes are scored by first counting the total number of nonduplicated words listed by the student in the "Important Words" section. Next, the words listed by the students are compared to the words listed by the teachers on the Content Planning Worksheet, and exact matches between the two are counted.

To score the section on most important ideas, the number of ideas written, the number of words matching those identified by the teacher on the Content Planning Worksheet, and the total number of words per idea are calculated. An "idea" is defined as any sequence of two or more recognizable words. The final section of the perception probe, where students describe the relation between ideas, is scored by examining whether the student wrote a paragraph or drew a picture. Again, the number of matches between the words students used in their responses and teacher-targeted concepts is calculated.

Essays

Essays consist of three parts: introduction, knowledge form, and intellectual operation stem. The introduction establishes the context or setting of the problem, the topic of the question, and the context of the task. Subsequent sentences establish the knowledge forms and intellectual operations to be used by the student.

In forming the essay task, the teacher must give special consideration to the words used in the stem. These words direct the student to use the correct intellectual operation. For example, if one wishes the student to use the operation of *reiteration,* the prompts need to include words such as repeat the exact words, recite, state the definition, give a verbatim re-

Pretend that you have to tell a friend what you have learned in class today. You would want to tell your friend about the most important words and ideas discussed. You also would want to tell your friend why these words and ideas are important to remember.

IMPORTANT WORDS

List the words you think are most important to help your friend understand the material discussed in class today. You may list new words you learned for the first time in this chapter or unit or you may list words we have talked about in previous classes. List as many important words as you can remember.

1. _____   5. _____   9. _____

2. _____   6. _____   10. _____

3. _____   7. _____   11. _____

4. _____   8. _____   12. _____

IMPORTANT IDEAS

Tell your friend three important ideas that were discussed today. You may write a phrase or a complete sentence, but be sure to provide your friend with enough information for them to know what you mean.

1. _____

_____

2. _____

_____

3. _____

_____

PUTTING IT ALL TOGETHER

Tell how the words and ideas you listed above are related to one another. You may write a short paragraph or you may draw a sketch that shows how these ideas and words are connected. Use as many words and ideas from your lists as you like. If you need more room, use the back of this page.

FIGURE 8.3. Perception Probe.

TABLE 8.4. Words That Prompt Intellectual Operations for Essay Responses

Intellectual operation	Words
Reiteration	Repeat the exact words, recite, state the definition, give a verbatim response.
Summarization	Paraphrase the content, retell what you read, summarize what was said, describe the main issue.
Illustration	Provide an example, present a comparable issue, relate an analogous incident.
Evaluation	Decide which alternative, determine the correct choice, consider which option, compare and determine, select one and justify.
Prediction	Tell what will happen, make a prediction, guess an outcome, describe subsequent events.
Application	Explain the outcomes, give some reasons.

sponse. An example of a reiteration questions would be: State the definition of inertia. Words that would prompt other intellectual operations are presented in Table 8.4.

Tindal and Nolet (1995) have developed both quantitative and qualitative methods for scoring essays. Quantitatively, they have counted the number of words written and the number of "thought units" produced in student responses. A thought unit is a grammatical group of words (i.e., reflecting correct usage) that can stand alone. Thought units have the minimal elements of subject, verb, and object. Qualitatively, Tindal and Nolet have developed flowcharts that lead the teachers through a number of steps in scoring student responses. For an example of a flowchart for rating the quality of an evaluation essay, see Tindal and Nolet (1995).

Validity of CTMs

Tindal and Nolet have conducted several studies to examine the use of CTMs in the curriculum. They have focused their studies on the validity of the measures by examining whether the measures permit the teacher to answer the question, "Did the students learn what I wanted them to learn?" (Nolet, Tindal, & Blake, 1993). To answer this question, they have examined (1) differences in performance between general education students and "special needs" (i.e., Chapter 1 and special education) students, (2) the relation between student performance on the CTMs and teacher identification of important content via the Content Planning Worksheet, and (3) the relation between student performance on the CTMs and student performance on end-of-chapter or end-of-unit tests.

Perception Probes

Three studies examined the use of perception probes for assessing students' understanding of the curriculum. The first (Nolet & Tindal, 1993) examined the use of perception probes in a sixth-grade science class. Prior to instruction, teachers completed a Content Planning Worksheet. Following completion of the unit, students completed perception probes and an end-of-the-unit achievement test designed by the teacher.

Results of the study revealed differences in the responses between general education and special needs students. General education students wrote more words on the "Important Words" section of the probe, and these words more closely matched teacher-targeted concepts than did those of the special needs students. The two groups did not differ in the number of ideas they produced on the probe, nor did they differ on the number of targeted words included in these ideas. Finally, special education and Chapter 1 students used drawings more frequently than writing to illustrate relations between concepts.

Two subsequent studies supported the findings related to group differences on perception probes. In the first, Tindal and Nolet (1996) found that general education students in seventh grade wrote more important words and listed more important ideas on their perception probes than did the special needs students. In the second, Nolet and Tindal (1994) found that, although general and special needs students did not differ on the *number* of concepts listed on their perception probes, they did differ on the *type* of concepts listed. Virtually all of the concepts listed by general education students were those identified by the teacher as an "important idea" on the Content Planning Worksheet. In contrast, only about one-fourth of the concepts listed by the special education students had been identified by the teacher as important.

The relation between performance on the perception probes and the end-of-unit achievement tests was also examined in the studies described, but the results are less consistent than those related to group differences. Nolet and Tindal (1993) found that the more often a concept was listed on the perception probe, the more likely it was to be answered correctly on the end-of-the-unit test ($r = .82$). The authors noted that the end-of-the-unit test in this case closely matched the teachers' instruction.

Nolet and Tindal (1994), however, found a different pattern of results. In this study, there was no reliable relation between performance on the perception probes and performance on the end-of-chapter test. The authors note that the end-of-chapter test created by the teacher for this study did not match the teacher's instruction, whereas the perception probes and essay test did. As a result, the more often a concept was summarized or illustrated in the class, the more likely students were to use the concept in their essays, with correlations of .67 and .60, respectively, for general education students, and .59 and .65, respectively, for special education students. In addition, for the general education students, the more often a concept was summarized or illustrated, the more likely it was to be included in their perception probes ($r = .61$ and .60, respectively).

In summary, results of the research on perception probes reveal consistent group differences in performance, with general education students identifying words and concepts on their probes that more closely match the words and concepts listed by the teacher on the Content Planning Worksheet. In addition, the information listed by students on the perception probes relates to student performance on end-of-chapter or unit tests, but only when the tests reflected the concepts and ideas presented during instruction. These results support the use of perception probes to get a "quick take" on whether students are learning the material that has been taught by the teachers, and for predicting how students will do on end-of-chapter or end-of-unit tests. Essays, the second CTM developed by Tindal and Nolet, can be used to provide the teacher with more in-depth information about students' ability to use critical thinking skills as they relate to content material.

Essays

Three studies investigated the use of essays as measures of critical thinking. In the first (Nolet & Tindal, 1994), students completed an evaluation essay in which they wrote a letter to the inhabitants of an imaginary planet where fossil fuels were recently discovered. The students had to make a recommendation about whether fossil fuels should be developed on the planet and had to provide a rationale for their answer. The study examined group differences on the measures, as well as the relation between performance on the measures and an end-of-unit teacher-made test.

Results of the study revealed differences in performance between general and special needs students. General education students spelled a greater percentage of words correctly on their essays than did special needs students. In addition, general education students used significantly more concept labels in their essays and produced responses that had greater logical soundness than did the special needs students. Finally, general and special needs students differed on the number of teacher-targeted concepts used in the essays. General education students mentioned 9 out of the 11 teacher-targeted concepts, whereas the special needs students mentioned only 2 out of the 11.

As with the perception probes, no reliable relation between performance on the essay and performance on the end-of-chapter test was found, most likely due to the lack of correspondence between the end-of-chapter test and teacher instruction.

In the second study (Nolet & Tindal, 1995), the use of two different types of essays—evaluation essays and compare-and-contrast essays—for measuring student performance was examined. The study took place in a seventh-grade science class. Students covered two units during the study. The first was on the use of the scientific method. The second was on classifying organisms. Again, prior to instruction, the teacher completed a Content Planning Worksheet. Following instruction, students completed three essays (two evaluation and one compare-and-contrast essay) and two criterion-referenced tests. The essays and criterion-referenced tests were based on the information provided by the teacher in the Content Planning Worksheet. The criterion-referenced tests were constructed by the teacher.

Essays were scored in terms of the total number of words written, the percentage of words spelled correctly, the average length of thought units, the number of teacher-targeted concepts, the number of attributes written for each teacher-targeted concept, the number of examples given for each teacher-targeted concept, and a qualitative rating of critical thinking.

Results of the study supported the use of the evaluation essay for measuring critical thinking skills. Reliable and moderately strong correlations were found between the number of teacher-targeted concepts and concept-related attributes listed by the student in the essay and qualitative ratings of critical thinking ($r = .54$ and $.50$, respectively). In addition, there was a significant relation between performance on one of the two criterion-referenced tests and the number of concepts included in the essay ($r = .35$).

Results did not support the use of the compare-and-contrast essay for measuring critical thinking. Although, a positive correlation was found between the number of concepts listed in the essay and qualitative ratings of critical thinking ($r = .50$), the number of concept-related attributes and qualitative ratings of critical thinking were negative ($r = -.31$) In addition, qualitative ratings of critical thinking were related to typical indices of writing, including the total number of words written by the student ($r = .43$) and the average length of the thought units in the essay ($r = -.70$), implying that the ratings were more affected by students' writing ability than by their content knowledge.

The utility of the evaluation essay over other types of essays was supported in the third study (Tindal, Rebar, Nolet, & McCollum, 1995) with students in an eighth-grade social studies classes. In this study, students completed both short and extended essays that tapped application, prediction, and evaluation operations. Reliable between-group differences were found only for the extended evaluation essay. None of the other CTMs resulted in group difference.

The results of the essay studies lend support to the use of an evaluation essay for measuring students' critical thinking skills. In scoring the evaluation essay, the most useful indices of performance seem to be the number of concepts and concept-related attributes written by students.

Summary

Research conducted on the validity of CTMs lends support to the use of the measures to help teachers determine students' ability to use critical thinking skills as they relate to content-area material. Support was found for the use of perception probes for getting a "take" on what students are learning and for determining whether students are understanding and correctly interpreting the information presented in the text and in class. In addition, support was found for the use of the evaluation essays for examining students' ability to manipulate concepts and attributes related to the content material presented during instruction. Student performance on the CTMs did not relate, however, to student performance on teacher-made tests when those tests did not match the teacher's instruction.

A COMPARISON OF CBMs AND CTMs

Two different approaches to developing progress measures in the content areas have been discussed in this chapter: (1) the development of reading measures as critical indicators of performance in the content areas by Espin, Deno, and colleagues; and (2) the development of CTMs by Tindal, Nolet, and colleagues. The two approaches are complementary to each other.

Espin, Deno, and colleagues have tried to identify critical indicators of students' performance in the content areas; that is, they have examined the use of reading measures from content-area material as indicators of students' general performance in content-area learning. Probes are developed so that they can be used on a frequent basis (one to three times per week) to monitor student progress over time. The probes are not designed to offer the teacher information regarding what to change when instruction is not working. In addition, the probes provide little information about how much students are learning in a particular lesson or unit.

The measures developed by Tindal, Nolet, and colleagues, in contrast, offer the teacher information about what modifications to make when students are not learning. In addition, because the measures are tied to the material presented in a lesson or unit, they provide teachers with information regarding how much the student has learned from recent instruction. This close tie to the curriculum, however, also places limitations on the measures. It is difficult to use the measures to examine growth across an extended period of time (e.g., 1 year), because with the beginning of each new unit, the student's performance dips (see Tindal & Nolet, 1995). A graph of student performance does not show a gradual increase over time as students gain knowledge and information in a content area. In addition, the measures developed by Tindal, Nolet, and colleagues are more time consuming to develop and score than typical CBMs. This makes it difficult to measure student performance as often as one would with a typical CBM.

As we will illustrate in the case study that follows, the two types of measures can be used together to help the teacher gain a rich and full picture of student performance. The critical indicators developed by Espin, Deno, and colleagues can be used to help monitor students' growth and progress over time in reading or in the content areas. The CTMs developed by Tindal, Nolet, and colleagues can provide the teacher with immediate feedback regarding students' understanding and perceptions about what has been taught, and can be used to evaluate students' critical thinking skills related to content-area material. Evaluation of students' critical thinking skills can then help the teacher determine what type of changes to make when students are not progressing or learning.

Most of the work conducted thus far on CBM at the secondary level has focused on the development of measures; little has addressed programmatic implementation. In the case study that follows, we illustrate how the measures might be used for decision making in both basic skill and content areas.

Case Study: Use of CBMs at the Secondary Level

Ms. Jappers is the special education teacher at East High. Part of her job has been to work with students with disabilities to ensure that they successfully pass the reading and written expression portion of the state graduation test. The other part of her job has been to work closely with the ninth-grade science teachers to help students with disabilities succeed in their science classes.

Ms. Jappers would like to have a systematic method for determining which students will need extra help to pass the reading and written-expression portions of the state graduation test. In addition, Ms. Jappers and the science teachers would like to have a systematic method for determining the best science class placement for the special education students prior to the beginning of the school year. The general policy of East High is to include all students in general education classes. Most of Ms. Jappers's students are in a basic science class, which is designed for students who are not planning to attend college. Other students, however, are in advanced science classes or in separate, special education science classes.

Ms. Jappers and the science teachers decide to implement CBM procedures to help them in their decision making. At the beginning of the academic year, Ms. Jappers and the science teachers collect data on all ninth graders using CBM procedures. In reading, students read aloud for 1 minute from narrative texts selected from the ninth-grade English literature textbook, and the number of words read correctly is recorded. In written expression, students are given story starters and compose for 3 minutes on the computer. The number of sentences written and number of characters per word are scored by the students at the end of the 3 minutes using the grammar-check component of the word-processing component. The number of correct word sequences are scored by hand by Ms. Jappers and the paraprofessionals who work with her.

In science, students complete vocabulary-matching probes. The vocabulary-matching probes are 5-minute probes in which students match 20 words with their definitions. Words and definitions are randomly selected from the glossary of textbooks used in the special education, basic, and advanced science classes. Probes are scored according to the number of correct matches.

Ms. Jappers and the science teachers work with the school psychologist to establish levels of performance on the CBM probes that predict success on the state graduation test and in science classes. During the academic year, students' scores on the state graduation tests are recorded. In addition, their grades in science classes are recorded. At the end of the year, the school psychologist uses the data to create a table of "likely success" (see Table 8.5). The left-hand column in Table 8.5 represents students' scores on CBMs in reading. The right-hand column indicates the percent of students who are likely to earn a passing grade on the state graduation test. To illustrate further, one can use the table to determine that 30% of students who read 81 words in 1 minute on the CBM probes are likely to pass the state graduation test. The table of "likely success" provides the teachers with guidelines to use in decision making for the coming year.

The following year, Ms. Jappers and the science teachers administer CBMs to incoming ninth graders. Using the tables created in the previous year, Ms. Jappers and the science teachers target students who are likely to experience difficulty passing the state graduation test or difficulty achieving success in the basic science class. For example, Ms. Jappers targets stu-

TABLE 8.5. Hypothetical Example of a Table of Likely Success on State Graduation Test for Ninth-Grade Students at "East High"

Scores on Curriculum-Based Measures in reading	Percentage of students likely to pass reading portion of state graduation test
41	10
64	20
81	30
94	40
108	50
121	60
134	70
151	80
174	90

Note. Data are fictitious.

dents who read 81 words or less in 1 minute on the CBM probes for extra help in reading. Ms. Jappers then monitors the progress of the targeted students.

In reading, students read from narrative text for 1 minute and Ms. Jappers graphs the number of words read correctly. In written expression, students write for 3 minutes, and Ms. Jappers graphs the number of correct minus incorrect word sequences written. Ms. Jappers is able to use the data from Table 8.5 to establish long-range goals for her students. For example, she knows that 70% of students who score 134 on the CBM reading probes are likely to pass the reading portion of the state graduation exam. She sets this level as her goal for the students with whom she is working. Ms. Jappers follows the same procedures for goal setting in written expression.

To monitor the progress of students in science, Ms. Jappers and the science teachers administer weekly vocabulary probes and graph the number of correct matches made. When students seem to be struggling, Ms. Jappers intervenes in collaboration with the science teachers. The science teachers also collect data related to students' critical thinking skills. At the end of each week, the teachers administer perception probes to all of their students. The perception probes tell the teachers how well students have understood the information that was covered that week. Once a month, the science teachers administer an essay to the students related to the content they have covered that month. The essay reveals the students' ability to use critical thinking skills in science. Ms. Jappers places the perception probes and essays for the special education students in portfolios. Ms. Jappers uses the information in the portfolios to identify exactly where students are experiencing problems and to determine how to intervene.

If the results of the progress-monitoring data, the perception probes, and the essays reveal that an individual student is not learning in the basic science class, Ms. Jappers confers with the parents, student, and science teacher to discuss the possibility of placing that student in a special education science class.

This case study illustrates the potential use of CBM in basic skills and content areas. It also illustrates the overlap between the two areas at the secondary level. The validity of this system for informing instruction and making decisions (Messick, 1989) has yet to be tested.

CONCLUSION

The majority of work conducted on the use of CBM at the secondary level has been conducted in the area of content-area learning and reading. A small body of work has been conducted in written expression and mathematics.

The work in the area of written expression indicates that progress monitoring in written expression may require more complex measurement procedures than those used at the elementary level. One indicator trait that consistently appears as a useful measure is the number of correct word sequences, especially as it relates to the number of incorrect word sequences. In mathematics, support was found for the use of a basic operation task, as well as for an estimation task in which students are given a probe consisting of computation and word problems, and asked to select the nearest correct answer.

The work conducted on reading and content-area learning has overlapped. Under the heading of reading, we reviewed research on the use of CBMs in reading to determine not only students' reading proficiency but also to determine their content-area learning. A vocabulary-matching measure proved to be a good predictor of student performance on reading comprehension and content-learning tasks; however, its usefulness as a progress-monitoring measure is not known. Reading-aloud and maze measures also may be appropriate CBMs, especially for students at the lower ends of the achievement continuum.

In the area of content learning, work has been conducted on the development of CTMs. The measures examined included perception probes and essays. Both measures show promise for identifying what students have learned, and for measuring critical thinking skills. Their utility as measures of progress over time is unknown.

Due to the space limitations, we were not able to review in this chapter a related body of research on the development of CBM for use in adult literacy programs (see Bean et al., 1989; Bean & Lane, 1990; Bean et al., 1996). This research may have application to the development of measures at the secondary level, and we recommend that readers who are interested review this research.

The majority of work conducted thus far at the secondary level has focused on establishing the criterion-related validity of measures in reading, mathematics, written expression, and content-area learning. Two general conclusions can be drawn from the research reviewed in this chapter.

First, valid and reliable indicators of student performance *can* be developed for secondary students, although several questions remained unanswered: (1) Which indicators will prove useful for progress monitoring? (2) Are there differences in the validity of the measures for low-achieving/special education students and average/above-average students? (3) Are there differences in the validity of the measures for middle- and high school students? These issues must be examined more closely.

Second, we cannot assume that the indicators used at the elementary-school level will also be appropriate for use at the middle- and high school level. For example, one of the simple indicators of performance in written expression at the elementary-school level is to count the number of words written by the student. At the secondary level, the number of words written does not predict student performance when used with a range of typical secondary students. Slightly more complex measures, such as number of correct and incorrect word sequences show more promise as measures of performance.

The work conducted thus far at the secondary-school level has focused on the questions of "what to measure." In that sense, the primary purpose has been to identify valid and reliable indicators of performance. Much work remains to be done related to the use of CBM for progress monitoring and decision making. We have examined the use of the measures to assess students' performance and progress in the basic skill areas of written expression, mathematics, and reading, as well as in the content areas. Our work in developing measures at the secondary-school level will always be driven by the curricular and educational decision we make for these students. Thus, it is will be necessary for us to continuously step back and evaluate our goals and assumptions regarding the education of secondary-school students with mild disabilities.

REFERENCES

Alley, G. R., & Deshler, D. D. (1979). *Teaching the learning disabled adolescent: Strategies and methods.* Denver: Love Publishing.

Baumann, J. F., & Kameenui, E. J. (1991). Research on vocabulary instruction: Ode to Voltaire. In J. Flood, J. M. Jensen, D. Lap, & J. R. Squire (Eds.), *Hand-*

book of research on teaching the English language arts (pp. 604–632). New York: Macmillan.

Bean, R. M., Burns, D. D., Cox, R. C., Johnson, R., Lane, S., & Zigmond, N. (1989). *Identifying valid measures of reading, mathematics, and writing for workplace environments* (Technical report). Pittsburgh, PA: University of Pittsburgh, Institute for Practice and Research in Education.

Bean, R., & Lane, S. (1990). Implementing curriculum-based measures of reading in an adult literacy program. *Remedial and Special Education, 11,* 39–46.

Bean, R. M., Lazar, M. K., Johnson, R. S., Burns, D. D., Cox, R. C., Lane, S., & Zigmond, N. (1996). The ALERT: One answer to literacy screening. Literacy Assessment for Tomorrow's Schools. In *Literacy assessment for today's schools* (pp. 217–226). Greeley, CO: College Reading Association.

Beck, J., & McKeown, M. (1991). Conditions of vocabulary acquisition. In R. Barr, M. L. Kamil, P. B. Mosenthal, & P. D. Pearson (Eds.), *Handbook of reading research* (Vol. II, pp. 789–814). White Plains, NY: Longman.

CTB/McGraw-Hill. (1985). *California Achievement Test.* Monterey, CA: Author.

deBettencourt, L. U., Zigmond, N., & Thornton, H. (1989). Follow-up of postsecondary-age rural learning disabled graduates and dropouts. *Exceptional Children, 56,* 40–49.

Deno, S. L. (1985). Curriculum-based measurement: The emerging alternative. *Exceptional Children, 52,* 219–232.

Deno, S. L., & Fuchs, L. S. (1987). Developing curriculum-based measurement systems for data-based special education problem solving. *Focus on Exceptional Children, 19*(8), 1–16.

Deshler, D., Lowrey, N., & Alley, G. (1979). Programming alternatives for learning disabled adolescents: A nationwide survey. *Academic Therapy, 14,* 54–63.

Deshler, D. D., Schumaker, J. B., Alley, G. B., Warner, M. M., & Clark, F. L. (1982). Learning disabilities in adolescent and young adult populations: Research implication. *Focus on Exceptional Children, 15*(1), 1–12.

Deshler, D. D., Warner, M. M., Schumaker, J. B., & Alley, G. R. (1983). The learning strategies intervention model: Key components and current status. In J. D. McKinney & L. Feagans (Eds.), *Current topics in learning disabilities* (Vol. 1, pp. 245–283). Norwood, NJ: Ablex.

Espin, C. A. (1997, February). *Validity and reliability of curriculum-based measures in written expression for middle-school students.* Paper presented at the annual meeting of the Pacific Coast Research Conference, La Jolla, CA.

Espin, C. A. (1990). *Reading aloud from text as an indicator of achievement in the content areas.* Unpublished doctoral dissertation, University of Minnesota, Minneapolis.

Espin, C. A. (1994, February). *Combining curriculum-based measurement and portfolio assessment.* Paper presented at the annual meeting of the Pacific Coast Research Conference, La Jolla, CA.

Espin, C. A., & Deno, S. L. (1993a). Content specific and general reading disabilities of secondary-level students: Identification and educational relevance. *Journal of Special Education, 27*(3), 321–337.

Espin, C. A., & Deno, S. L. (1993b). Performance in reading from content area text as an indicator of achievement. *Remedial and Special Education, 14*(6), 47–59.

Espin, C. A., & Deno, S. L. (1994–1995). Curriculum-based measures for secondary students: Utility and task specificity of text-based reading and vocabulary measures for predicting performance on content-area tasks. *Diagnostique, 20*(1–4), 121–142.

Espin, C. A., & Foegen, A. (1996). Curriculum-based measures at the secondary level: Validity of three general outcome measures for predicting performance on content-area tasks. *Exceptional Children, 62,* 497–514.

Espin, C. A., Scierka, B. J., Skare, S., & Halverson, N. (in press). Curriculum-based measures in writing for secondary students. *Reading and Writing Quarterly.*

Foegen, A. (1995). *Reliability and validity of three general outcome measures for low-achieving students in secondary mathematics.* Unpublished doctoral dissertation, University of Minnesota, Minneapolis.

Fuchs, L. S., & Deno, S. L. (1994). Must instructionally useful performance assessment be based in the curriculum? *Exceptional Children, 61,* 15–24.

Fuchs, L. S., Fuchs, D., & Maxwell, L. (1988). The validity of informal reading comprehension measures. *Remedial and Special Education, 9*(2), 20–28.

Halpern, A. S., & Benz, M. R. (1987). A statewide examination of secondary special education for students with mild disabilities: Implications for the high school curriculum. *Exceptional Children, 54,* 122–129.

Levin, E. K., Zigmond, N., & Birch, J. W. (1985). A follow up study of 52 learning disabled adolescents. *Journal of Learning Disabilities, 18,* 2–7.

McKenzie, R. G. (1991a). Content area instruction by secondary learning disabilities teachers: A national survey. *Learning Disability Quarterly, 14,* 115–122.

McKenzie, R. G. (1991b). The form and substance of secondary resource models: Content area versus skill instruction. *Journal of Learning Disabilities, 24,* 467–470.

Mercer, C. D. (1997). *Students with learning disabilities* (5th ed.). Upper Saddle River, NJ: Prentice-Hall.

Messick, S. (1989). Validity. In R. L. Linn (Ed.), *Educational measurement* (3rd ed., pp. 13–104). New York: Macmillan.

Mikulecky, L., & Diehl, W. (1980). *Job literacy: Reading Research Center technical report.* Bloomington: Indiana University Press.

Nolet, V., & Tindal, G. (1993). Special education in content area classes: Development of a model and practical procedures. *Remedial and Special Education, 14*(1), 36–48.

Nolet, V., & Tindal, G. (1994). Instruction and learning in middle school science classes: Implications for students with disabilities. *Journal of Special Education, 28,* 166–187.

Nolet, V., & Tindal, G. (1995). Essays as valid measures of learning in middle school science classes. *Learning Disabilities Quarterly, 18,* 311–324.

Nolet, V., Tindal, G., & Blake, G. (1993). *Focus on assessment and learning in content classes* (Training Module No. 4). Eugene: University of Oregon, Research, Consultation, and Teaching Program.

Parker, R., Tindal, G., & Hasbrouck, J. (1991). Countable indices of writing quality: Their suitability for screening-eligibility decisions. *Exceptionality, 2,* 1–17.

Roid, G. H., & Haladyna, T. M. (1982). *A technology of test item writing.* New York: Academic Press.

Schumaker, J. B., & Deshler, D. (1988). Implementing the Regular Education Initiative in secondary schools: A different ball game. *Journal of Learning Disabilities, 21*(1), 36–42.

Scruggs, T. E., & Mastropieri, M. A. (1993). Current approaches to science education: Implications for mainstream instruction of students with disabilities. *Remedial and Special Education, 14,* 15–24.

Sitlington, P. L., & Frank, A. R. (1990). Are adolescents with learning disabilities successfully crossing the bridge into adult life? *Learning Disability Quarterly, 13,* 97–111.

Tindal, G., & Nolet, V. (1995). Curriculum-based measurement in middle and high schools: Critical thinking skills in content areas. *Focus on Exceptional Children, 27*(7), 1–22.

Tindal, G., & Nolet, V. (1996). Serving students in middle school content classes: A heuristic study of critical variables linking instruction and assessment. *Journal of Special Education, 29,* 414–432.

Tindal, G., Nolet, V., & Blake, G. (1992). *Focus on teaching and learning in content classes* (Training Module No. 3). Eugene: University of Oregon, Research, Consultation, and Teaching Program.

Tindal, G., & Parker, R. (1989). Assessment of written expression for students in compensatory and special education programs. *Journal of Special Education, 23,* 169–183.

Tindal, G., Rebar, M., Nolet, V., & McCollum, S. (1995). Understanding instructional outcome options for students with special needs in content classes. *Learning Disabilities Research and Practice, 10,* 72–84.

Videen, J., Deno, S., & Marston, D. (1982). *Correct word sequences: A valid indicator of writing proficiency in written expression* (Research Report No. 84). Minneapolis, MN: Institute for Research on Learning Disabilities.

Wagner, M. (1990, April). *The school programs and school performance of secondary students classified as learning disabled: Findings from the National Longitudinal Transition Study of Special Education Students.* Paper presented at the annual meeting of the America Educational Research Association, Boston, MA.

Wagner, M., Blackorby, J., & Hebbeler, K. (1993). *Beyond the report card: The multiple dimensions of secondary school performance of students with disabilities. A report from the National Longitudinal Study of Special Education Students.* Menlo Park, CA: SRI International. (ERIC Document Reproduction Service No. ED 365 088)

Warner, M. M., Schumaker, J. B., Alley, G. R., & Deshler, D. D. (1980). Learning disabled adolescents in the public schools: Are they different from other low achievers? *Exceptional Education Quarterly, 1*(2), 27–36.

Zigmond, N. (1990). Rethinking secondary school programs for students with learning disabilities. *Focus on Exceptional Children, 23*(1), 1–22.

CHAPTER 9

◆◆◆

The Use of Curriculum-Based Measurement in the Reintegration of Students with Mild Disabilities

◆

KELLY A. POWELL-SMITH
LISA HABEDANK STEWART

Special education can be thought of as a "problem-solving system" for general education. In a problem-solving system, special education exists to solve the problems of a subset of students whose performance is severely discrepant from their general education peers (Deno, 1989). Special education services are based on the premise that individualized instruction can reduce this discrepancy, and when it is reduced to a satisfactory level, students should be returned to general education (Allen, 1989). The continuum of services available in special education ranges from special education support provided to a student instructed in a general education classroom to part-time and full-time "pull-out" programs within a school to residential or homebound programs. This continuum is intended to assist in addressing the unique needs of students with disabilities and moving them toward short- and long-term goals, including eventual "problem solution" and return to general education without an Individualized Education Plan (IEP).

Too often, however, students who receive special education services get "stuck" in a service delivery system that is not designed to recognize when the discrepancy has been reduced and has few procedures for systematically moving students toward instruction in the general education classroom and eventual exit from special education (Fuchs & Fuchs, 1992). According to the Seventeenth Annual Report to Congress on the Implementation of the Individuals with Disabilities Education Act (U.S. Department of Education, 1995), over 2.4 million children 6–21 years old receive special education services for students with learning disabilities. Yet it is estimated that as few as 2% (Lytle & Penn, 1986) to 8% (Shinn, 1986) of these special education students will return to general education classrooms over the course of the school year. Indeed, an accurate picture of whether and how students are moving toward general education placements or exiting special education is very difficult to obtain. Federal reporting procedures only recently have started collecting data on special education exit to general education (U.S. Department of Education, 1995).

RECENT ATTENTION TO THE
LEAST RESTRICTIVE ENVIRONMENT

The Least Restrictive Environment (LRE) clause of the Individuals with Disabilities Act (IDEA; 1991) has gained a lot of attention in recent years and has brought the issue of the special education student's instructional setting to the forefront of public and professional consciousness. The LRE clause states that

> to the maximum extent appropriate, handicapped children, including children in public or private institutions or other care facilities, [should be] educated with children who are not handicapped, and that separate schooling or other removal of handicapped children from the regular educational environment [should] occur only when the nature or severity of the handicap is such that education in regular classes with the use of supplementary aids and services cannot be achieved satisfactorily (20 U.S.C. §1412(5)(B); 34 C.F.R. § 300.551).

The LRE clause means that whenever educational teams are making decisions about where and how a child with a disability will receive services, the restrictiveness of the setting and consideration of changes in placement should be a part of the decision-making process.

Although the LRE clause has been in special education legislation since the 1970s, focus on the LRE began in earnest in the late 1980s after then Assistant Secretary of Education Madeline Will issued a white paper in 1986 on the regular education initiative. The white paper carried the message that (1) too many students in special education were receiving services in programs outside their general education classrooms, and (2) increased effort must be made to educate students with disabilities in the general education setting by restructuring special and general education

(Will, 1986). This kind of attention to the LRE provision has made an impact on both general and special education, including an increase in research and rhetoric on the effects of integrating special and general education students and political and legal pressure to include students with disabilities in general education settings in neighborhood schools (Fuchs & Fuchs, 1994; McLesky & Pacchiano, 1994; Sawyer, McLaughlin, & Winglee, 1994).

However, despite the amount of attention being focused on the LRE for students in special education, questions about how to make accountable, data-based decisions about what constitutes the LRE for students with mild disabilities largely remain unanswered. For example, Houck and Rogers (1994) reported that, according to their sample of 788 teachers and administrators in the state of Virginia, there were "active efforts to increase the amount of time students with Specific Learning Disabilities spend in general classroom settings; however, limited program change-related guidelines or category-specific outcome-monitoring measures were reported" (p. 435). The presence of "active efforts" to change the instructional placement for students with mild disabilities in the absence of guidelines or outcome measures indicates a reaction to recent rhetoric about "inclusion" and the LRE without a firm underpinning of exactly how to implement sound LRE decision making.

A MODEL FOR RESPONSIBLE REINTEGRATION

A program of research by Shinn and colleagues at the University of Oregon has provided one research-based model for making case-by-case LRE decisions for students with mild disabilities (e.g., Shinn, Habedank, Rodden-Nord, & Knutson, 1993). Their model, the Responsible Reintegration of Academically Competent Students (RReACS), provides a data-based process for identifying students with mild disabilities, who may be potential candidates for reintegration, and then monitoring the effects of reintegrating those students. The term "reintegration" in this model refers to the process of moving students with mild disabilities from a pull-out program (e.g., resource room) to the general education classroom for instruction in an academic area(s).

The RReACS model is in contrast to a "full inclusion" philosophy (Fuchs & Fuchs, 1990; Fuchs, Fuchs, & Fernstrom, 1993). Instead of *widespread* return of students in special education to general education, decisions about where students should receive their education are made on a case-by-case basis using systematic, data-based, decision-making strategies. Curriculum-Based Measurement (CBM) plays an integral role in this systematic decision-making model. CBM provides individual student and comparison data relevant to (1) identifying candidates for reintegration and (2) evaluating and monitoring the effects of reintegration. The model is composed of six steps:

1. Identifying potential candidates to be considered for reintegration.
2. Comparing the academic performance of reintegration candidates to a comparison group using CBM.
3. Reintegration decision making by an educational team.
4. Planning for successful reintegration.
5. Actual reintegration into general education.
6. Evaluating the effects of reintegration.

The remainder of this chapter discusses the foundation of the RReACS model, details the six implementation steps, and reviews research on the model to date.

FOUNDATION OF THE RReACS MODEL

The RReACS model incorporates validated practices that operationalize key philosophical (e.g., ecological and data-based perspectives) and legal concepts (e.g., LRE) to reintegrate students and monitor the effects of reintegration. The RReACS model is based on (1) the concept of "satisfactory achievement" emphasized in the LRE and case law; (2) a data-based, ecological approach to decision making; and (3) the use of direct and sensitive measurement.

Emphasis on "Satisfactory Achievement" in LRE Clause and Case Law

The LRE clause of IDEA states that children are to be educated in the least restrictive setting where satisfactory achievement can be shown. Along a continuum of potential placements, the general education classroom is on the least restrictive end of the continuum of possible instructional settings. However, if a more restrictive setting, such as a resource room or self-contained classroom is proven necessary for the child to achieve satisfactorily, then that setting is the LRE for the student at that point in time.

The courts have upheld the importance of the LRE clause in educational decision making. Several cases, (e.g., *Daniel R. R. v. State Board of Education*, 1989; *Greer v. Rome City School District*, 1991; *Oberti v. Board of Education of Clementon School District*, 1993; and *Sacramento City Unified School District v. Rachel H.*, 1994; from the 5th, 11th, 3rd, and 9th U.S. Court of Appeals, respectively) have addressed the importance of the LRE clause of IDEA directly. For example, in *Oberti v. Board of Education of Clementon School District* (1993), the federal court stated that children with disabilities had the right to be educated in regular classrooms with their peers without disabilities and, that if school districts advocated for the removal of a child from regular classes, the burden of proof was on the district to prove a more restrictive setting was necessary.

Exactly what constitutes "proof" also has been addressed by the courts. In *Hendrick Hudson District Board of Education v. Rowley* (1982), special education students were defined as benefiting from general education if their achievement was satisfactory by the grading and achievement system within the general education setting. This court interpretation indicates that one approach to determining benefit is to compare directly the achievement of the student with disabilities to the achievement of general education students using "general education" standards for what constitutes satisfactory achievement.

A key concept that drives decisions about the LRE is "satisfactory achievement." It is difficult to operationalize "satisfactory achievement," however. One starting point, supported by the *Hendrick Hudson District Board of Education v. Rowley* (1982) ruling, is to use the performance of other children in the general education environment as a guide. Marston (1988) and Allen (1989) describe an approach to operationalizing the LRE and satisfactory achievement that uses the achievement of peers without disabilities as a comparison. When students' academic skills fall in the range of their peers without disabilities, they may be ready to return to the general education classroom. In fact, Marston (1988) stated that students in special education should be compared to lower-performing students in general education, because this represents the minimum general education expectation. He argued that students in special education should not have to perform to a higher standard than students in general education to be placed in the general education environment for instruction.

The RReACS model incorporates the idea of "satisfactory achievement" into reintegration decision making. It does this by using lower-performing students in general education as a comparison when providing data to teams making decisions about the potential appropriateness of reintegration. General education students also serve as a basis for evaluating the effects of reintegration. The RReACS model operationalizes satisfactory achievement in general education as the lowest *level* of skills and *rate of progress* considered acceptable for general education students. If a child with a disability can attain the same level of skill and rate of progress as his or her general education peers who are benefiting from school, then the general education classroom is the LRE for that student.

Tied to a Data-Based, Ecological Approach

Operationalizing satisfactory achievement based on the academic skills of general education students implies the collection of academic skills data. Within the educational context, data can impact how and when decisions are made. For example, without objective achievement data, there is no evidence that general education teachers are willing to accept special education students into their classrooms for instruction. With data suggesting acceptable performance, general education teachers appear to be willing to reintegrate special education students (Rodden-Nord, Shinn, & Good, 1992). Furthermore, without *ongoing* data collection, the effects of reintegration are either assumed to be positive or are determined by subjective judgment. To responsibly reintegrate students and accurately evaluate the effects of reintegration, systematic monitoring of student outcomes is necessary.

However, academic data alone do not provide an adequate basis for evaluating the context where the child receives instruction. The LRE clause and court cases both imply that decisions about *where* a child should receive his or her education should take into account the *educational context.* The educational context is more than just the academic achievement of other students. Success in any setting depends on many things: the instructional environment, student behavior, teacher attitudes, and curricular materials, to name a few (Ysseldyke & Christenson, 1987a). An ecological approach to educational decision making, then, needs to incorporate knowledge of the behavior and progress of general education students, critical instructional factors that can impede or facilitate success for a student with a disability, as well as what supplemental aids and supports may be appropriate. A true ecological approach needs to be individualized to *each* particular student and situation (Burden & Fraser, 1993; Ysseldyke & Christenson, 1987a). It must allow for a way to gather information on an ongoing basis to determine if the decisions that were made are leading to benefit for the student, and at what point changes in the student's instructional plan—even a change in instructional placement toward a more or less restrictive environment—need to be made (Tindal & Marston, 1990).

The RReACS model is a data-based, ecological approach. It incorporates systematic data collection of academic achievement, attitudes, behavior, and the instructional environment. These data are used at various steps in the model, such as identification of reintegration candidates, planning for reintegration, and evaluating the effects of reintegration. Without ongoing data collection of many facets of the educational context, the RReACS model would not be "responsible."

Use of Sensitive and Direct Measurement

The evaluation of the educational context and ongoing evaluation of reintegration effects necessitate measurement tools that are reliable, valid, and efficient for these purposes. Importantly, measurement tools must be sensitive to changes in student achievement over time so that reintegration effects can be evaluated in a timely manner. Traditionally, the data that are collected for team decision making are not directly relevant to decisions about the LRE and may not be sensitive to short-term changes in achievement. Published, nationally norm-referenced achievement tests, intelligence tests, behavior rating scales, and personality measures are the most common assessment tools used in eligibility and initial placement decisions (Goh, Teslow, & Fuller, 1981; Hutton, Dubes, & Muir, 1992).

These tools do not provide information about how the student compares to *local* peers and therefore would be difficult to use in determining whether a special education student's skills fall within the range of local expectations. For example, information that a special education student's reading score is at the 15th percentile compared to a national norm sample does not necessarily tell the general education teacher whether the student reads as well as or better than some of the general education students in her classroom. Also, the content validity of published, norm-referenced achievement tests has been criticized widely (e.g., Bell, Lentz, & Graden, 1992; Good & Salvia, 1988; Jenkins & Pany, 1978; Shapiro & Derr, 1987). If the overlap between what is taught and what is tested is questionable, the utility of these tests for making decisions about how a student performs in a specific general education curriculum is limited, and examining changes in achievement across time is problematic. Furthermore, nationally norm-referenced tests were never designed to be given at frequent intervals and evaluate student progress. They are lengthy, sample various skills at many levels, often utilize indirect methods such as pointing or editing, and do not have a large number of items at any particular age or grade level. According to Shapiro (1996), "Norm-referenced tests cannot be sensitive to small changes in student behavior, were never designed to contribute to the development of intervention procedures, and may not relate closely to what is actually being taught" (p. 11).

CBM provides direct measurement of students' basic academic skills in the local curriculum and is sensitive to student progress over time. Curriculum-Based Measures (CBMs) serve as dynamic indicators of student academic "health" in the basic skills areas of reading, mathematics computation, spelling, and written expression (Shinn, 1989). These measures can be used in a frequent, ongoing manner (e.g., biweekly) to facilitate timely, data-based decisions about a student's achievement. CBM has been validated for the purpose of identifying where a student's skills fall compared to local peers in the local curriculum (Habedank, 1995; Shinn, 1988) and for evaluating the effects of instructional interventions (Fuchs, 1989; Fuchs & Fuchs, 1986).

In the RReACS model, CBM is used to operationalize "satisfactory achievement" in general education by measuring the level of skills and rate of progress of students in general education. The special education student's level of skills and rate of progress over time are then compared to this general education standard when determining whether the special education student is a good potential candidate for reintegration and whether reintegration is successful.

Measurement tools and techniques such as interviews, behavior and attitudinal rating scales, and direct observations also assist in evaluating the instructional environment and student behavior. Many of these tools may already be used by teams for eligibility and LRE decisions, but could be used on an ongoing basis within a coherent decision-making framework for determining the effects of those decisions and what changes need to be made. The RReACS model incorporates attitude questionnaires and instructional planning forms that are useful in reintegration decision making. Suggestions for additional data-collection instruments also are made at critical decision-making points.

The RReACS model implementation steps stem directly from the conceptual foundations. In the following section, the steps of the model are detailed, including how and when CBM data are collected, as well as when attitudinal questionnaires and instructional planning forms are employed.

RReACS MODEL IMPLEMENTATION STEPS

The six steps of the RReACS model are summarized in Table 9.1. These steps outline a responsible procedure for taking a student with mild disabilities who is receiving instruction outside of the general education classroom and reintegrating that student into the general education classroom for instruction in a specific academic area(s). Throughout this chapter, reintegration examples will be in the area of reading. Most of the research on the systematic implementation of the RReACS model has been conducted in the area of reading. However, strategies similar to those discussed throughout the chapter have been applied in math (see Fuchs et al., 1993).

TABLE 9.1. Overview of RReACS Implementation Steps, Data Collected, and Actions Taken

Step	Data collected	Action taken
1. Identification of potential reintegration candidates	• Special education teacher nomination form with names of reintegration nominees, identified curriculum materials, and names of low-reading peers (LRPs) for comparison group.	• Nominated students proceed to Step 2.
2. Reintegration candidate and comparison group CBM data collection	• Three randomly selected CBM oral reading probes and one CBM reading maze from nominated students and LRPs.	• Summarize CBM data for each nominated student and LRPs. • Potential candidates (students with reading skills within the range of LRPs) identified.
3. Reintegration decision making by the educational team	• Attitude questionnaires completed by team members after seeing data summary and graph.	• Team decides whether to reintegrate student.
4. Planning and consultation for successful reintegration	• Instructional Planning Form. • Observations of instructional environment as directed by educational team. • Requests for consultation.	• Adjustments in instructional environment made as needed. • Consultation provided when requested.
5. Actual reintegration into general education		• Reintegration timing coordinated with all involved parties.
6. Evaluating the effects of reintegration	• CBM testing on reintegrated students and LRPs for a minimum of 12 weeks (e.g., oral reading probes twice weekly and maze once per month).	• Monthly checkup reports created and provided to parents, teachers, and students with attitudinal questionnaires. • Additional consultation provided upon request. • Instructional changes made when necessary.

Step 1: Identification of Potential Reintegration Candidates

The process of identifying students for reintegration begins by asking special education teachers to consider all of the students with mild disabilities on their caseload and nominate students who they believe are good candidates for reintegration. This nomination process could be done as part of the periodic and annual review procedures already in place for these students, or during established times throughout the school year (e.g., quarterly). Regardless of when this process occurs, it should be a thoughtful and intentional opportunity for the special education teacher to nominate students for reintegration. A form to facilitate this process is provided in Appendix 9.1. On this nomination form, special education teachers list the students in their classrooms they believe may have skills within the range of low-reading peers (LRPs) in their general education classroom. Also, space is provided for listing the general education teacher's name and the LRPs' teacher's name, if different from the general education teacher (i.e., low readers move to another classroom for reading instruction). Finally, the form provides space to list information on the materials used for reading instruction for the general education LRPs and a list of four to seven LRPs.

A special education teacher nomination process similar to the one described here was used in a study by Shinn, Powell-Smith, Good, and Baker (1997). Special education teachers were asked to nominate students for reintegration. Thirty students were nominated and subsequently were tested using the CBM procedures and LRP comparison described in Step 2. Of those 30 students, 18 students (60%) read within the range of LRPs from their classroom. School-based teams decided it was appropriate to reintegrate 17 of the 18 students. For the 12 students tested who read below the range of their LRPs, school-based teams decided it was appropriate to reintegrate six of these students despite reading skills below the range of their LRPs. Based on this research, it appears that special education teachers are reasonably accurate at nominating students for reintegration who have good reading skills and/or other factors that the teams believe are necessary for reintegration.

It also is possible to identify potential candidates for reintegration by screening all of the students with mild disabilities and determining that students whose CBM scores fall within the range of their general education LRPs are potential candidates. This procedure was used in research conducted by Rodden-Nord et al. (1992) and Shinn, Baker, Habedank, and Good (1993) on identifying potential candidates for reintegration, discussed in detail later in this chapter. This process would be facilitated in a school system where ongoing CBM progress-monitoring data for special education and/or general education students already were being collected and used for decision making.

Step 2: Reintegration-Candidate and Comparison-Group CBM Data Collection

After a potential reintegration candidate has been nominated, initial testing using CBM occurs. The nominated special education student and a group of appropriate comparison peers would be tested in the academic areas where reintegration was being considered. The comparison group should be based on the lowest level of acceptable performance in the classroom(s) where the student likely would be placed. For example, the low reading group or lowest readers (e.g., four to six students) in a student's general education classroom may be chosen for comparison purposes. Also, the low reading groups across all classrooms at the student's grade level could make up the comparison group (Shinn et al., 1993).

When students are reintegrated in reading, CBM testing consists of having reintegration candidates and the comparison general education LRPs complete two types of reading tasks; CBM oral reading and CBM maze reading. CBM oral reading tasks are standardized tests where students read aloud passages developed from their reading curriculum. Research has provided strong support for CBM oral reading as a reliable and valid measure of general reading skill, including comprehension (Deno, Mirkin, & Chiang, 1982; Fuchs, Fuchs, & Maxwell, 1988; Marston, 1989; Shinn, Good, Knutson, Tilly, & Collins, 1992).

To conduct the CBM oral reading testing, students read aloud at least three randomly selected passages taken from a pool of 18–20 passages developed from the lowest level of the reading series used in the classroom where they are being considered for placement. Passages should be developed, administered, and scored according to standardized procedures (for details of these procedures see Shinn, 1989, 1993). The median number of words read correctly across all three passages is calculated.

The reintegration candidate and LRPs also complete a 5-minute CBM maze-reading task developed from another passage from the same curriculum level. Maze is a multiple-choice cloze reading test developed according to procedures suggested by Fuchs and Fuchs (1992), Guthrie (1973), and Howell and Morehead (1987). Maze passages are about 250 words long and have every seventh word deleted and replaced by a blank. Three response choices are provided under the blank. One of the choices is the correct word. The other two choices are distracters chosen systematically from the same story from which the passage was drawn. One of these distracters is any randomly chosen word from the passage, while the other distracter is the same part of speech (e.g., verb, noun) and tense as the correct word. Research has established that CBM maze-reading tasks as reliable and valid measures of reading comprehension (Espin, Deno, Maruyama, & Cohen, 1989; Fuchs & Fuchs, 1992).

Maze passages are administered to reintegration candidates and LRPs according to standardized procedures. Maze can be administered on either a group or individual basis. Students are instructed to read the story and circle the correct word that goes in each blank. Students are given 5 minutes to complete this task. The measure is scored by counting the number of correct selections (words circled).

Once these CBM data are collected, they are graphed and summarized so that decision-making teams (e.g., IEP or multidisciplinary team [MDT]) can examine the information and identify which candidates for reintegration displayed reading skills within the range of their peer comparison group. Students with skills in the range of their comparison peers generally would be considered potential candidates for reintegration. The graph of student data in Figure 9.1 is an example of how these data can be displayed. The reintegration candidate, Cody, a fourth-grade student, and his four peers were tested using three CBM oral-reading passages from Scribner's *Find Your Way* (1987). The graph displays Cody's median score (the dark circle) in relation to the LRPs' performance (the dark

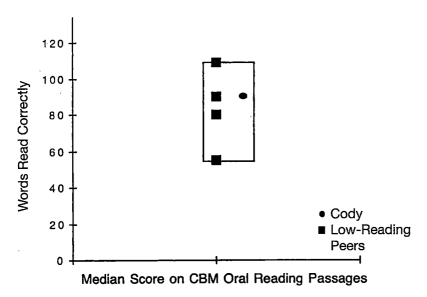

FIGURE 9.1. A special education student (Cody) compared to his low-reading peers (LRPs) in general education: A potential reintegration candidate.

squares). The range of general education LRP performance is shown by the box around the scores. Cody would be considered a potential candidate for reintegration, because his scores were within the range of his LRPs.

A second example is displayed in Figure 9.2. In this example however, the reintegration candidate, Steven, also a fourth-grade student, was tested along with four LRPs using three CBM oral-reading passages from Scribner's *Find Your Way*. The dark circle on the graph represents Steven's median score, and the dark squares on the graph represent the median scores of the LRPs. The box around the scores represents the range of the LRPs' scores. Steven's scores fell below the range of the LRPs; thus, he would be considered an unlikely candidate for reintegration.

Step 3: Reintegration Decision Making by the Educational Team

Reintegrating a student who currently receives instruction in a pull-out, resource-room setting into instructional delivery in the general education classroom is a change-in-placement decision that typically requires a team meeting (e.g., IEP or MDT team). Prior to the team meeting, team mem-

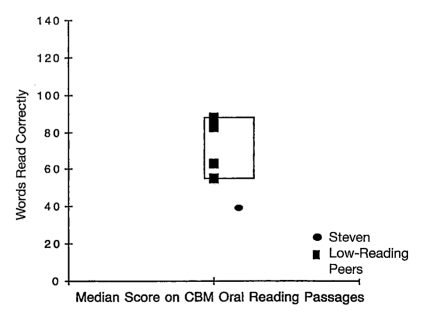

FIGURE 9.2. A special education student (Steven) compared to his low-reading peers (LRPs) in general education: An unlikely reintegration candidate.

bers (e.g., the special education teacher, general education teacher, parent, and special education student) examine a report showing the CBM data graph and a written summary (e.g., see Figure 9.3) and indicate their attitudes toward reintegration. Questionnaires have been developed to assess respondents' beliefs about how much progress the student would make if the change in placement/reintegration were to occur, the appropriateness of making a change in placement or reintegration, the most appropriate placement for the student, the likelihood of success if the student were to change placement or be reintegrated, and the need for supplemental services (e.g., tutoring, instructional or behavioral consultation, study skills, etc.) to make the change in placement or reintegration successful. A sample teacher questionnaire and a sample student questionnaire are found in Appendices 9.2 and 9.3, respectively. These questionnaires may assist the team in (1) identifying areas of consensus, disagreement, and concern; (2) determining if additional information needs to be collected before the team is confident in making a decision about whether to reintegrate the student; (3) planning the transition to the general education classroom; and (4) establishing a baseline of attitudes toward reintegration that can help determine if reintegration has been successful down the line. The teacher and parent questionnaires were based upon the Teacher Attitudes toward Reintegration questionnaire (TATR; Rodden-Nord et al., 1992) and the Parent Attitudes toward Reintegration questionnaire (PATR; Shinn, Baker, et al., 1993), respectively. The student questionnaire was modeled after interviews and questionnaires used by Fuchs, Fuchs, and Fernstrom (1992) and Jenkins and Heinen (1989).

Once the surveys are collected and summarized, typically by the case manager, the team meets to discuss all of the data collected, add any additional information the team members can bring to the meeting that they believe is relevant to a reintegration decision, and reach a decision about whether the student should be reintegrated. The impact the reintegrated student would have on the general education classroom (e.g., effects on other students) could be another consideration discussed by the MDT. Notably, consideration of the impact the reintegrated student may have on other students is consistent with recent case law (e.g., *Oberti v. Board of Education of Clementon School District,* 1993).

At this time, the team may decide it needs to meet again after collecting additional data. For example, the team members may decide that a potential candidate's study skills, academic survival skills (e.g., question asking), and rates of academic engagement need to be examined to see if they are within the range of acceptable performance. The team may decide they need more information about general education instruction before making the reintegration decision. Analysis of the instructional environment could include an examination of the degree to which elements of

GENERAL EDUCATION TEACHER REPORT:
BEFORE CODY MOVED TO THE GENERAL EDUCATION CLASSROOM FOR READING

Initial Reading Test
Recently, Cody was given a brief reading test. Cody read three stories out loud for the test. The stories were from the Scribner reading book *Find Your Way*. A group of four readers from your classroom, Cody's low-reading peers (LRPs), read the same stories out loud. This type of reading test has been shown to give a good measure of student's reading skills.

The picture below shows Cody's median score on the reading tests compared to the other students. By looking at the picture, you can see if Cody's score is similar to or below the other students. The circle is Cody's reading score. The squares are the reading scores of the LRPs. The box shows the range of reading skills of the four LRPs tested from your classroom. Scores near the top of the box mean more words were read correctly than scores near the bottom of the box.

Cody and General Education Low-Reading Peers (LRPS) from Mrs. Cooper's Fourth-Grade Class Reading in Scribner's *Find Your Way*

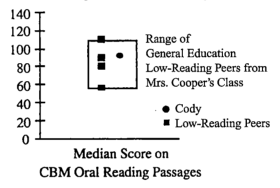

Median Score on
CBM Oral Reading Passages

Cody's median, or middle, score on the three stories was 91 words read correctly in 1 minute. The highest score earned by the four LRPs was 109 words read correctly in 1 minute and the lowest score was 55 words read correctly in 1 minute. So Cody's score was within the range of scores of the low readers in your classroom.

Maze Test
Cody and the low readers also took a test to see how well they understood what they read. This test is called a Maze Test. To make the Maze Test, a story was chosen from the reading book, *Find Your Way*. The story was retyped so every seventh word was replaced by a blank. Three words were typed under the blank. Only one word under the blank was correct. The student's job was to read the story silently and circle the correct word for each blank. Students were given 5 minutes to do the Maze Test. Cody answered 22 words correctly. The highest Maze score earned by the low readers was 27 words correct. Their lowest score was 19 words correct. So Cody's Maze score was within the range of the low readers.

FIGURE 9.3. Data summary provided to the general education teacher before reintegration decision is made.

effective teaching are present in the classroom (e.g., sufficient opportunities for practice and feedback). Although potentially important information, this additional data was not provided to MDTs in previous research on the RReACS model. Instead, the CBM data were used in the context of the knowledge of students' study skills and academic survival skills as the teachers and parents have experienced them.

Step 4: Planning and Consultation for Successful Reintegration

Once a decision has been made that a trial reintegration is appropriate, then the classroom instructional environment needs to be examined by using an instructional planning interview and possibly packaged observation codes. Also, consultation to the teacher and/or parent is offered during this step of the RReACS process.

A brief (20–30 minute) interview with the classroom teacher is conducted to obtain information about instructional planning. During this interview an *Instructional Planning Form* (IPF) is completed. The IPF is a modified version of the Instructional Plan Form (Wesson & Deno, 1989) and is used to assess elements of effective instruction present in a specific instructional area (e.g., reading). The IPF is a one-page form divided into six sections. The first section describes the *focus* or activity/skill. For example, in the area of reading, this could be vocabulary, oral reading, or silent reading. The second section describes the *teaching strategy* (e.g., teacher modeling, lecture, discussion). The third section is where *instructional materials* are described (e.g., basal readers, library books, study guides, worksheets). In the fourth section, the *arrangement* of the classroom during instruction is described (e.g., whole class, small group, independent). The fifth section delineates the *time allocated* for each activity, while the sixth section of the IPF describes the *motivational strategies* used during instruction (e.g., teacher praise, points). (See Figures 9.4 and 9.5 for a sample blank IPF and a sample completed IPF.)

The IPF is used to describe the instructional environment as well as the components of instruction. This information serves two purposes. First, it serves as documentation of the instruction the student receives. If the instruction is working well for the student, this information may be helpful to the student's future teachers. Second, should the student not be successful in the classroom, the information can serve as a starting point in consulting with the teacher around potential changes that could be made in the student's instruction or instructional environment.

In addition to the IPF, tools such as packaged observation codes may be used to facilitate the evaluation of the instructional environment if the MDT desires additional, or more detailed, information. Two examples of packaged observation codes that could be used are the Ecobehavioral Assessment Systems Software (EBASS; Greenwood, Carta, Kamps, &

Instructional Planning Form

Student: _____ Grade: _____ Date: _____

Teacher: _____ School: _____

Focus or skill	Activity				
	Teaching strategy	Materials	Arrangements	Time	Motivational strategies

FIGURE 9.4. Instructional Planning Form (IPF). From "An analysis of long-term instructional plans in reading for elementary resource room students" by C. L. Wesson and S. L. Deno, *Remedial and Special Education, 10*(1), 21–28. Copyright 1989 by PRO-ED, Inc. Adapted and reprinted by permission.

Instructional Planning Form

Student: Hannah
Teacher: Mrs. Joseph
Grade: 3rd
School: Anytown Elementary
Date: 10/8/96

Activity		Materials	Arrangements	Time	Motivational strategies
Focus or skill	Teaching strategy				
Oral reading	Round robin Choral responding Teacher modeling	Better Reading Series Book III Literature books	Teacher-led Small Group (5 students) or whole class (20 students)	9:00–9:30 each day	Teacher praise Stickers
Silent reading	Modeling Read for 20 minutes each night at home	Better Reading Series Book III Literature books	Independent	12:00–12:30 each day	Teacher praise "Rocket Chart" of pages read.
Vocabulary —definitions —spelling	Teacher-led instruction; modeling; use words in sentence; use keyword strategy; play spelling games	Vocabulary list from Better Series Book III	Teacher-led; whole class (20 students) Practice with peer	20 min. daily 10 min. daily	Teacher praise Whole class chart of progress
Phonics skills/ decoding —vowel sounds —blends	Teacher-led instruction with choral responding Independent practice and teacher feedback	Better Reading Series Book III skills exercises and worksheets	Teacher-led; whole class (20 students) Independent	20 min. daily 15 min. 2× weekly	Teacher praise Stickers and pencils
Comprehension —literal facts —inference —opinion	Teacher-led discussion; question and answer; students take turns	Better Reading Series Book III Study guides and skills book	Teacher-led; whole class (20 students) and small group (5 students)	15 minutes daily after oral reading time	Teacher praise

FIGURE 9.5. Sample completed Instructional Planning Form (IPF). From "An analysis of long-term instructional plans in reading for elementary resource room students" by C. L. Wesson and S. L. Deno, *Remedial and Special Education, 10*(1), 21–28. Copyright 1989 by PRO-ED, Inc. Adapted and reprinted by permission.

Delquadri, 1992) or The Instructional Environment Scale · (TIES; Ysseldyke & Christenson, 1987b). Research on the RReACS model to date has not utilized formal classroom observations as part of the planning process, however.

As a final component of the planning process, the general education teacher (or teacher of the classroom where the child will be placed) is given the opportunity to request consultation services. For example, as part of the questionnaire given during the "decision-making" stage of the process, teachers and parents are given the opportunity to indicate what additional support the child needs to experience success in the new placement (see Appendix B). Furthermore, teachers and parents are given the opportunity to indicate with what supports they would like assistance. Supports are listed out in the form of a menu including items such as (1) instructional consultation (e.g., suggestions for curriculum modifications); (2) tutoring (e.g., peer tutoring); (3) intervention to improve study skills (e.g., using an assignment calendar); and (4) interventions for appropriate classroom behavior (e.g., following directions). Once items are selected, the team could decide who was the most appropriate person (e.g., school psychologist, school counselor, special education teacher) to consult with the teacher or parent regarding the item(s) indicated.

Step 5: Actual Reintegration into General Education

Some coordination needs to occur prior to the actual reintegration of the student candidate. This coordination should include, at a minimum, making sure parents and the student are aware of how and when reintegration will occur, as well as coordinating the timing of reintegration with the classroom teacher. This coordination ideally would be covered during the team meeting described in Step 3 and then reviewed in communication to the parents and child prior to actual reintegration.

Step 6: Evaluating Effects of Changes in Placement

Because there is no way to know with certainty that a child will be successful in any particular educational placement, evaluating the effects of reintegration is perhaps the most essential step of the RReACS process and is consistent with a problem-solving approach to educational service delivery (Deno, 1989, 1990; Shinn, 1995; Stoner & Green, 1992). Evaluating the effects of reintegration, or change in placement, involves primarily two processes. First, continuous and frequent monitoring of the student's academic achievement is needed so as much as possible can be known about reintegrated students' progress within a short period of time. Second, these data then are provided to concerned parties (teachers, parents) so their opinions regarding the change in placement can be evaluated and additional concerns can be addressed if necessary (e.g., through consultation).

To conduct the ongoing monitoring and evaluate reintegration outcomes in reading, twice each week, reintegrated students and their LRPs are administered two randomly selected CBM oral reading probes for a total of four probes per week. In addition to the twice weekly CBM oral reading testing, once per month, reintegrated students and LRPs are tested using one randomly selected CBM maze-reading task. These data then are summarized in narrative form and the oral-reading data are graphed. The oral-reading data typically are displayed in two ways. First, the median of the last three passages is calculated and plotted on a box plot graph similar to those used in Step 2. Second, the *slope* of reading progress since the change in placement is calculated and graphed for both the reintegrated student and the LRPs. To calculate the slope, either the ordinary least squares (OLS) method (for details see Good & Shinn, 1990) or the split-middle method (Barlow & Hersen, 1984; White, 1974) is used. Maze-reading data are provided in narrative form. This information forms the basis of what is referred to as monthly progress "checkups" for the reintegrated student. An example of a monthly checkup is shown in Figure 9.6.

These checkups are provided to parents and teachers along with another questionnaire asking them about most appropriate placement, success of reintegration, likelihood that the child will continue to make progress, success of the current reading program, their confidence the child will make reading progress equal to or greater than the LRPs, and their requests for consultation. Additional questions on this follow-up questionnaire ask about the student's behavior during instruction and assignment completion. A sample questionnaire is found in Appendix 9.4.

In the example (Figure 9.6), Cody's reading performance after 4 weeks of reintegration is shown, along with a narrative explanation of the data. As shown in the figure, during week 4 of reintegration, Cody's reading skills were within the range of his peers. Both Cody and three of his LRPs were not making progress, however, as indicated by the downward or flat trend in their slopes. Only one of the LRPs was making progress after 4 weeks in this example. Notably, Cody's rate of progress was roughly commensurate with two of the LRPs, as indicated by the nearly parallel slopes for both Cody and two of the LRPs.

The academic progress "checkup" is provided to parents, students, and teachers on a monthly basis. It is suggested that the student remain in the new placement (remain reintegrated) for *at least* 8 weeks before any decisions about the success of the reintegration or change in placement are made. This suggestion is based on the findings of previous research on the RReACS model (e.g., Shinn, Powell-Smith, Good, & Baker, 1997). An

GENERAL EDUCATION TEACHER REPORT:
4 WEEKS AFTER CODY MOVED TO THE GENERAL EDUCATION CLASSROOM FOR READING

Two times per week for the past 4 weeks, Cody was given a brief reading test. Each time, Cody read 2 stories out loud for 1 minute. The stories were from the Scribner reading book *Find Your Way.* A group of four readers from your classroom, Cody's low-reading peers (LRPs), read the same stories out loud. This type of reading test has been shown to give a good measure of students' reading skills.

Reading Level at Week 4
The picture below on the left shows Cody's median score on the reading tests given during week 4 compared to the other students. By looking at the picture, you can see if Cody's score is similar to or below the other students. The circle is Cody's reading score. The squares are the reading scores of the LRPs. The box shows the range of reading skills of the four LRPs tested from your classroom. Scores near the top of the box mean more words were read correctly than scores near the bottom of the box.

Cody read 82 words correctly in 1 minute. The highest score earned by the four LRPs was 117 words read correctly in 1 minute and the lowest score was 58 words read correctly in 1 minute. So, Cody's score was within the range of scores of the low readers in your classroom.

Cody and General Education Low-Reading Peers (LRPs) from Mrs. Cooper's Fourth-Grade Class
Reading in Scribner's *Find Your Way,* 4 Weeks after Reintegration

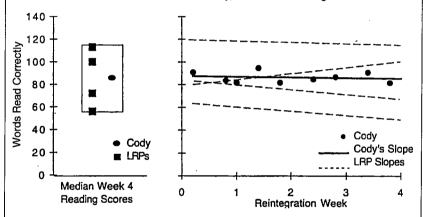

Reading Progress (Slope) after 4 Weeks
The graph above on the right shows Cody's reading progress compared to the other low readers over the last 4 weeks. Cody's scores are the dark circles. The thick straight line is Cody's slope of reading progress of the past 4 weeks. The dashed lines are the progress of the three low readers. A line that *goes up* means that the student's reading is improving. The more the line goes up, the more the student's reading is improving. A line that is *flat* or *goes down* means that the student's reading is not improving.

Cody's slope of reading progress is almost flat. That means that Cody's reading is not improving. One of the low readers in your classroom is showing improvement. The other three low readers from your classroom do not show improvement over the last 4 weeks.

Maze Test
During week 4, Cody and the low readers also took a test to see how well they understood what they read. This test is called a Maze Test. To make the Maze Test, a story was chosen from the reading book, *Find Your Way.* The story was retyped so every seventh word was replaced by a blank. Three words were typed under the blank. Only one word under the blank was correct. The student's job was to read the story silently and circle the correct word for each blank. Students were given 5 minutes to do the Maze Test. On the Maze Test, Cody answered 28 words correctly. The highest Maze score earned by the low readers was 30 words correct. Their lowest score was 25 words correct. So Cody's Maze score was within the range of the low readers.

FIGURE 9.6. Monthly checkup report provided to the general education teacher to evaluate the effectiveness of reintegration after 4 weeks of reintegration.

unanticipated outcome of the research was that several students (both reintegrated and LRP) were found to not be making progress after 4 weeks of reintegration, much like Cody and his LRPs. However, this pattern of performance changed after 8 weeks of reintegration. Shinn, Powell-Smith, Good, and Baker hypothesized that teachers, upon seeing the data after 4 weeks, realized that their students were not benefiting from instruction and made changes that benefited *both* the reintegrated student and LRPs. Thus, to allow for the evaluation of adjustments in instruction, which may occur after initial changes in placement are made, reintegration or change in placement trials should be at least 8 weeks and preferably longer (i.e., 12 weeks) before decisions about their success are made.

Consider once again the case of Cody. Cody's progress after 8 and 12 weeks is displayed in Figure 9.7. As is clear from the graphs, although Cody was not making progress (flat or downward trend) at week 4, at weeks 8 and 12, Cody *is* making progress. Cody also maintained his relative academic standing when compared to LRPs (i.e., median score within the range of LRPs and a slope that was parallel to LRPs).

At the end of the 12-week reintegration trial the educational team can choose to proceed in a number of ways. For example, the team may decide how frequently to continue monitoring the reintegrated student. It may be reasonable to reduce the frequency of monitoring with CBM to every other week, or once per month, if the child has experienced success with the reintegration. If the student has not benefited from the reintegration, or has not been achieving satisfactorily, then the team may choose to reconvene to review the entire process (e.g., determine if interventions were implemented with integrity) and decide a course of action.

RESEARCH OUTCOMES OF THE RReACS MODEL

Research supporting the six steps of the RReACS model has been ongoing since 1991. This research has concentrated on a number of aspects of the model, beginning with the identification of potential reintegration candidates. Next, teacher and parent attitudes toward reintegration were investigated. Finally, the achievement outcomes of reintegrated students were investigated. Much of this research occurred with the support of two grants from the U.S. Department of Education, Office of Special Education Research, Field-Initiated Research Grant No. H023C10151 and Student-Initiated Research Grant No. H023B10033.

Identifying Potential Candidates

The specific question of how many students would meet the satisfactory achievement standard established in the LRE was examined by Shinn,

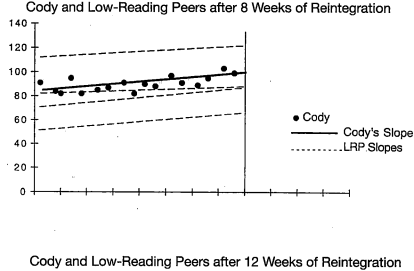

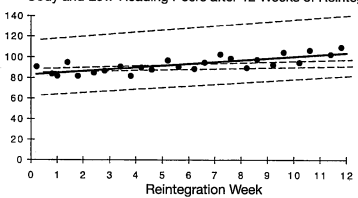

FIGURE 9.7. Oral-reading data graphs 8 and 12 weeks after reintegration: Cody and his low-reading peers (LRPs).

Habedank, et al. (1993). These authors examined the utility of CBM oral reading for examining the skills of special education students and low-achieving general education peers to determine how many students in special education would meet the satisfactory achievement standard (i.e., read within the range of general education LRPs). Two studies were undertaken to investigate two interpretations of the LRE. In the first study, special education students were compared to low-achieving general education students in multiple classrooms at their grade level. In the second study, special education students were compared to low-achieving general education students from the specific general education classroom in which the special education student was already receiving some instruction. In both studies, the sample of special education students tested was restricted to those who had an IEP in reading and were placed in special education for instruction for no more than one-half the school day. Thus, the focus was on students with mild disabilities.

Study 1

Subjects were 85 special education students and 244 general education students from grades three through five. All subjects were from 51 classrooms in a rural school district in the Northwest. The general education students, who served as comparisons for the special education students, were all identified by their teachers as being in the low reading group (LRG) in their classroom. All subjects were tested with two passages from the lowest level of their basal reader used across all general education classrooms at a particular grade level. Standardized administration and scoring procedures for CBM reading were used.

Data were analyzed using two approaches, one using idiographic methods, and the other using more traditional nomothetic methods. In the idiographic approach, special education students who had CBM reading scores within or above the range of their LRG peers within their school and grade were considered potential candidates for reintegration. Both the total number of potential candidates and the percentage of potential candidates relative to the total number of special education students who participated were calculated. Using this approach, an average 44% (range = 10–85%) of the special education students across schools and grade levels read as well or better than at least one LRG peer.

For the nomothetic analysis, students reading scores were transformed to z-scores. Each z-score corresponded to the number of standard deviation units the special education student was discrepant from LRG peers. A discriminant function analysis was conducted to determine if there was a clear differential of students' skills based upon whether they were a LRG peer or a special education student. Nearly half (48%) of the special education students were determined to have reading scores more consistent with LRG peers than with special education students. Thus, regardless of the approach used (idiographic or nomothetic), this study indicated that a large percentage of students in special education had reading skills within the range of their general education peers, evidence of meeting the satisfactory achievement standard.

Study 2

In this study, 190 children (140 LRG, 50 special education) in grades one through five from a suburban Northwest school district served as subjects.

The materials and procedures used in Study 2 were much like those for Study 1, except the reading materials were drawn from the lowest level of reading book used in each classroom instead of each grade level, and three passages were used instead of two. Again, both an idiographic analysis and a nomothetic analysis using the discriminant function were used. However, in Study 2, special education students' skills were compared to LRG peers from their specific classroom instead of all classrooms at their grade level. Results were similar to Study 1.

The idiographic analysis identified 36% of special education students as potential candidates (PCs) that is, read as well or better than at least one LRG peer from their classroom. There were differences in the percentage of students identified at some grade levels. For example, most first-grade students in special education read within the range of the LRG, but few second-grade students in special education read within the range of the LRG. Percentages of students meeting the PC criteria for the other grades were more uniform. The discriminant function analysis yielded results very similar to those in Study 1; 42% of special education students had reading scores more like those of the LRG than special education students.

Identifying Potential Candidates Research Summary

The lessons learned from this research are undeniably important when considering the push toward paying more attention to the LRE. These studies identified large percentages of special education students with mild disabilities who read within the range of their general education peers, regardless of the method used (across grade or within class; idiographic or nomothetic). It seems clear that large numbers of special education students may have skills within an acceptable performance range (i.e., that of low-achieving general education peers). Also, it is evident that CBM is a viable tool for use in this identification process.

Teacher and Parent Attitudes toward Changes in Placement

Positive teacher and parent attitudes toward changes in placement are essential for making the team decisions that are part of the current educational system and are embedded within the RReACS model. General education teachers who are reluctant to take instructional responsibility for a student with a mild disability may not only affect the determination of whether or when the student is reintegrated, but also may be less effective in teaching a reintegrated student (Bender, Vail, & Scott, 1995). In studies examining school personnel attitudes toward the educational placement of students with disabilities, general education teachers typically have reported they believe that general education is *not* the best instructional environment for students with mild disabilities (Bender et al., 1995; Garver-Pinhas & Schmelkin, 1989; Knoff, 1985; Schumm & Vaughn, 1995; Semmel, Abernathy, Butera, & Lesar, 1991). However, the research on teacher attitudes generally has been conducted using hypothetical situations and students, or asking about global attitudes toward groups of students (e.g., students with mild disabilities) rather than asking teachers about students in their classrooms and providing actual data and placement alternatives. This lack of context when assessing teacher attitudes was considered a major limitation to generalizing existing attitudinal research to the attitudes of the teachers using the RReACS procedures (Rodden-Nord et al., 1992).

Parents also are a crucial part of the determination of whether and when to make changes in placement for their children and are the best advocates for continued accountability for their children's education. Parental acceptance and participation in the reintegration process has been correlated with more successful outcomes for students with learning disabilities (Myles & Simpson, 1990). The research on the attitudes of parents of students with disabilities indicates a somewhat more positive attitude toward the possibility and desirability of educating students with disabilities with their peers without disabilities (e.g., Abramson, Willson, Yoshida, & Hagerty, 1983; Lowenbraun, Madge, & Afflect, 1990; Myles & Simpson, 1990; Simpson & Myles, 1989). However, once again, context is important to interpreting the research. Parents, in particular, tended to have more guarded opinions about instruction in the general education setting when the questions specifically addressed their own child. In a study by Abramson et al. (1983), 74% of parents of students in special education agreed that educating students with and without disabilities in the same classroom would improve the academic skills of the children with disabilities. In that same study, however, only 14% of the parents indicated that they believed *their* child would show improvement in an integrated setting.

Under the assumption that attitudes will and do affect the feasibility and integrity of implementing any framework for reintegration decision making and to examine the attitudes of teachers and parents under more "real-world" situations that could include relevant, contextualized assessment information, a series of studies was conducted utilizing the RReACS model procedures and data.

Study 1

Rodden-Nord et al. (1992) studied the attitudes of general education teachers toward reintegrating specific students with disabilities who were in their general education classroom for at least half of the school day already. The Rodden-Nord et al. study examined the attitudes of the general education teachers before being given any specific information about the student with a disability (predata willingness to reintegrate) and after being given a combination of written and graphically represented information about the student's reading achievement and the special education teacher's reintegration readiness rating (postdata willingness to reintegrate). Twenty-six teachers participated in the study. Half of the teachers ($n = 13$) had a student in their classroom who received special education services in a part-time, pull-out program, and who had been identified as a PC for reintegration for reading instruction based on CBM reading scores that were above the scores of at least one student in a group of low-performing general education peers from the same classroom. The other group of teachers ($n = 13$) each had a student in his or her classroom who received similar special education services, but who had been identified as an unlikely candidate (UC) for reintegration for reading instruction based on CBM reading scores that were below his or her low-performing general education peers. The teachers were unaware of which "group" they were a part. All teachers were asked to indicate their willingness to reintegrate the special education student from their classroom for reading instruction. The teacher's indicated their willingness on a scale ranging from 1 (*Very Unwilling*) to 7 (*Very Willing*).

At first, the teachers were given only the student's name and then were asked to indicate their willingness to reintegrate. Two weeks later, the teachers were given a packet of information on the student that included (1) written and graphic representation of the student's oral reading scores in the general education curriculum compared with low-performing general education readers from the same classroom, (2) Woodcock–Johnson Broad Reading Cluster scores (Woodcock & Johnson, 1989) for the special education student, and (3) the special education teacher's rating of that student's readiness for reintegration. After reading the information, the general education teachers were asked to rate their willingness to reintegrate the student in their classroom for reading.

As expected from previous studies of general education teacher's attitudes toward reintegration, the general education teachers ratings on the first survey (predata willingness) were primarily in the unwilling to neutral range ($M = 4$, neutral) and there was little difference between the two groups of teachers. However, after being provided with the reading achievement information and special-education-teacher readiness rating, the general education teachers' ratings changed substantially and in the direction predicted by the reading data provided. General education teachers who had PC students became significantly more willing to reintegrate, with a mean rating of 6 (*Willing*), and teachers who had UC students became significantly less willing to reintegrate, with a mean rating of 2 (*Unwilling*; $F[1,23] = 84.55$, $p < .05$).

Furthermore, multiple regression analysis was employed to determine what variables best accounted for the changes in postdata willingness. The final regression model accounted for 89% of the variance in teacher ratings and included four variables: predata willingness, PC/UC status, behavior problem magnitude, and the Woodcock–Johnson Broad Reading score. Whether the student was PC or UC (i.e., read within or outside of the range of LRPs) accounted for 58% of the variance. The Woodcock–Johnson scores and special education teacher ratings did not account for significant additional variance in the final regression model.

Study 2

In a second study, Shinn, Baker, et al. (1993) expanded the external validity of the Rodden-Nord et al. (1992) study through a modified replication. They also expanded the investigation of reintegration attitudes to include the attitudes of parents. Twenty-three general education teachers and 40 parents served as subjects in this study. Using similar methodology, the general education teachers and parents were given pre- and postdata questionnaires assessing their willingness to reintegrate a student in the general education classroom for reading instruction.

As expected, the mean predata willingness ratings of the general education teachers was on the unwilling end of the scale (*M* = 3.6, with 4 being neutral). Similar to the Rodden-Nord et al. (1992) study, general education teachers' willingness ratings diverged on the postdata questionnaire and reflected the PC or UC status of the student. The average ratings of general education teachers with PC students increased from 3.5 to 4.6 (*Somewhat Willing*) whereas those with UC students decreased from 3.7 to 2.9 (*Somewhat Unwilling*). These results are not as robust as the Rodden-Nord and Shinn findings but do indicate, again, that general education teacher attitudes are not unchangeable.

A multiple regression analysis was conducted to gain insight into what accounted for the change in this study in teacher ratings on the pre- to postdata questionnaires. The analysis accounted for 59% of the variance in teacher ratings. Furthermore, in this study, "special education teacher readiness rating accounted for the most variance in post-data willingness ratings of general education teachers (37%)" (Shinn, Baker, et al., 1993, p. 225).

The 40 parents in the study were given modified pre- and postdata questionnaires, the PATR questionnaires. Like the general education teachers, the parent predata willingness ratings fell between the somewhat unwilling to neutral points on the rating scale (*M* = 3.1, with 4 being neutral). Unlike the general education teacher ratings, however, the parent ratings of both PC and UC students remained the same after being provided with data on their child's reading performance ($M = 2.9$).

Study 3

In an effort to understand what drives parent attitudes about changes in placement, particularly within the context of the RReACS model, Green and Shinn (1994) conducted a qualitative study examining the attitudes of 21 parents of students with mild disabilities currently served in part-time resource room programs. Using a combination of attitude scales and interviews, Green and Shinn found that the parents in their study reported being reluctant to place their child in the regular classroom for reading instruction ($M = 2.6$ on a scale ranging from 1 [Most Negative] to 5 [Most Positive]), accompanied by a high overall degree of satisfaction with the services their children received ($M = 4.8$). The basis for this satisfaction appeared to be "derived primarily from subjective perceptions (such as teacher's caring), rather than academic performance data" (p. 269).

Green and Shinn (1994) concluded that these findings constitute a "good news, bad news" situation. The good news is that parents in this study appeared satisfied with special education services. The bad news is that the parents were often unaware of how their own children actually were achieving, particularly in comparison to typical peers, did not recall discussing exit criteria with special education staff, and did not appear to base their satisfaction on academic outcomes. This state of affairs is bad news if the field of education wants to shift the focus of special education from categories and procedure to flexible service-delivery systems and outcomes. As educators, we want parents to be knowledgeable about student academic goals and outcomes, and value those outcomes. If parents base their attitudes and decisions solely on issues of perceived individualization of services, teacher friendliness, or student self-esteem, for example, a very important aspect of the child's education, namely academic outcomes, is left entirely up to the school system. In the words of Green and Shinn, "Although parents report a great deal of satisfaction, it is not based explicitly on the academic performance of their children and their reasons for satisfaction may be at cross purposes with special education reform. Strategies for making parents more effective advocates for appropriate education exist, and parents express interest in learning more about them" (p. 279).

Attitude Research Summary

The RReACS research suggests that general education teacher attitudes toward changes in placement may be somewhat negative initially but can change in the context of relevant data comparing a special education student in their classroom to his or her low-performing general education peers. This information is encouraging news for the feasibility of the RReACS model. Parents, of course, also should play an important role in educational decision making. The data from Shinn, Baker, et al. (1993) and Green and Shinn (1994) indicate that parents initially may be reluctant to reintegrate their children, although studies by other educational researchers (e.g., Lowenbraun et al., 1990) indicate that parent attitudes toward reintegration are generally positive once reintegration has occurred. Green and Shinn (1994) also reported that although parents were very interested in academic performance information on their children, they typically did not have a good picture of where their child was performing compared to typical peers. To implement the RReACS model successfully, parents must be provided with clear information about the concept of satisfactory achievement and understandable, ongoing data about how their children are achieving academically. Perhaps in this context, parental attitudes toward changes in placement will be based on more objective information and less on subjective factors, thereby allowing the parents to be more effective advocates for their children.

Benefits of Reintegration

Given the empirical support for reintegration-candidate identification practices and encouraging results from the teacher attitude studies, research was conducted to determine if reintegrated students benefited from reintegration practices based upon the RReACS model. Three primary studies have investigated the outcomes of reintegrating special education students into their general education classroom for reading instruction. The first study (Shinn, Powell-Smith, Good, & Baker, 1997) focused on the achievement outcomes for 23 elementary-school-aged students with mild disabilities, who had been receiving services in special education pull-out programs for reading, and who were reintegrated into their general education classroom for reading instruction for a 12-week trial period. The second study (Shinn, Powell-Smith, & Good, 1997) reported the results of using expert judges to evaluate the benefits and outcomes of reintegrating 18 elementary-school-aged students with mild disabilities, who were served in special education pull-out programs on a case-by-case basis. The third study (Habedank, 1994) examined the instructional environment, classroom behavior, and reading achievement for 6 reintegrated students before and after reintegration.

Study 1

Shinn, Powell-Smith, Good, and Baker (1997) investigated the effects of reintegrating 23 students into their general education classrooms for reading. The 23 students had all been receiving special education services in pull-out programs (e.g., resource rooms) for no more than half the school day. All students had been receiving their reading instruction in the special education setting, and all had IEP goals in reading. Subjects were from five elementary schools in three Pacific Northwest school districts. The communities in which the schools were located ranged from a small, rural community to a suburb of a large city and were diverse socioeconomically, ranging from below average SES to well above average SES. All students had social competence skills in teacher-preferred, peer-preferred, and school adjustment behavior within the average range according to their teacher's ratings on the *Walker–McConnell Social Skills Rating Scale* (Walker & McConnell, 1988).

Each of the 23 students was reintegrated into his or her general education classroom for a trial period of about 12 weeks. Prior to reintegration taking place, each student was tested using the identification procedures described in this chapter. First, students were nominated by their special education teachers. Thirty-four students were nominated, and 4 dropped out for various reasons (e.g., moved out of the school district). The 30 remaining students were tested, along with 3–6 LRPs per classroom, using three CBM oral-reading tests and one CBM maze-reading task. The scores were summarized and provided to parents, general education teachers, and special education teachers in both narrative and graphic form. Students also saw their graphs and had the data explained to them. Students, parents, and teachers all completed questionnaires regarding their opinions about reintegration. School-based teams decided to reintegrate 23 of the 30 students who were tested.

During the 12-week reintegration trial, each reintegrated student and his or her LRPs were monitored using CBM. As described earlier in this chapter, students were tested twice weekly using two CBM oral-reading probes each time. Once per month, students completed another maze task. These data were summarized monthly in "checkup" reports, which were provided along with another questionnaire to parents and teachers of the reintegrated student. The reintegrated students also completed another questionnaire, although whether they saw their graph depended upon whether they were performing near or within the range of their peers.

Data analyses examined student reading achievement, student reading progress, parent and teacher opinions about reintegration, and student "comfort" with reintegration over the course of the four measurement points in the 12-week trial reintegration (i.e., prereintegration and after 4, 8, and 12 weeks of reintegration). Reading achievement was examined using CBM oral-reading and CBM maze. For CBM oral reading, the median of the final three oral-reading probes administered within each phase was used as the metric for comparison. Reading progress was examined by comparing the slope of reintegrated students' reading scores to the slopes of their LRPs over the course of each measurement phase (i.e., at 4-, 8-, and 10- to 12-week time periods).

Reintegrated students' skills were compared to the mean reading performance of their LRPs on both CBM oral reading and CBM maze reading using a series of two-way, within-classroom analyses of variance (ANOVAs). Before reintegration, students read approximately 12 words correctly per minute less than their LRPs. After 4 weeks of reintegration, neither reintegrated students nor their LRPs had increased their oral reading skills significantly. Also, reading skills of the reintegrated students still were lower, on the average, than their LRPs. However, reintegrated students *maintained their relative position* after 4 weeks of reintegration, meaning that they had neither fallen further behind nor caught up to their LRPs. In contrast, reintegrated students and their LRPs both increased their CBM maze performance from initial reintegration to 4 weeks after reintegration. The reading progress data at week 4 also are important to consider, because they provide information beyond a one-point-in-time assessment of the student's reading skills. At the end of 4 weeks of reintegration, neither group of students was making much progress, as their slopes were near 0 words read correctly gained per week.

In contrast to week 4, both reintegrated students and their LRPs show increases in reading achievement after 8 weeks. Reading outcomes after 8 weeks of reintegration were much more positive than after 4 weeks of reintegration. Reintegrated students still were making progress commensurate with their LRPs, but now both groups of students were making significantly more improvement in their reading over time than they were after 4 weeks of reintegration. Slopes after 8 weeks of reintegration were about 1.5 words read correctly gained per week. Similar to week 4, LRPs continued to perform better on the CBM oral-reading task than the reintegrated students, but reintegrated students maintained their position relative to their LRPs and earned scores similar to the LRPs on CBM maze.

At the end of the reintegration trial (i.e., after 10–12 weeks), reintegrated students and their LRPs were earning scores on the CBM oral-reading task that were no longer significantly different. Both groups increased their oral-reading skills significantly from prereintegration to 10–12 weeks after reintegration. Reading progress data for the final measurement phase indicated that reintegrated students and their LRPs made about the same rate of progress, about 1.5 words read correctly gained per week.

Teachers', parents', and students' opinions about reintegration also provided additional information with regard to the success or benefits of reintegration. Both parents and teachers rated the success of the reading program as *Neutral* to *Somewhat Successful,* and these ratings did not change significantly over the course of the 12 weeks of reintegration. Similarly, parent and teacher ratings of their confidence that the reintegrated student would make progress fell in the *Neutral* to *Somewhat Confident* range. Again, these ratings did not change significantly over the course of the reintegration trial. For both of these questions, no significant differences existed between parent and teacher ratings. However, differences between raters were found regarding their responses to the question of most appropriate placement. General education teachers indicated that *general education* alone was the most appropriate placement, whereas parents indicated that *general education with assistance from the special education teacher* was preferred. Special education teachers' ratings fell in between the ratings given by parents and general education teachers. These ratings did not differ significantly over the course of the reintegration trial.

Five questions from the student questionnaire were summarized as a measure of student "comfort" with reintegration. Results of a series of pairwise comparisons indicated that students were significantly more comfortable with reintegration after 4 weeks than they were initially.

Overall, the results of the Shinn, Powell-Smith, Good, and Baker study indicate that the reintegrated students may achieve satisfactorily or maintain academic achievement levels and rates of progress commensurate with their LRPs. The study also demonstrated the lack of sensitivity of the subjective judgments to evaluate the success of reintegration and the importance of systematic, ongoing progress monitoring of academic outcomes for reintegrated students using tools like CBM.

Study 2

The benefits of reintegration were investigated further by Shinn, Powell-Smith, and Good (1997) by having a pool of expert judges answer a series of questions about the success of reintegration and academic benefits to the reintegrated students. In their study, the achievement gains of 18 reintegrated students were evaluated on a case-by-case basis by 10 expert judges. The 18 reintegrated students also were participants in Study 1, described previously. The judges were persons with expertise in using CBM to make student academic-progress decisions, as well as expertise in single-subject research.

The 18 students were reintegrated using procedures described in this chapter and in Study 1. Their reading achievement in the general education classroom was monitored weekly using the CBM procedures described in this chapter. Three to six LRPs from each reintegrated student's classroom were monitored as well. These data were summarized graphically at each phase of reintegration (i.e., prereintegration, at week 4, week 8, and final). Both a box-plot graph showing the reintegrated students' reading level compared to LRPs and a progress graph showing the slope or rate of progress compared to LRPs were produced at each point in time except for prereintegration.

Each expert judge was sent a set of packet of materials that included a set of graphs for each of the 18 reintegrated students, a series of questions about the graphs, and directions for how to complete the judgments. The expert judges were asked to answer a series of questions regarding the benefits and success of reintegration. For example, for the prereintegration graph, the expert judges were asked if the student should be reintegrated. For week 4 through the final week (10–12 weeks after reintegration), experts were asked first if the reintegrated student was benefiting from reintegration and second, if changes in reading instruction were necessary. Questions about each student's graph were to be answered sequentially, meaning that judges were asked only to view graphs up to the phase of reintegration for which they were answering questions. For example, when answering questions about benefit of reintegration at week 4, judges were to only view the prereintegration box-plot graph and the box-plot graph and slope graph for week 4. Finally, experts were asked not to change any of their previous answers after viewing later graphs for a student. Analyses of interjudge agreement showed that the judges were reliable in making their ratings. Using the overall agreement method described by Sulzer-Azaroff and Mayer (1977), interjudge agreement ranged from 80% to 93%. Using coefficient kappa (Fleiss, 1981), interjudge agreement was "fair" to "excellent" overall, with a median kappa coefficient of .49. Finally, for judges to be considered in consensus on a particular question, 7 of the 10 judges (70%) had to respond with either a "yes" or a "no." Questions on which less than 70% of the judges reached consensus were considered mixed judgments.

For the question of whether a student should be reintegrated, expert judges reached consensus that 14 of the 18 students should be reintegrated. These judgments were related strongly to whether the students' reading skills were within the range of the LRPs. Eleven students performed within or above the range of their LRPs prior to reintegration. Each of these 11 were rated by the judges as appropriate for reintegration, along with 3 additional students who read below the range of their LRPs. Performance patterns of the reintegrated students revealed two primary outcomes. Prior to and throughout the reintegration, as a group, the reintegrated students' *level of reading skills was lower* than their LRPs. However, by week 4 and throughout the rest of the reintegration trial, the reintegrated students as a group had *faster rates of progress* than their LRPs.

Judgments of benefit at week 4 indicated unanimous agreement that one-third (6) of the 18 students were benefiting from reintegration. However, judges also were in consensus that 10 students were not benefiting.

Furthermore, the judges unanimously responded that a change in reading program was necessary for 12 of the 18 students. Importantly, judges' written comments indicated that changes in reading instruction were needed for *both* the reintegrated student and the LRPs. Judgments of benefit at week 8 indicated that the judges believed more students were benefiting from reintegration. However, although judges reached consensus that 10 of the 18 students were benefiting, for only 4 of these 10 students was the response unanimous. Notably, the judges again were consistent in indicating a need for changes in reading instruction for *both* reintegrated students and LRPs. On the final week ratings, judges reached consensus that 8 of the 18 students were benefiting and 5 of the 18 were not benefiting. A marked increase in the number of "mixed" judgments was noted. The judges continued in their consensus that instructional changes were needed in most cases (13 of 18).

Finally, when asked to make a final summative judgment about the overall reintegration success, consensus (70% of judges agreed) was reached that reintegration was successful for half (9) of the 18 reintegrated students, and unsuccessful for one-sixth (3) of the 18 reintegrated students. Mixed judgments were noted for the remaining 6 students. When the reading performance of the students was examined, two features became evident. Most (6) of the 9 students rated as successful read more words correctly than their LRPs, and 8 of these 9 had slopes of progress equal to or greater than their LRPs. Slope of improvement for 6 of the 9 students were two words correct per week. However, for the 3 students rated as not successful, reading performance levels were all at least one-third lower than their LRPs, and slopes of improvement for these 3 reintegrated students *and* their peers were less than one word per week. For students on which "mixed" ratings were obtained, these two reading-performance features also were notable. Overall, these students' reading levels were lower than their LRPs, yet their slopes were about one word correct improvement per week and typically greater than or equal to the slopes of their LRPs.

The Shinn, Powell-Smith, and Good (1997) study provided a case-by-case examination of reintegration appropriateness and benefit through the use of expert ratings of these issues. The results indicated that despite the concern of some educators that reintegration cannot work without major changes in general education, a relatively high proportion of reintegrated students were judged to be successful, and relatively few were judged to be clearly unsuccessful. Further evidence for using LRPs for comparison was provided also. When the LRPs' reading skills were improving, the reintegrated student often improved. However, when LRPs were not improving as a group, the reintegrated student often did not improve either. In such cases, an ethical concern arises whereby changes in instruction for all students (both reintegrated student and LRPs) are warranted. Importantly, it could be argued that the general education classroom still is the LRE for the potential reintegration candidate. Finally, continued support for the use of CBM to identify reintegration candidates and evaluate the success of reintegration, as well as the apparent necessity of an extended period of evaluation, was provided.

Study 3

A replicated, single-subject design was used by Habedank (1994) to study the effects of reintegrating six students with mild disabilities in grades four to six more intensively. The study included a 3- to 5-week baseline phase and a 5-week (minimum) reintegration phase. CBM was used to identify potential candidates and monitor the reading achievement of the candidates and their general education LRPs. The TATR, PATR and student surveys (e.g., Shinn, Baker, et al., 1993; Shinn, Powell-Smith, Good, & Baker, 1997) also were used to assess attitudes toward reintegration and aid in reintegration decision making. In addition to the tools used in earlier research, however, Habedank (1994) utilized seatwork accuracy checks and multiple observations using the Classroom Activities Recording Form (CARF; Sindelar, Smith, & Harriman, 1986) to assess classroom behavior and the instructional environment.

According to the observational data, the six reintegrated students' instructional activities in general education were significantly different from their instructional activities in special education. Special education instruction consisted almost entirely of independent seatwork (88.8%). When teacher-directed group instruction did take place in special education, the instructional groups were much smaller ($M = 8.6$ students) than the instruction groups in general education ($M = 25.4$ students). General education reading instruction was primarily teacher-directed (96.3%), and the whole class was given the same materials and instruction. The change in instructional environment was accompanied by lower academic engagement and seatwork accuracy for four of the six students, though the drop did not appear to be a significant issue. In fact, three of the four students who had lower engagement in general education than in special education still had engagement rates higher than their general education comparison peers.

As a group, the reintegrated students' average CBM reading slope in general education was positive ($M = 0.9$ words per week) and actually was higher than the average LRP reading slope. Visual analysis of the individual student graphs and summary statistics, however, indicated that reintegration effects on reading achievement varied from student to student. According to visual analysis conducted by a panel of 13 experts, three of the six reintegrated students benefited from general education reading instruction, and the change from special education to general education did not have a significant impact on their reading achievement. These three students were doing well in the resource room and continued to do well when they were reintegrated. The remaining three reintegrated students did not benefit from general education reading instruction. These students also were doing well in the resource room, but the change from pull-out instruction in the resource room to instruction in general education negatively affected the reading achievement for these three students.

The results of the Habedank (1994) study indicate that students previously served in pull-out special education programs *can* be reintegrated successfully into general education, even when general education instruction is very different from resource room instruction. However, there are no guarantees of success. Ongoing evaluation is essential for responsible reintegration. The ongoing CBM monitoring used in this study provided a data base for making decisions about the success of reintegration and if modifications in general education, or even a return to the special education resource room, were needed. Modifications in general education also may benefit the LRPs given their lack of progress.

Furthermore, study results indicated that the 13 visual analysis judges had high interrater agreement on which students benefited from reintegration. The judges opinions were based on graphs of reintegrated student CBM reading data in the context of low reading peer CBM slopes of progress. The interjudge kappa coefficient was .84, meaning that interjudge agreement was 84% better than chance. This coefficient indicates excellent agreement according to Fleiss (1981; $p < .1$). This high agreement indicates that determinations of benefit from the type of data used in this study can be made reliably.

CONCLUSIONS FROM THE RESEARCH ON BENEFITS OF REINTEGRATION

The research thus far on the outcomes of reintegration, specifically the benefits to the reintegrated student, generally have been positive. Many reintegrated students demonstrated positive academic outcomes by sustaining achievement commensurate with their LRPs. These results are in contrast to some previous research (see Fuchs, Fuchs, & Fernstrom, 1992; Fuchs, Fuchs, & Fernstrom, 1993; Fuchs, Dempsey, Roberts, & Kintsch, 1995). Further, reintegration may be successful even if general education instruction is very different from resource room instruction. However, some individual students did not demonstrate these positive outcomes. Notably, the research summarized here points out the individual nature of reintegration effects and shows clearly the need for systematic ongoing monitoring of reintegration outcomes at the *individual* child level. The studies on the benefits of reintegration also point out the continued need for measures like CBM that are sensitive to determining reintegration benefit. While teacher and parent opinions are important, measures of them do not appear to be sensitive enough for evaluating reintegration success. Finally, many of the LRPs did not appear to be making progress at some point during the reintegration period. The notion that changes in instruction may be needed for the reintegrated student as well as the LRPs was a consistent theme. Whether the LRPs lack of progress should impact reintegration decision making may prompt continued debate with regard to reintegration. It also may prompt continued discussions relative to providing effective instruction for *all* students.

DIRECTIONS FOR FUTURE RESEARCH AND PRACTICE

Future research efforts should focus first on replicating the results found in the research summarized in this chapter. Future research efforts also should extend the database supporting the RReACS model by implementing the RReACS reintegration strategies in other academic areas (e.g., mathematics), examining students' rates of progress prior to changes in placement occurring, and gathering longitudinal data (e.g., achievement and social–emotional) on students who have been reintegrated (Shinn, 1995). This research could examine more closely the positive effects of seeing student performance data and the provision of consultation on the academic performance of the LRPs. Additionally, future research could examine the cultural and linguistic variables that need to be considered for successful reintegration or for changes in placement to occur, as well as student preferences with regard to placement (Smith & Bassett, 1990). Student preferences and attitudes toward reintegration could be evaluated relative to whether they are benefiting academically from instruction in the new placement (e.g., general education classroom).

Finally, the impact of additions to the RReACS model, such as the use of more detailed analyses of the general education instructional environment and student academic survival skills (see Fuchs, Dempsey, Roberts, & Kintsch, 1995) and the use of packaged observation codes, could be investigated. As noted by Shinn, Habedank, et al. (1993), good reintegration decision making may not rest solely upon the notion of establishing that a student's academic skills are within the range of a group of low-achieving general education students. Although these data have established social validity, with teachers responding favorably to being provided with this type of information (Shinn, Habedank, et al., 1993c), as has been made clear in this chapter, other elements that could have an impact on the process may need serious consideration. For example, it may be important to examine students' study skills or skills in sustaining attention during academic tasks and work completion (Gleason, Colvin, & Archer, 1991; Grossen & Carnine, 1991).

CONCLUSIONS

Because special education involves uncertainty and risk, it should be monitored carefully, with the notion of flexibility in placement and programming depending upon the data obtained from monitoring children's achievement. Serious questions about the effectiveness and role of special education have led to discussions relative to the Regular Education Initiative and inclusion. Arguments along a continuum from abolishing special education to conserving special education (with proposed reforms) have ensued (Fuchs & Fuchs, 1990). It has been said that "the reintegration of handicapped students from special classes into the mainstream of education has stimulated much interest at legal, philosophical, social, and educational levels" (Morsink, Thomas, & Smith-Davis, 1987, p. 299). Interest in this topic likely will continue in these arenas. However, without a data-based decision-making model such as the RReACS model, it seems unlikely that much progress will be made in the debate about how and why to make such decisions.

The decision-making model outlined in this chapter gives educators a systematic strategy built upon solid conceptual, legal, and measurement principles. This model provides a basis for deciding when reintegration to a less restrictive environment is appropriate for a student with mild disabilities and evaluating the outcomes of these decisions. The RReACS research supports the use of low-achieving peers as a standard for establishing the "satisfactory achievement" component of the LRE. Furthermore, research evidence supports the need to collect ongoing progress-monitoring data on reintegration effects. Ultimately, the truest test of reintegration success comes in the form of beneficial academic and social outcomes for reintegrated students. Our hope is that by providing published guidelines for a data-based decision-making model, the debate over inclusion practices will become more focused on educational outcomes and less focused on rhetoric.

ACKNOWLEDGMENTS

This research was supported in part by two grants from the U.S. Department of Education (USDE), Field-Initiated Research Grant No. H023C10151 and Student-Initiated Research Grant No. H023B10033. The views expressed within this chapter are not necessarily those of the USDE. We would like to thank Mark R. Shinn for his contributions to both the development of the RReACS model and this chapter. We also would like to thank Carolyn Meyer Durda, Michelle Fedak, and Nicole Ligori, school psychology graduate students at the University of South Florida and Lynnette Bailey, school psychology graduate student at Moorhead State University, for their assistance.

REFERENCES

Abramson, M., Willson, B., Yoshida, R. K., & Hagerty, G. (1983). Parents' perceptions of their learning disabled child's performance. *Learning Disability Quarterly, 6,* 184–194.

Allen, D. (1989). Periodic and annual reviews and decisions to terminate special education services. In M. R. Shinn (Ed.), *Curriculum-based measurement: Assessing special children* (pp. 182–201). New York: Guilford Press.

Barlow, D. H., & Hersen, M. (1984). *Single-case experimental designs: Strategies for studying behavior change* (2nd ed.). Boston: Allyn & Bacon.

Bell, P. F., Lentz, F. E., & Graden, J. L. (1992). Effects of curriculum–test overlap on standardized test scores: Identifying systematic confounds in educational decision making. *School Psychology Review, 21,* 644–655.

Bender, W. N., Vail, C., & Scott, K. (1995). Teachers' attitudes toward increased mainstreaming: Implementing effective instruction for students with learning disabilities. *Journal of Learning Disabilities, 28*(2), 87–94.

Burden, R. L., & Fraser, B. L. (1989). Use of classroom environment assessment in school psychology. *Psychology in the Schools, 30,* 232–240.

Daniel R. R. v. State Board of Education, 874 F.2d 1036, 1046 (5th Cir. 1989).

Deno, S. L. (1989). Curriculum-based measurement and special education services: A fundamental and direct relationship. In M. R. Shinn (Ed.), *Curriculum-based measurement: Assessing special children* (pp. 1–17). New York: Guilford Press.

Deno, S. L. (1990). Individual differences and individual difference: The essential difference of special education. *Journal of Special Education, 24*(2), 160–173.

Deno, S. L., Mirkin, P., & Chiang, B. (1982). Identifying valid measures of reading. *Exceptional Children, 49*(1), 36–45.

Espin, C., Deno, S. L., Maruyama, G., & Cohen, C. (1989, April). *The basic academic skills samples (BASS): An instrument for the screening and identification of children at-risk for failure in regular education classrooms.* Paper presented at the annual meeting of the American Educational Research Association, San Francisco.

Fleiss, J. L. (1981). *Statistical methods for rates and proportions* (2nd ed.). New York: Wiley.

Fuchs, D., Dempsey, S., Roberts, H., & Kintsch, A. (1995). Best practices in school reintegration. In A. Thomas & J. Grimes (Eds.), *Best practices in school psychology—III* (pp. 879–891). Washington, DC: National Association of School Psychologists.

Fuchs, D., & Fuchs, L. S. (1990). Framing the REI debate: Abolitionists versus conservationists. In J. W. Lloyd, N. N. Singh, & A. C. Repp (Eds.), *The regular education initiative: Alternative perspectives on concepts, issues, and models* (pp. 241–255). Sycamore, IL: Sycamore.

Fuchs, D., & Fuchs, L. S. (1994). Inclusive schools movement and the radicalization of special education reform. *Exceptional Children, 60,* 294–309.

Fuchs, D., Fuchs, L. S., & Fernstrom, P. (1992). Case-by-case reintegration of students with learning disabilities [Special issue: Integrating learners with disabilities in regular education programs]. *Elementary School Journal, 92*(3), 261–281.

Fuchs, D., Fuchs, L. S., & Fernstrom, P. (1993). A conservative approach to special education reform: Mainstreaming through transenvironmental programming and curriculum-based measurement. *American Educational Research Journal, 30*(1), 149–177.

Fuchs, L. S. (1989). Evaluating solutions: Monitoring progress and revising intervention plans. In M. R. Shinn (Ed.), *Curriculum-based measurement: Assessing special children* (pp. 153–181). New York: Guilford Press.

Fuchs, L. S., & Fuchs, D. (1986). Effects of systematic formative evaluation: A meta-analysis. *Exceptional Children, 53,* 199–209.

Fuchs, L. S., & Fuchs, D. (1992). Identifying a valid measure for monitoring student reading progress. *School Psychology Review, 21*(1), 45–58.

Fuchs, L. S., Fuchs, D., & Maxwell, L. (1988). The validity of informal reading comprehension measures. *Remedial and Special Education, 9,* 20–28.

Garver-Pinhas, A., & Schmelkin, L. P. (1989). Administrators' and teachers' attitudes toward mainstreaming. *Remedial and Special Education, 10,* 38–43.

Gleason, M. M., Colvin, G., & Archer, A. L. (1991). Interventions for improving study skills. In G. Stoner, M. R. Shinn, & H. M. Walker (Eds.), *Interventions for achievement and behavior problems* (pp. 137–160). Silver Spring, MD: National Association of School Psychologists.

Goh, D. S., Teslow, C. J., & Fuller, G. B. (1981). The practices of psychological assessment among school psychologists. *Professional Psychology, 12,* 699–706.

Good, R. H., & Salvia, J. (1988). Curriculum bias in published, norm-referenced tests: Demonstrable effects. *School Psychology Review, 17,* 51–60.

Good, R. H., & Shinn, M. R. (1990). Forecasting accuracy of slope estimates for reading curriculum-based measurement: Empirical evidence. *Behavioral Assessment, 12,* 179–193.

Green, S., & Shinn, M. R. (1994). Parent attitudes about special education and reintegration: What is the role of student outcomes? *Exceptional Children, 61*(3), 269–281.

Greenwood, C. R., Carta, J. J., Kamps, D., & Delquadri, J. (1992). *Ecobehavioral Assessment Systems Software (EBASS): Practitioner's manual.* Kansas City: Juniper Gardens Children's Project, University of Kansas.

Greer v. Rome City School District, 950 F.2d 688 (11th Cir. 1991).

Grossen, B., & Carnine, D. (1991). Strategies for maximizing reading success in the regular education classroom. In G. Stoner, M. R. Shinn, & H. M. Walker (Eds.), *Interventions for achievement and behavior problems* (pp. 333–356). Silver Spring, MD: National Association of School Psychologists.

Guthrie, J. (1973). Reading comprehension and syntactic responses in good and poor readers. *Journal of Educational Psychology, 65,* 294–299.

Habedank, L. (1995). Developing local norms for problem solving in the schools. In A. Thomas & J. Grimes (Eds.), *Best practices in school psychology* (3rd ed., pp. 701–716). Washington, DC: National Association of School Psychologists.

Habedank, L. (1994). *The effects of reintegrating students with mild disabilities in reading.* Unpublished doctoral dissertation, University of Oregon, Eugene.

Hendrick Hudson District Board of Education v. Rowley, 458 (U.S. 176, 1982).

Houck, C. K., & Rogers, C. J. (1994). The special/general education integration initiative for students with specific learning disabilities: A "snapshot" of program change. *Journal of Learning Disabilities, 27,* 435–453.

Howell, K. W., & Morehead, M. K. (1987). *Curriculum-based evaluation for special and remedial education.* Columbus, OH: Merrill.

Hutton, J. B., Dubes, R., & Muir, S. (1992). Assessment practices of school psychologists: Ten years later. *School Psychology Review, 21,* 271–284.

Individuals with Disabilities Education Act, Pub. L. No. 101-476, Sec. 1400 *et. seq.,* 104 Stat. 1142, 34 C.F.R. 300.4(a), (b), (c). (1991).

Jenkins, J. R., & Pany, D. (1978). Standardized achievement tests: How useful for special education? *Exceptional Children, 44,* 448–453.

Jenkins, J., & Heinen, A. (1989). Student's preferences for service delivery: Pullout, in-class, or integrated models. *Exceptional Children, 55*(6), 516–523.

Knoff, H. M. (1985). Attitudes toward mainstreaming: A status report and comparison of regular and special educators in New York and Massachusetts. *Psychology in the Schools, 22,* 411–418.

Lowenbraun, S., Madge, S., & Afflect, J. (1990). Parental satisfaction with integrated class placement of special education and general education students. *Remedial and Special Education, 11*(4), 37–40.

Lytle, J., & Penn, W. (1986). *Special education: Views from America's cities.* Philadelphia: Research for Better Schools.

Marston, D. B. (1988). The effectiveness of special education: A time-series analysis of reading performance in regular and special education settings. *Journal of Special Education, 21,* 13–26.

Marston, D. B. (1989). Curriculum-based measurement: What is it and why do it? In M. R. Shinn (Ed.), *Curriculum-based measurement: Assessing special children* (pp. 18–78). New York: Guilford Press.

McLeskey, J. & Pacchiano, D. (1994). Mainstreaming students with learning disabilities: Are we making progress? *Exceptional Children, 60,* 508–517.

Morsink, C. V., Thomas, C. C., & Smith-Davis, J. (1987). Noncategorical special education programs: Processes and outcomes. In M. C. Wang, M. C. Reynolds, & H. J. Walberg (Eds.), *The handbook of special education: Research and practice* (Vol. 1, pp. 287–311). Oxford, UK: Pergamon.

Myles, B. S., & Simpson, R. L. (1990). Mainstreaming modification preferences of elementary-age children with learning disabilities. *Journal of Learning Disabilities, 23*(4), 234–239.

Oberti v. Board of Education of Clementon School District, 995 F.2d 1204 (3rd Cir. 1993).

Rodden-Nord, K., Shinn, M. R., & Good, R. H. (1992). Effects of classroom performance data on general education teacher's attitudes toward reintegrating students with learning disabilities. *School Psychology Review, 21*(1), 138–154.

Sacramento City Unified School District v. Rachel H., 14 F.3d 1398 (9th Cir. 1994).

Sawyer, R. J., McLaughlin, M. J., & Winglee, M. (1994). Is integration of students with disabilities happening? *Remedial and Special Education, 15,* 281–287.

Schumm, J. S., & Vaughn, S. (1995). Getting ready for inclusion: Is the stage set? *Learning Disability Research and Practice, 10*(3), 169–179.

Scribner Educational Publishers. (1987). *Find your way.* New York: Author.

Semmel, M. I., Abernathy, T. V., Butera, G., & Lesar, S. (1991). Teacher perceptions of the Regular Education Initiative. *Exceptional Children, 58,* 9–23.

Shapiro, E. S. (1996). *Academic skills problems: Direct assessment and intervention* (2nd ed.). New York: Guilford Press.

Shapiro, E. S., & Derr, T. F. (1987). An examination of overlap between reading curricula and standardized achievement tests. *Journal of Special Education, 21,* 59–67.

Shinn, M. R. (1986). Does anyone care what happens after the referral–test–placement process? The systematic evaluation of special education effectiveness. *School Psychology Review, 15,* 49–58.

Shinn, M. R. (1988). Development of curriculum-based local norms for use in special education decision making. *School Psychology Review, 17,* 61–80.

Shinn, M. R. (Ed.). (1989). *Curriculum-based measurement: Assessing special children.* New York: Guilford Press.

Shinn, M. R. (Ed.). (1993). *Curriculum-based measurement and problem-solving assessment: Training modules* (4th ed.). (Available from School Psychology Program, College of Education, 5208 University of Oregon, Eugene, Oregon 97403-5208)

Shinn, M. R. (1995). Best practices in curriculum-based measurement and its use in a problem-solving model. In A. Thomas & J. Grimes (Eds.), *Best practices in school psychology—III* (pp. 547–567). Washington, DC: National Association of School Psychologists.

Shinn, M. R., Baker, S., Habedank, L., & Good, R. H. (1993). The effects of classroom reading performance data on general education teachers' and parents' attitudes about reintegration. *Exceptionality, 4*(4), 205–228.

Shinn, M. R., Good, R. H., Knutson, N., Tilly, W. D., & Collins, V. (1992). Curriculum-based reading fluency: A confirmatory analysis of its relation to reading. *School Psychology Review, 21*(3), 458–478.

Shinn, M. R., Habedank, L., Rodden-Nord, K., & Knutson, N. (1993). Using curriculum-based measurement to identify potential candidates for reintegration into general education. *Journal of Special Education, 27*(2), 202–221.

Shinn, M. R., Powell-Smith, K. A., & Good, R. H. (1997). Evaluating the effects of responsible reintegration into general education for students with mild disabilities on a case-by-case basis. *School Psychology Review.*

Shinn, M. R., Powell-Smith, K. A., Good, R. H., & Baker, S. (1997). The effects of reintegration into general education reading instruction for students with mild disabilities. *Exceptional Children, 64*(1), 59–78.

Simpson, R. L., & Myles, B. S. (1989). Parents' mainstreaming modification preferences for children with educable mental handicaps, behavior disorders, and learning disabilities. *Psychology in the Schools, 26,* 292–301.

Sindelar, P. T., Smith, M. A., & Harriman, N. E. (1986). *The classroom activity recording form: An instrument for evaluating teaching in special education programs.* (Available from Paul Sindelar, Florida State University, Gainesville).

Smith, D. D., & Bassett, D. S. (1990). The REI debate: A time for systematic research agendas. In J. W. Lloyd, N. N. Singh, & A. C. Repp (Eds.), *The regular education initiative: Alternative perspectives on concepts, issues, and models* (pp. 149–160). Sycamore, IL: Sycamore.

Stoner, G., & Green, S. K. (1992). Reconsidering the scientist–practitioner model for school psychology practice. *School Psychology Review, 21*(1), 155–166.

Sulzer-Azaroff, B., & Mayer, G. R. (1977). *Applying behavior analysis procedures with children and youth.* New York: Holt, Reinhart, & Winston.

Tindal, G. A., & Marston, D. B. (1990). *Classroom-based assessment: Evaluating instructional outcomes.* Columbus, OH: Merrill.

U.S. Department of Education. (1995). *Seventeenth annual report a to Congress on the implementation of the Individuals with Disabilities Education Act.* Washington, DC: Author.

Walker, H. M., & McConnell, S. R. (1988). *The Walker–McConnell Scale of Social Competence and School Adjustment.* Austin, TX: PRO-ED.

Wesson, C. L., & Deno, S. L. (1989). An analysis of long-term instructional plans in reading for elementary resource room students. *Remedial and Special Education, 10*(1), 21–28.

White, O. R. (1974). *The "split middle": A "quickie" method of trend estimation.* Seattle, WA: University of Washington, Experimental Education Unit, Child Development and Mental Retardation Center.

Will, M. (1986). Educating students with learning problems: A shared responsibility. *Exceptional Children, 52,* 411–415.

Woodcock, R. W., & Johnson, M. D. (1989). *Woodcock–Johnson Tests of Achievement— Revised: Standard and supplemental batteries.* Allen, TX: DLM Teaching Resources.

Yell, M. (1995). The law and inclusion: Analysis and commentary. *Preventing School Failure, 39,* 45–49.

Ysseldyke, J. E., & Christenson, S. L. (1987a). Evaluating student's instructional environments. *Remedial and Special Education, 8,* 17–24.

Ysseldyke, J. E., & Christenson, S. L. (1987b). *The Instructional Environment Scale.* Austin, TX: PRO-ED.

APPENDIX 9.1

Special Education Teacher Nomination Form

Your name: _____

Date: _____

SPECIAL EDUCATION TEACHER NOMINATIONS FOR REINTEGRATION

Directions

Please fill out the columns in the chart below as follows:

Column 1: Please list three to five students whom you believe may be good candidates for reintegration. These students must have an IEP for reading and spend at least half of each school day in the *general education* classroom.

Column 2: Please indicate their general education teacher's name.

Column 3: If the teacher for the low readers in the student's general education class is different from the person listed in column 2, please indicate so by writing in that teacher's name. If the teacher is the same write in "same."

Column 1 Student name	Column 2 General ed. teacher name	Column 3 Low-reading teacher name
1.		
2.		
3.		
4.		
5.		

For each special education student listed in the chart above, please complete a general education low-reading peer information form. These forms are found on the attached pages. Thank you for your time and effort.

GENERAL EDUCATION LOW-READING
PEER INFORMATION FORM

Special education student: _____.

1. Reading material used for instruction with the low readers is: (Circle your answer.)
   (a) Basal reader (b) Whole language/literature (c) Mixture of (a) and (b)

2. If you circled (a) or (c) in question 1 above, please list the basal material used with the general education low readers. Please write in publisher, series, and book (e.g., Scott-Foresman, *Focus* series, *Rough and Ready*).

   _____

   _____

3. Please list the names of the students in the general education low-reading group. If there are no reading groups, please list the lowest four to seven readers in the general education classroom.

   _____

   _____

   _____

   _____

   _____

   _____

   _____

4. Are any of the students listed in number 3 above in Chapter 1? If yes, please list their names here.

   _____

   _____

   _____

   _____

5. Are any of the students listed in number 3 above in special education with IEPs *in reading*? If yes, please list their names here.

   _____

   _____

   _____

   _____

APPENDIX 9.2

Sample General Education Teacher Questionnaire

GENERAL EDUCATION TEACHER OPINION SURVEY (BEFORE REINTEGRATION)

Student name: _____   Grade: _____

Teacher name: _____   School: _____

Date completed: _____

Reintegration decision and date: _____

1. Compared to *other students in your low-reading group or other low readers in your classroom,* please rate the student on their current level of reading skill.

Below average			Average			Above average
1	2	3	4	5	6	7

2. Given what you now know about this student, what do you currently believe is the most appropriate reading placement? (Circle one.)

   a. The lowest reading group in my classroom.
   b. The lowest reading group in my classroom supplemented by Chapter 1 services.
   c. The lowest reading group in my classroom with collaboration from the special education teacher.
   d. A special education resource room.
   e. A self-contained special education placement.
   f. Other (please specify) _____.

3. If the student is reintegrated, how successful is the reading program likely to be in meeting the student's needs?

Very unsuccessful	Unsuccessful	Somewhat unsuccessful	Neutral	Somewhat successful	Successful	Very successful
1	2	3	4	5	6	7

4. If the student is reintegrated, how confident are you that the student would make reading progress equal to or greater than other students in your low-reading group (or other low readers in your classroom)?

Not confident			Neutral			Very confident
1	2	3	4	5	6	7

FACILITATING SUCCESSFUL REINTEGRATION EFFORTS

5. What would be needed to make the student's reintegration more successful? Please *circle* all that apply.

   a. Instructional consultation (e.g., specific skills analysis, suggestions for curriculum modifications, alternative instructional curricula)
   b. Tutoring (e.g., peer/same age, cross grade, classwide; parent)
   c. Study skills (e.g., note taking, using an assignment calendar, organizing desk and materials)
   d. Interventions for appropriate classroom behavior (e.g., following directions, completing assignments, improving peer and teacher interactions)

6. Circle the letter(s) indicating the areas in which you would like assistance with this student.

   a. Instructional consultation (e.g., specific skills analysis, suggestions for curriculum modifications, alternative instructional curricula)
   b. Tutoring (e.g., peer/same age, cross grade, classwide; parent)
   c. Study skills (e.g., note taking, using an assignment calendar, organizing desk and materials)
   d. Interventions for appropriate classroom behavior (e.g., following directions, completing assignments, improving peer and teacher interactions)

APPENDIX 9.3

Sample Student Questionnaire

RReACS STUDENT QUESTIONNAIRE

Reintegration Trial

Date: _____

Student: _____

School:_____

Special education teacher: _____

General education teacher: _____

Timing of questionnaire (circle): Before reintegration/week 4/week 8/final

1. Do you read better now than last month?

1	2	3	4	5
Definitely yes	Probably yes	Sometimes	Probably not	Definitely not

2. Do you think you read as well as other kids in Ms./Mr._____ (GE)_____'s classroom?

1	2	3	4	5
Definitely yes	Probably yes	Sometimes	Probably not	Definitely not

3. Do you get along with *most* of the other kids in Ms./Mr. _____ (GE)_____'s classroom?

1	2	3	4	5
Definitely yes	Probably yes	Sometimes	Probably not	Definitely not

4. Do you like learning to read in Mr./Ms. _____ (GE)_____'s classroom?

1	2	3	4	5
Definitely yes	Probably yes	Sometimes	Probably not	Definitely not

5. Do you know how Mr./Ms. _____ (GE) _____ wants you to behave in class?

1	2	3	4	5
Definitely yes	Probably yes	Sometimes	Probably not	Definitely not

6. Can you do the reading work in Ms./Mr. _____ (GE) _____'s class-room?

1	2	3	4	5
Definitely yes	Probably yes	Sometimes	Probably not	Definitely not

7. Do you think you belong in Mr./Ms. _____ (GE) _____'s classroom for reading?

1	2	3	4	5
Definitely yes	Probably yes	Sometimes	Probably not	Definitely not

8. Do you have problems getting along with *some* of the other kids in Ms./Mr. _____ (GE) _____'s classroom?

1	2	3	4	5
Definitely yes	Probably yes	Sometimes	Probably not	Definitely not

9. Do you think you are a good reader?

1	2	3	4	5
Definitely yes	Probably yes	Sometimes	Probably not	Definitely not

Remove the student's 5-point scale and say: "Now I'm going to ask you some questions about school where you have to pick the answer that best fits how you feel."

10. Do you think you learn to read better in Mr./Ms. _____ (SE's) _____ class or in Ms./Mr. _____ (GE's) _____ class?

    Circle one: SE teacher   GE teacher

11. If you were having a lot of problems in reading and needed extra help would you rather:
    (a) Get extra help from Mr./Ms. _____ SE _____, or
    (b) Get extra help from Mr./Ms. _____ GE _____?
    Why would you rather get extra help from (insert a or b, depending on the student's response)?

    _____

    _____

    _____

If the Student chooses answer (a) (would rather get help from the SE teacher), ask:

12. If you were having a lot of problems in reading and needed extra help, would you rather:
    (a) Go to Mr./Ms. _____ SE's _____ classroom for help, or
    (b) Have Mr./Ms._____ SE's _____ come to your classroom to help you?

Why would you rather (insert a or b, depending on student response)?

_____

_____

_____

Note. Questions 11 and 12 are adapted from "Students' preferences for service delivery: Pull-out, in-class, or integrated models" by J. R. Jenkins and A. Heinen, *Exceptional Children, 55*(6), 1989, pp. 516–523. Copyright 1989 by The Council for Exceptional Children. Adapted and reprinted with permission.

APPENDIX 9.4

◆◆◆

Sample General Education Teacher Follow-Up Questionnaire

GENERAL EDUCATION TEACHER OPINION SURVEY (MONITORING)

Student name: _____ Grade: _____

Teacher name: _____ School: _____

Date reintegrated: _____ Report for week #: _____

Date: _____

1. Compared to *other students in your low-reading group or other low readers in your classroom,* please rate the reintegrated student on the following items:

	Below average		Average			Above average	
a. Current level of reading skill	1	2	3	4	5	6	7
b. Reading progress since reintegration	1	2	3	4	5	6	7
c. Behavior during reading instruction	1	2	3	4	5	6	7
d. Quality of peer interactions during reading instruction	1	2	3	4	5	6	7
e. Quality of teacher interactions during reading instruction	1	2	3	4	5	6	7
f. Number of reading assignments completed	1	2	3	4	5	6	7
g. Quality of reading assignments completed	1	2	3	4	5	6	7

2. Given what you now know about this student, what do you currently believe is the most appropriate reading placement? (Circle one).

   a. The lowest reading group in my classroom.
   b. The lowest reading group in my classroom supplemented by Chapter 1 services.
   c. The lowest reading group in my classroom with collaboration from the special education teacher.
   d. A special education resource room.
   e. A self-contained special education placement.
   f. Other (please specify) _____.

3. How successful is the reading program in meeting the student's needs?

Very unsuccessful	Unsuccessful	Somewhat unsuccessful	Neutral	Somewhat successful	Successful	Very successful
1	2	3	4	5	6	7

4. How confident are you that the student will make reading progress equal to or greater than other students in your low-reading group (or other low readers in your classroom)?

Not confident			Neutral			Very confident
1	2	3	4	5	6	7

FACILITATING SUCCESSFUL REINTEGRATION EFFORTS

5. What would be needed to make the student's reintegration more successful? Please *circle* all that apply.

   a. Instructional consultation (e.g., specific skills analysis, suggestions for curriculum modifications, alternative instructional curricula)
   b. Tutoring (e.g., peer/same age, cross grade, classwide; parent)
   c. Study skills (e.g., note taking, using an assignment calendar, organizing desk and materials)
   d. Interventions for appropriate classroom behavior (e.g., following directions, completing assignments, improving peer and teacher interactions)

6. Circle the letter(s) indicating the areas in which you would like assistance with this student.

   a. Instructional consultation (e.g., specific skills analysis, suggestions for curriculum modifications, alternative instructional curricula)

b. Tutoring (e.g., peer/same age, cross grade, classwide; parent)
c. Study skills (e.g., note taking, using an assignment calendar, organizing desk and materials)
d. Interventions for appropriate classroom behavior (e.g., following directions, completing assignments, improving peer and teacher interactions)

7. List or describe any major changes that have been made in the student's reading program since you completed the last survey (e.g., the length of reading instruction, curriculum materials, motivational strategies, instructional arrangements—instructional strategies, group or individual instruction, etc.).

_____

_____

_____

_____

_____

OPTIONAL

8. Describe your impressions of the reintegration's success. Please include suggestions that could make this reintegration and future reintegration efforts more successful.

_____

_____

_____

_____

_____

Index

♦